Chinese Adolescents in Hong Kong

Quality of Life in Asia

Volume 5

Series Editors:

ALEX C. MICHALOS

DANIEL T.L. SHEK
The Hong Kong Polytechnic University, Hunghom, P.R.C.

DOH CHULL SHIN
University of Missouri, Columbia, MI, U.S.A.

MING-CHANG TSAI
National Taipei University, Taipei, Taiwan

This series, the first of its kind, will examine both the objective and subjective dimensions of life quality in Asia, especially East Asia. It will unravel and compare the contours, dynamics and patterns of building nations, offering innovative works that discuss basic and applied research, emphasizing inter- and multi-disciplinary approaches to the various domains of life quality. Thus, the series will appeal to a variety of fields in humanities, social sciences and other professional disciplines. Asia is the largest, most populous continent on Earth, and it is home to the world's most dynamic region, East Asia. In the past three decades, East Asia has been the most successful region in the world in expanding its economies and integrating them into the global economy, offering lessons on how poor countries, even with limited natural resources, can achieve rapid economic development. Yet while scholars and policymakers have focused on why East Asia has prospered, little has been written on how its economic expansion has affected the quality of life of its citizens. The series will publish several volumes a year, either single or multiple-authored monographs or collections of essays.

More information about this series at http://www.springer.com/series/8416

Daniel T.L. Shek • Rachel C.F. Sun
Cecilia M.S. Ma
Editors

Chinese Adolescents in Hong Kong

Family Life, Psychological Well-Being and Risk Behavior

Springer

Editors
Daniel T.L. Shek
Cecilia M.S. Ma
Department of Applied Social Sciences
The Hong Kong Polytechnic University
Hunghom, Hong Kong

Rachel C.F. Sun
Faculty of Education
The University of Hong Kong
Hong Kong, Hong Kong

ISSN 2211-0550 ISSN 2211-0569 (electronic)
ISBN 978-981-10-1197-9 ISBN 978-981-287-143-5 (eBook)
DOI 10.1007/978-981-287-143-5
Springer Singapore Heidelberg New York Dordrecht London

Softcover reprint of the hardcover 1st edition 2014

Printed on acid-free paper

Springer is part of Springer Science+Business Media (www.springer.com)

Preface

Most of the existing theories on the personal well-being of adolescents have been developed in the West. Similarly, most of the existing studies have been conducted in the West. One important question that social scientists should ask is whether Western theories and research findings are applicable to adolescents in non-Western cultural contexts. Obviously, the answer to this question depends on the availability of empirical evidence. Unfortunately, studies on adolescent personal well-being are grossly inadequate in the scientific literature. Using the search term "adolescents," computer search in March 2014 using PsycINFO showed 87,601 citations. When we used "Chinese" and "adolescents," there were only 2,102 citations. In other words, 2.4 % of the citations were related to Chinese adolescents. As the Chinese population roughly constitutes one-fifth of the world's population, this percentage of research on adolescents is definitely out of proportion.

There are several questions one should ask as far as adolescent well-being is concerned. The first question is how well-being changes during the adolescent years. In other words, what are the developmental trajectories associated with personal well-being during adolescence? While numerous cross-sectional studies have been conducted to understand this problem, only longitudinal data can provide us with a more comprehensive picture. Unfortunately, longitudinal studies are grossly inadequate in Chinese societies. In this book, we report the developmental trajectories of personal well-being indexed by different indicators in junior secondary school students in Hong Kong.

The next question is what sociodemographic factors are related to adolescent well-being. Several sociodemographic factors have been found to be closely related to the personal well-being of adolescents. For example, compared with adolescent girls, adolescent boys are more likely to exhibit suicidal behavior. Regarding age effect, adolescent risk behavior is linearly related to age during adolescence. Some family risk factors also impair adolescent well-being. Findings from studies reveal that adolescents with economic disadvantage develop unfavorably when compared with adolescents who do not experience economic disadvantage. Compared to adolescents in intact families, adolescents in non-intact families show poorer well-being. Again, we are not sure whether the effects of such sociodemographic factors continue during adolescence. In the chapters of this book, special emphasis is placed on the influence of economic disadvantage and family non-intactness on adolescent well-being in the junior secondary school years.

The next question is what factors can protect adolescents from poor well-being, such as risk behavior, during the adolescent years. Using an ecological perspective, factors in different systems influence adolescent well-being. Besides personality traits, developmental assets within an individual, such as emotional control, resilience, spirituality, self-confidence, and compassion for other people, definitely shape the well-being of adolescents. In other words, inner resources shape adolescent well-being. The 3-year longitudinal study covered in this book addressed the question of how positive youth development attributes are related to measures of adolescent well-being across the junior high school years.

Besides developmental assets within an individual, factors in the environment also determine adolescent well-being. Among the influences of different environmental systems, family plays a crucial role in the process of socialization. There are both systemic and dyadic family processes in the family. For systemic family processes, family functioning attributes such as communication and emotional expressiveness are important parameters. For dyadic parent-child relationship, processes such as parenting, conflicts, and relational quality have been widely examined. In the sociological literature, numerous studies have underscored the importance of family social capital in adolescent development. In the psychological literature, the role of parenting and parent-child relationship on child and adolescent development has been widely documented. In our longitudinal study spanning across 3 years, another research question addressed is how systemic and dyadic parent-child relational qualities influence adolescent well-being in the junior high school years.

How can the research findings related to positive youth development and family processes function as protective factors to help adolescent development? The obvious answer is to apply the related findings to youth enhancement programs, although the process is not easy and straightforward. As far as youth enhancement programs are concerned, while there are numerous positive youth development programs in the West, very few validated programs exist in different Chinese communities. One notable exception is the Project P.A.T.H.S. in Hong Kong, which utilizes positive youth development constructs identified in the successful programs in the field. Obviously, the collection of data in the Chinese context is important as far as the development of positive youth development programs for Chinese adolescents is concerned. Regarding programs which aim at promoting the quality of family life, literature review shows that while there are many programs in the West, there are only very few validated programs in Chinese societies. Based on the findings reported in the various chapters of this book, the theoretical basis for promoting family quality of life is formed. It is hoped that such findings can facilitate helping professionals to develop family quality of life enhancement programs for Chinese adolescents.

In the Confucian thought, one popular doctrine is "cultivation of oneself, regulation of one's family, governing one's country and creating peace and harmony for the world" ('xiu shen, qi jia, zhi guo, ping tian xia'). Basically, it means that

> Before one can create peace and harmony for the world, one must be able to govern one's country. Before one can govern one's country, one must be able to regulate one's family. Before one can regulate one's family, one must be able to cultivate one's virtues and character.

Conceptually speaking, Confucianism emphasizes self-cultivation which is consistent with the notion of positive youth development. Both focus on the importance of "inner strengths," particularly character and moral codes. Similarly, the notion of family regulation is in line with the Western notion of family functioning, particularly in the area of family rules and leadership. Through the findings reported in the chapters of this book, we earnestly hope that we will be able to integrate scientific theories and findings from the West in the Chinese context.

I also wish to take this opportunity to thank all the schools, parents, and students who have participated in this longitudinal study. Without their unfailing support, this groundbreaking attempt will not be possible.

Hunghom, Hong Kong Daniel T.L. Shek

Contents

Contributors

Ben M.F. Law is currently Assistant Professor of the Department of Social Work and Social Administration at the University of Hong Kong. Before joining the tertiary education field, Dr. Law has been a social worker for more than 15 years in the areas of school social work, family social work, and special education. He is currently one of the coprincipal investigators for the positive youth development program P.A.T.H.S. and a member of the Committee on Services for Youth at Risk under the Social Welfare Department, HKSAR. His research interests are prosocial behavior, volunteerism, coping among youth, and special education.

Moon Y.M. Law is an Instructor of the Department of Applied Social Sciences at the Hong Kong Polytechnic University and the Project Manager of a positive youth development project. She is currently a doctoral student in social work. Apart from providing training for teachers and social workers in Hong Kong and mainland China, she has taught different courses for university students, including counseling, leadership, and service learning. Her research interests include positive youth development, leadership, and Internet addiction. Her current research projects focus on positive youth development programs and adolescents' Internet addiction.

Tak Yan Lee is an Associate Professor in the Department of Applied Social Sciences at the City University of Hong Kong. His teaching interests cover social work research and evaluation, group work, and practice teaching and learning methods. He is currently one of the coprincipal investigators of a large-scale applied research study on the development and evaluation of a positive youth development program for junior secondary school students in Hong Kong and in mainland China. His recent research covers adolescent prostitution, positive youth development, resilience of children, adolescents, adults, and the elderly as well as the process and outcomes of practicum teaching and learning.

Hildie Leung is a Research Assistant Professor in the Department of Applied Social Sciences at the Hong Kong Polytechnic University. She earned her undergraduate degree in Psychology from the Australian National University and obtained her

Ph.D. degree in Psychology at the Chinese University of Hong Kong. Her research centers on positive youth development and its application to the promotion of healthy adolescent development and the prevention of problem behaviors among children and adolescents. She is also interested in teaching and research on service leadership, positive psychology, and prosocial decision making.

Janet T.Y. Leung is an Assistant Professor of the Department of Applied Social Sciences at the City University of Hong Kong. She is a registered social worker and has been working in the social welfare field for over 20 years. She was a service supervisor in a social service organization and was responsible to supervise a wide range of services such as children and youth services, school counseling services, training projects for dyslexic children, family support programs, service for the homeless people, community development projects, etc. Her areas of interests include poverty, adolescent development, family processes, and parent education.

Xiang Li is a Postdoctoral Research Fellow in the Department of Applied Social Sciences, the Hong Kong Polytechnic University. She obtained her Ph.D. degree from the Department of Applied Social Sciences, City University of Hong Kong. Her research and working experience in social work and psychology generate strong interest in child and adolescent development for her. In particular, her research interests involve behavioral and mental health, subjective well-being, aggression and victimization, training and intervention, and psychometric assessment.

Li Lin is an Instructor in the Department of Applied Social Sciences, The Hong Kong Polytechnic University. She currently teaches leadership course for university students. Her research interests largely involve development of adolescence and emerging adulthood, particularly parent-child relationship, positive youth development, and sociocultural influence. Her publications cover many adolescent issues, such as positive youth development and adolescent materialism, as well as program evaluation.

Cecilia M.S. Ma is an Assistant Professor in the Department of Applied Social Sciences at the Hong Kong Polytechnic University. She received her Ph.D. from the University of South Carolina. Her research interests include psychometrics, structural equation modeling, and program evaluation. She has published peer-reviewed papers in journals such as *Research on Social Work Practice*, *Social Indicators Research*, and *International Journal on Disability and Human Development*. She has also coauthored book chapters and articles in the area of Chinese adolescents' psychological development. Her current research projects focus on positive youth development programs and the development of a university leadership program.

Catalina S.M. Ng is a Research Assistant Professor in the Department of Applied Social Sciences at the Polytechnic University of Hong Kong. She holds a Ph.D. in Psychology from the University of London focusing on adolescent self-harm behavior. Prior to joining the Hong Kong Polytechnic University, Catalina was trained as a health psychologist. Her research interests and existing publications cover several psychology-related and health-related subjects, including positive youth development and adolescent development, with a particular focus on internalizing disorders/ self-harm and addictions such as smoking and alcohol use. She is currently working for the Project P.A.T.H.S. in Hong Kong.

Daniel T.L. Shek is Associate Vice President (Undergraduate Program) and Chair Professor of Applied Social Sciences at the Hong Kong Polytechnic University, Advisory Professor of East China Normal University, and Honorary Professor of Kiang Wu Nursing College of Macau. He is Chief Editor of *Journal of Youth Studies* and Editorial Board Member of several international refereed journals, including *Journal of Adolescent Health*, *Social Indicator Research*, *International Journal of Behavioral Development*, and *International Journal of Adolescent Medicine and Health*. He is Chairman of the Action Committee Against Narcotics and Family Council of the Government of Hong Kong Special Administrative Region, P.R.C.

Rachel C.F. Sun got her BSocSc and Ph.D. at The University of Hong Kong, Hong Kong. She is an Assistant Professor, Faculty of Education at The University of Hong Kong. She is a principal investigator of school misbehavior research studies and coprincipal investigator of the positive youth development programs and a service leadership program in Hong Kong. Her research areas include academic achievement motivation, school satisfaction, life satisfaction, positive youth development, problem behavior, school misbehavior, adolescent suicidal ideation, and psychological health. She is a member of the editorial boards of *Research on Social Work* and *Frontiers in Child Health and Human Development.*

Florence K.Y. Wu has dedicated her early career as a frontline teacher and was in various leading roles in school to nurture students' whole-person development. Upon her completion of the doctorate degree in 2013, Florence becomes a Research Assistant Professor in the Hong Kong Polytechnic University, dedicating her research areas in positive youth development prevention of substance abuse guidance curriculum designs, implementation, and effectiveness. Incorporating the frontline experiences, she has developed the track records and published papers in investigating the effectiveness of the positive youth development programs implemented in secondary school settings and leadership trainings in the university arenas.

Lu Yu is an Assistant Professor of the Department of Applied Social Studies, The Hong Kong Polytechnic University. She was trained in clinical medicine, psychiatry, education, and positive psychology. Her research interests include positive youth development, leadership, cross-cultural studies, gender development, mental health, and program evaluation. Her work appeared in *Personality and Individual Differences*, *Archives of Sexual Behaviors*, *BMC Public Health*, *International Journal on Disability and Human Development*, *Journal of Pediatric and Adolescent Gynecology, Journal of Sex Research, Sex Roles, The Scientific World Journal, Asian Journal of Counseling, and International Journal of Child Health and Human Development.*

Family Quality of Life, Personal Well-Being, and Risk Behavior in Early Adolescents in Hong Kong: Related Phenomena and Research Gaps

Daniel T.L. Shek and Catalina S.M. Ng

Abstract Family processes and positive youth development attributes are salient determinants of adolescent development. In this chapter, the influences of family factors (family functioning, parent-child relationship, parenting style, parent-child communication, parental marital problems, and economic disadvantage) and positive youth development attributes on the personal well-being of Chinese adolescents are reviewed. The review demonstrates that there are several limitations of the existing scientific literature in the Chinese context. First, in contrast to the abundance of Western studies, there is a lack of Chinese studies. Second, more emphasis should be put on understanding families from an ecological perspective. Third, few studies have examined both systemic and dyadic family processes in a single study. Fourth, positive youth development research is still in its infancy in different Chinese contexts. Fifth, there are few Chinese validated measures of personal well-being and family quality of life in the field. Sixth, there are few longitudinal studies in different Chinese societies. Finally, there are few studies in which multiple positive and negative measures of personal well-being are employed in one single study.

Keywords Family processes • Positive youth development • Personal well-being • Family quality of life • Chinese adolescents

Introduction

Local studies consistently report that risk behavior among early adolescents in Hong Kong is growing (e.g., Law & Shek, 2013; Lee & Shek, 2013; Shek, 2013). For instance, using a large sample of Hong Kong primary and secondary students (N=26,111), a study investigating youth risk behavior found that 18.1 % of the

D.T.L. Shek, Ph.D., B.B.S., S.B.S., J.P. (✉) • C.S.M. Ng, Ph.D.
Department of Applied Social Sciences, The Hong Kong Polytechnic University, Hunghom, Hong Kong
e-mail: daniel.shek@polyu.edu.hk

D.T.L. Shek et al. (eds.), *Chinese Adolescents in Hong Kong*, Quality of Life in Asia 5, DOI 10.1007/978-981-287-143-5_1

participants had experimented with smoking and 45.2 % reported lifetime alcohol consumption (Lee & Tsang, 2004). In another study utilizing three waves of longitudinal data, Yu and Shek (2013) reported that about 22.5 % of the participants could be classified as having Internet addiction. This increase in youth risk behavior has led local researchers to explore the risk and protective factors of adolescent problem behavior because getting a deeper understanding of the factors that lead to youth risk behavior can help develop effective and targeted intervention strategies.

Since numerous Western studies have reported that family plays a key role in adolescent development, it would be theoretically and practically useful to analyze how different family processes such as parenting and family functioning influence the development of adolescent risk behavior in the Chinese context. The Department of Child and Adolescent Health and Development of the World Health Organization (2001) analyzed research findings on risk and protective factors for substance use from more than 50 countries and concluded that conflicts in families are risk factors for adolescent substance use in Asia, whereas having positive parent-child relationships as well as having parents who provide structure and boundaries are protective factors for substance use. Likewise, Yip and associates (2011) found that Hong Kong Chinese adolescents who took drugs were influenced by dysfunctional families, with problems such as unstable family condition, low income, long working hours of family members, and poor/ineffective communication between young people and their family, which is consistent with Shek's (1993) perspective that family plays an important role in shaping adolescent development.

Although family is the basic form of social capital (Putnam, 1995), family quality of life has been a neglected topic (Shek, 2008a). As Hoffman, Marquis, Poston, Summers, and Turnbull (2006) pointed out, "research on quality of life has traditionally focused on individuals rather than families" (p. 1069), suggesting that family quality of life is under-researched. In particular, there is an urgent need to understand how different family processes influence adolescent development. Although there are several family theories (e.g., structural family theories) which assert the importance of family processes on adolescent development, ecological models have been commonly utilized to understand the development of individuals within their environments. The primary assertion of ecological models is that human behavior is influenced by different individual and environmental factors in different systems, particularly processes within the family. Therefore, ecological models are commonly used as a theoretical model to help us understand the complex nature of the interactions between an individual and its environment.

Apart from family processes, developmental assets within adolescents are also critical determinants of the personal well-being of teenagers. In the literature on positive youth development, there are views asserting that developmental assets can protect adolescents from risk behavior. For example, in a series of studies based on Chinese adolescents in Hong Kong, Sun and Shek (2010, 2012, 2013) showed that positive youth development attributes negatively predicted adolescent problem behavior via the mediating effects of life satisfaction.

Positive youth development is a promising approach in preventing youth problems as it not only thwarts problems but also strengthens adolescent developmental assets (Catalano, Hawkins, Berglund, Pollard, & Arthur, 2002). Programs utilizing positive youth development principles can help adolescents avoid risky behavior, ensure young people become healthy adults, and promote a positive personal and psychological development. Overall, positive youth development is expected to enhance life satisfaction and reduce problem behavior.

According to Catalano, Berglund, Ryan, Lonczak, and Hawkins (2004), there are several attributes of the positive youth development approach, including (a) upholding the belief that "problem-free is not fully prepared," (b) emphasis on integrated youth development (i.e., focusing on a range of youth developmental possibilities and problems) rather than solely handling a single youth problem, (c) emphasis of person-in-environment perspective, and (d) focus on developmental models on how young people learn, grow, and change. The underlying assumption of positive youth development programs is that adolescent risk behavior will not be easily developed through the strengthening of psychosocial competencies in adolescents. Principles and theories of positive youth development have been utilized in youth enhancement programs as well.

Ample research results point to the effectiveness of positive youth development programs which successfully led to a reduction of problem behavior, such as substance abuse and delinquency. Catalano et al. (2004) found that 25 programs in the field in North America have provided support for the effectiveness of developing youth developmental assets in reducing youth risk behavior (Tremblay, Pagani-Kurtz, Masse, Vitaro, & Pihi, 1995). In the context of Hong Kong, Shek and his associates have implemented a positive youth development program entitled the Project P.A.T.H.S., with evaluation findings showing that the Project P.A.T.H.S. was able to promote positive youth development attributes and reduce risk behavior in adolescents (Shek & Ma, 2012; Shek & Yu, 2012).

Since family processes and positive youth development attributes are salient determinants of adolescent development, the purpose of this chapter is to review how family factors (such as family functioning, parent-child relationship, parenting style, parent-child communication, parental marital disruption, and economic disadvantage) and positive youth development attributes contribute to adolescent quality of life, including risk behavior. The limitations of the existing literature and the way forward are also discussed.

Family Factors and Adolescent Well-Being

Family Functioning and Adolescent Developmental Outcome

Family functioning is often used as an indicator of family life quality (Shek & Lee, 2007). It refers to "the quality of family life at the systemic level, such as wellness, competence, strengths, and weaknesses of a family" (Shek, 2005a, p. 518).

To understand how family functioning affects adolescent development, it is therefore important to understand how family operates at the systemic level.

For example, studies on family functioning often refer to the Circumplex Model proposed by Olson, Sprenkle, and Russell (1979) and Olson, Russell, and Sprenkle (1983) to explain family systems. According to the Circumplex Model, a family system needs cohesion and adaptability to be able to cope with change. However, as the presence of an adolescent in the family system naturally causes change, parents need to adjust to the adolescent's demand for independence (Parker, 2000), which not all parents successfully do. Parental failure to adjust to the adolescent's needs results in increased levels of tension, stress, and conflicts in the family, which affect children emotionally. Deprived from family support and understanding, the adolescent may therefore start to feel alone, unloved, and unsupported to face the developmental challenges brought by adolescence, which may lead him to engage in risk behavior.

Although the Circumplex Model is derived from research carried out in Western countries, similar observations have been made in the Chinese context. In a local study exploring the perspectives on family functioning among Chinese people, participants responded that harmony, mutuality, and the absence of conflicts are crucial attributes of a happy family (Shek, 2001a, 2001b). In addition, the Chinese culture places a strong emphasis on the concept of harmony which is captured by a popular saying "*jia he wan shi xing*" (everything will prosper if a family lives in harmony). Therefore, Chinese families experiencing a high level of conflicts are perceived as unhappy families, and unhappiness creates an environment that is certainly not optimal to the needs of a young person dealing with the challenges of adolescence. Data from longitudinal studies also reported similar findings. For instance, results from a study by Shek (2005a) showed that family functioning has an impact on early adolescent development as a lower level of perceived family functioning predicted poor adjustment in the domains of psychological distress, overall psychological health, delinquency, and well-being in female adolescents over time. Conversely, well-functioning families can positively influence adolescents, preventing them from engaging in risk behaviors. This positive influence may not only protect them from the negative outcomes of relationships with deviant friends, thereby reducing the possibility of getting involved in delinquency in the Chinese context (Gao, Yu, & Ng, 2013), but it can also prevent early adolescents from becoming Internet addicts (Yu & Shek, 2013) and buffer the negative effects of hopelessness which leads to suicidal ideation (Lai, 2007).

All of the above findings therefore suggest that family functioning can influence adolescent development. However, there are several limitations intrinsic to the existing literature on family functioning. First, existing studies on the relationship between family functioning and adolescent adjustment have been predominately conducted in the West. As Shek (1997) pointed out, "no scientific study to date has been done to examine how family functioning is related to adolescent adjustment in Chinese culture" (p. 468). This has not changed much over the past 15 years in such a way that only very few studies focusing on family functioning have been carried out in a Chinese context to date. However, since Chinese people might perceive family functioning in a different way than Westerners, it is important to explore family relationships in a Chinese context. Second, a large majority of local studies on family functioning are cross-sectional. Longitudinal studies are relatively sparse, which makes it difficult to firmly establish whether family functioning is causally related to adolescent adjustment in the Chinese context. Third, since validated measures for family functioning are scant, it is difficult to assess family functioning in an objective manner. For instance, there are only a few indigenously developed and validated family functioning measures, such as the Chinese Family Assessment Instrument (C-FAI) (Shek, 2002). Obviously, more efforts are needed to address the methodological issues related to family functioning.

Parent-Child Relationship and Adolescent Developmental Outcomes

Parent-child relationship can affect family functioning as poor parent-child relationship can be a source of tension within the family. Family can then constitute a stressful context for adolescents which can make them feel isolated and more vulnerable to risk behavior. On the other hand, the crucial role of good parent-child relationship in healthy youth development is well documented. Studies have shown consistently that good parent-child relationship serves as a buffer preventing adolescents from engaging in risk behavior (e.g., Korkeila et al., 2004).

Unfortunately, as teenagers seek greater autonomy from parental control, adolescence is often seen as a synonym for conflict, so conflicts tend to be expected or seen as normal in many adolescent families. Research is challenging this popular view though, as studies have shown that conflicts are not a necessity during adolescence and parents may in fact be more distressed by conflicts with their adolescent child than the adolescent themselves (Steinberg, 2001). As a result, the inability for parents to cope with the challenges brought by the transition of their child into adulthood may upset parents and cause long-lasting misunderstandings and an increased number of conflicts, which in turn can adversely affect the adolescent's developmental outcomes.

In general, children who have a good relationship with their parents show higher self-esteem (Cheung & Lau, 1985), whereas children who have a hostile relationship with parents show low self-esteem and higher delinquency tendency (Leung & Lau, 1989). High levels of parent-adolescent conflict have been found to be linked to depression and suicidal ideation in adolescents of both genders (Lee, Wong, Chow, & McBride-Chang, 2006). Overall, the existing literature indicates clearly that poor family relationships have a strong influence on the development of risk behavior in early adolescents while good family relationships can prevent the development of risk behavior.

However, it is important to note that there are more research studies on the global aspects (e.g., overall assessment of the relationship) rather than specific aspects of parent-child relational qualities (e.g., trust, satisfaction with parental control). In addition, most of the existing studies were cross-sectional, and there is a lack of longitudinal studies examining the changes and causal effects of parent-child relationships in the early adolescent years. Furthermore, there are only very few studies in which parenting and parent-child relational qualities are included in a single study.

Parenting Styles and Adolescent Developmental Outcomes

Another facet of parent-child relationship is parenting style, which is an important determinant of children's emotional and behavioral development. The most commonly cited model of parenting style was proposed by Baumrind (1991) who describes four main parenting types, namely, authoritative, authoritarian, permissive, and rejecting-neglecting with additional subtypes in adolescent families. In Western studies on parenting styles, the authoritative style is usually credited as the most effective in protecting adolescents from problem behaviors such as drug use, delinquent activities, and academic performance (Baumrind, 1991; Lamborn, Mounts, Steinberg, & Dornbusch, 1991; Steinberg, Lamborn, Dornbusch, & Darling, 1992; Steinberg, Mounts, Lamborn, & Dornbusch, 1991). However, the same findings may not be culturally relevant to the Chinese context (Fok & Shek, 2011). For example, a study by Kang and Moore (2011) reported that Mainland Chinese "students with authoritarian mothers scored significantly higher than those with authoritative and permissive mothers on the total of core courses (Chinese, English and Math)" (p. 136), which establishes the authoritarian parenting type as more desirable than the authoritative type in Chinese families. Furthermore, Fok and Shek observed that the Western categorization of parenting types may not be fully relevant to the Chinese context, since "in addition to authoritative and non-authoritative parenting styles, most Hong Kong parents also adopt psychologically controlling parenting styles" (p. 102).

Psychological control is a kind of parenting behavior which manipulates children through negative tactics, such as constraining verbal expression, guilt induction, personal attack, erratic emotional behavior, and love withdrawal, so that children adhere to parental standards (Boughton & Lumley, 2011). Psychological control is thought to be a parenting practice that can easily lead to family dysfunction and negative adolescent developmental outcomes. Boughton and Lumley argued that psychological control affects parent-child communication and the parents' ability to understand the child's emotional well-being. Empirically, excessive control over an adolescent's psychological world has detrimental effects on adolescent development, particularly internalizing and mood problems (e.g., Shek, 2006; Shek & Lee, 2005). Despite the fact that parenting style is a well-researched area, psychological control is still a "neglected construct," and "there is little research specifically measuring psychological control and its covariates" (Barber, 1996, p. 3313). With specific reference to Chinese culture, the topic of psychological control is under-researched (Shek, 2005b).

Alternatively, parenting practices can also be interpreted in terms of parental behavioral control which comprises five dimensions, namely, parental knowledge, expectations, monitoring, discipline, and demandingness (Shek & Lee, 2007). In a local study analyzing parental behavioral control, paternal behavioral control was perceived to be lower than maternal behavioral control (Shek, 2005b). This finding is interesting as it suggests that the popular saying "strict fathers, kind mothers" in the Chinese context needs to be changed to "strict mothers, kind fathers" in Hong Kong. This illustrates the need for conducting further research on different types of parental control in Chinese families, such as psychological control or behavioral control, to see how they contribute to adolescent developmental outcomes and potentially yield to further culturally relevant insight.

Parent-Child Communication and Adolescent Developmental Outcomes

Positive parent-child communication contributes to positive adolescent development. In a local study, Shek (1997) found that positive communication with parents was associated with better adolescent psychological well-being and less delinquent behavior. However, a large majority of Hong Kong working parents do not have positive communication with their children. Fathers in particular spend most of the time on working which results in the contemporary phenomenon of "detached fathers, involved mothers." A local survey even reported that about 47 % ($N=853$) communicated with their parents for less than 30 min per day and 68 % of their conversations focused on academic studies (Children Council, 2006).

Another macro factor which is not family-friendly is that in most Hong Kong families, both parents have to work to sustain the family. Therefore, it is common to employ foreign domestic helpers to alleviate household chores, which often include taking care of children. However, the excessive dependency on foreign domestic helpers undermines the development of children because children rely heavily on them. As a result, children cannot do even simple things such as tie up shoelaces and expect others to care for their every need. Some families even rely on foreign domestic helpers to educate their children. However, the role as a foreign domestic helper with low status in the family makes it almost impossible for her to teach or discipline the children. Domestic helpers playing the role of "surrogate mother" (Yip et al., 2011) result in loose parenting and adolescent behavioral problems.

Furthermore, in the traditional Chinese culture, Confucianism emphasized family harmony and family hierarchy (Ho, 1981). Therefore, non-confrontational communication was essential to avoid interpersonal conflicts. However, with the weakening of traditional collectivistic Chinese beliefs and growth of contemporary individualistic beliefs and youth culture in Hong Kong nowadays, there is a decline in the respect for parents and an increase in detachment between children and their parents. As a result, there are more conflicts between parents and children, and the quality of parent-adolescent communication is declining. Parent-adolescent conflict not only has detrimental effects on parent-child relationship but also makes adolescents feel distressed, emotionally distant, and stressful.

The aforementioned situation may also lead to further parent-child relationship difficulties. As parents do not feel respected by their adolescent child, they may resort to excessive parental control in an attempt to force respect. However, as adolescents need more independence, too much parental behavioral control may undermine their perceived ability to achieve independence, which may result in the adolescent feeling incompetent and may give them a sense of not being accepted, undermining their self-esteem, and potentially causing depression and other mental health issues or behavioral problems in their adolescent child. In addition, as adolescents fail to feel supported by their parents, they may develop difficulties in maintaining positive and long-term relationships with peers. All of those difficulties increase the likelihood for adolescents to engage in risk behavior (Beveridge & Berg, 2007).

Parental Marital Disruption and Adolescent Development

The number of divorce decrees granted in 2011 in Hong Kong was 18,374 (Census and Statistics Department, 2012). This number significantly soared from only 2,060 in 1981. As a result, more and more children have to grow up in single-parent or recomposed families and bear the consequence of parental marital disruption.

Marital disruption is seen as a stressor which causes parents to focus more on their problems than on their children. Family ecological theorists assert that marital disruption has negative effects on adolescent development due to changes in family processes. During adolescence, teenagers require support from families to meet their developmental needs. However, a study by Mechanic and Hansell (1989) suggests that "divorce and family conflict probably erode family member's capacity to nurture children's well-being by diverting time and attention from the children and by undermining the children's perceptions of parental interest" (p. 106). As parents focus on the conflict with their spouse instead of taking care of their children, they effectively become neglectful. As a result, children lack support, supervision, and other basic emotional and/or physical needs which may translate into the development of risky behavior during early adolescence.

Empirically, family processes in non-intact families in Hong Kong are comparatively poorer than those of intact families. Consistent results from a series of studies by Shek (2007, 2008a, 2008b) found that parent-child relational qualities, perceived parental behavioral control processes, and psychological well-being were worse in non-intact families than in intact families. Moreover, parenting qualities, such as parental control and parental warmth, were found to be lower in non-intact families when compared to intact families (Shek, 2007).

All of the above studies clearly indicate that parental divorce not only causes changes in the composition of a family but also affects parenting and parent-child relationships which in turn influence adolescent emotion and behavior.

Economic Disadvantage and Adolescent Well-Being

The stress induced by economic disadvantage affects parents not only financially but also emotionally, impacting the quality of parenting, parent-child communication, and parent-child relationship and therefore resulting in family dysfunction. According to the Family Stress Model of economic hardship, financial strain has negative influence on parents' emotions, behaviors, and relationships which may affect their parenting (Conger & Conger, 2002). Poverty reduces parent's capacity for being supportive as well as involved, and economically disadvantaged parents are more likely to use coercive discipline as opposed to negotiation and reasoning (McLoyd, 1990). Specifically, poverty causes emotional distress in parents which reduces warmth in parent-child relationships and increases parent-child conflicts. Those repeated conflicts in turn influence a child's well-being, emotional state, academic performance, and cognitive functioning (Conger, 2005), which all contribute to the development of adolescent risk behavior.

The above findings support previous findings from earlier research by Shek (e.g., 2003) that demonstrated that poverty was associated with lower levels of self-esteem, substance abuse, and problem behavior in adolescents. Based on the results from a series of studies (Shek & Lee, 2007; Shek & Tsui, 2012), Shek (2013) concluded that developmental outcomes of economically disadvantaged adolescents were comparatively poorer than those without economic disadvantage. Adolescents with economic disadvantage demonstrated lower levels of positive identity, family interaction, and perceived paternal parenting. Psychological well-being, which was assessed by hopelessness, mastery, life satisfaction, and self-esteem of adolescents experiencing economic disadvantage, was weaker than those not experiencing economic disadvantage.

Positive Youth Development Attributes and Adolescent Developmental Outcomes

As discussed above, positive youth development programs are highly needed for strengthening psychosocial competencies in adolescents and reduce adolescent risk behavior.

In their review of the effectiveness of positive youth development programs, Catalano et al. (2004) concluded that there are 15 basic youth development constructs which are related to a reduction in adolescent problem behavior (including bonding, social competence, emotional competence, cognitive competence, behavioral competence, moral competence, self-efficacy, prosocial norms, resilience, self-determination, spirituality, clear and positive identity, beliefs in the future, prosocial involvement, and recognition for positive behavior). Research showed that adolescents who developed positively are able to utilize their potential and contribute to their well-being (Rutter, 1987). Hence, positive developmental assets are indeed protective factors and can be conceived as personal strengths which help adolescents to become healthy individuals.

There are also theoretical propositions showing that positive youth development influences an individual's well-being. For instance, in Lent's model (2004), self-efficacy is one of the positive development attributes which influences life satisfaction. The social learning theory (Bandura, 1997) posits that self-efficacy affects positive health outcomes. In addition, based on the concepts of protective factors in resilience literature, internal resources such as psychosocial competencies and external resources such as bonding (e.g., Jessor et al., 2003) protect individuals from stresses in life.

Empirically, there are research findings showing that positive youth development qualities influence adolescent problem behavior via life satisfaction (Sun & Shek, 2013). Life satisfaction has been shown to be predicted by several positive youth development constructs, such as social and emotional competencies (Ciarrochi, Scott, Deane, and Heaven 2003), prosocial motivation and behavior (Gebauer, Riketta, Broemer, and Maio 2008), academic and social self-efficacy (Vecchio, Gerbino, Pastorelli, Del Bove, and Caprara 2007), as well as spirituality and religiosity (Laudet & White, 2008). The influence of positive youth development on problem behavior is direct during early adolescence, suggesting that promoting positive strengths to reduce problem behavior via the implementation of positive youth development programs is beneficial to early adolescents (Sun & Shek, 2013).

However, positive youth development theories and research are still in their infancy in different Chinese contexts (Shek & Sun, 2013). One possible exception is the Project P.A.T.H.S. in Hong Kong. While most positive youth development programs were developed and implemented in the West, the Project P.A.T.H.S. is a pioneering adolescent development program in Asia. Evaluation findings based on the Project P.A.T.H.S. showed that students who joined the program (experimental group) had significantly better positive outcomes in terms of psychosocial competencies, better academic performance, and higher global positive youth development and showed fewer delinquent behavior when compared to students who never participated in the program (control group) (Shek & Sun, 2010). Findings which support the effectiveness of the Project P.A.T.H.S. were consistently reported (e.g., Shek & Ma, 2011; Shek & Yu, 2011a). Overall, positive youth development programs have been shown to be effective in preventing adolescent risk behavior.

Research Gaps of the Existing Literature

There are several research gaps intrinsic to the existing studies pertaining to the influence of family quality of life (e.g., family functioning) and positive youth development attributes and individual well-being indexed by adolescent risk behavior. First, most of the existing studies on adolescent risk behavior have been predominantly conducted in Western societies. Using the search terms of "adolescence" and "risk behavior" to search relevant research studies up to November 2013, results indicated that there were 1,533 citations in the PsycINFO, 33 citations in the Sociological Abstracts, and 5 citations in the Academic Search Premier. However, utilizing search terms of "adolescence" and "risk behavior" and "Chinese," an identical search showed that there were only 14 citations in PsycINFO, whereas no publications were found in both Sociological Abstracts and Academic Search Premier. The dearth of relevant research data in the Chinese context would motivate one to ask whether the related phenomena are in congruence with those in the West. Furthermore, the low search figures suggest that there is an urgent need to exert more efforts to conduct adolescent risk behavior research in different Chinese communities. Since there is a lack of Chinese studies, it would be theoretically and practically crucial to investigate further the relationship between family and adolescent risk behavior in the Chinese context. Shek (2006) argued that since the Chinese population has constituted approximately one-fifth of the world's population, "the implication of these figures is that if any theory is claimed to be universally applicable, relevant data from Chinese people must be collected" (p. 276).

Second, the phenomena reviewed in this chapter underscore the importance of family in adolescent development. In contrast to individualistic explanations, such as genetic and psychological explanations, ecological models suggest that there is a need to explore how different contexts, such as family, might influence adolescent development (Bronfenbrenner, 1979). Ecological models can help explain the complex interactions between individual and family. With particular reference to the recent emergence of family issues and a dearth of Chinese studies examining family processes, there is an urgent need to understand adolescent risk behavior from an ecological perspective, particularly the family ecological perspective (Shek, 2003).

Third, there are only isolated studies in which dyadic and systemic family processes are simultaneously examined in a single study. Empirically, it would be interesting if the study incorporates both dyadic and systemic processes as this would be an advance in the field. For example, economic stress has adverse effects on the psychological well-being of parents which in turn disrupts dyadic family processes, such as parent-child relationship and spousal relationship, which in turn influence adolescent adjustment.

Fourth, there is a lack of positive youth development studies and programs in Chinese communities. After reviewing the recent adolescent studies and positive youth development programs in Macau, Luk (2010) concluded that there is a lack of theoretically sound and comprehensive programs for youth development. Similarly, based on a detailed review of adolescent prevention and positive youth development programs in Asia, Shek and Yu (2011b) arrived at the following conclusions: (a) when compared with the West, the number of validated programs in different Asian communities was very low; (b) the majority of programs focused on substance abuse than mental health problems; (c) positive youth development programs were sparse when compared with evaluated prevention programs; (d) rigorously designed evaluative studies of prevention and positive youth development programs over a long period of time were few. Therefore, there is an urgent need to develop positive youth development programs in different Asian communities (Shek & Yu, 2011b).

Luk (2011) asserted that positive youth development programs "can potentially help adolescents develop a positive growth and be better prepared for future challenges" (p. 35). Due to the limited number of positive youth development programs in Chinese communities, positive youth development research is in its infancy.

Fifth, some of the existing studies are methodologically inadequate. There is a lack of sound and validated psychosocial measurements and assessment tools for evaluating different aspects of positive youth development constructs in the field. Thus, some studies only utilized non-validated instruments with unclear psychometric properties. Irrespective of whether the measures of family and adolescent risk behavior are indigenously developed or imported from the West, the measures should first be validated. The use of non-validated instruments is problematic because their validity and reliability are unknown. Also, the measuring instruments may not be able to capture the essence of the Chinese culture if they are adapted from the West (Lai Kwok & Shek, 2010). In contrast, if indigenous Chinese measures are used, we can explore whether the research findings are consistent with previous research results conducted in the West. Additionally, the paucity of measures of positive youth development hampers program dissemination and widens the gap between research and practice (Ruth & Brooks-Gunn, 2003). Furthermore, along the line of research methodology, the sample size in some of the studies is small. For instance, Feldman, Wentzel, Weinberger, and Munson (1990) used 50 mothers and 43 fathers with 6th grade sons to investigate the relationship between marital satisfaction and family functioning. Bean, Barber, and Crane (2006) explored the relationship between psychological control and self-esteem in small samples of 75 African American and 80 European American adolescents. Chang, Mcbride-Chang, Stewart, and Au (2003) used 115 second graders and 74 eighth graders from Hong Kong to explore the relationships between self-concept, family relations, and life satisfaction. The major problems associated with small sample size are power (Kraemer & Thiemann, 1987) and generalizability. The use of multivariate statistical tests such as multiple regression analyses in small samples (e.g., Bean et al., 2006) increases the likelihood that the obtained data are due to chance effect. Tabachnick and Fidell (1989) warned that in multiple regression analyses, "power may be unacceptably low no matter the cases-to-IVs ratio if you have fewer than 100 cases" (pp. 128–129). Therefore, a large sample size will allow for a more precise estimation of the strength of the associations.

Sixth, with a few exceptions, a large majority of the existing research studies are primarily based on cross-sectional data. Data from longitudinal studies were scant. For instance, Shek (2001b) pointed out that "there is a severe lack of longitudinal studies" (p. 58). Although the existing cross-sectional studies can give us some ideas of the possible relationships between family functioning and adolescent risk behavior at a point of time, cross-sectional studies fail to unfold the causal relationships between family factors on adolescent development over time. For example, regarding the direction of influences between parent-child conflict and adolescent risk behavior, there are at least five possibilities: (1) parent-child conflict influences adolescent risk behavior, (2) adolescent risk behavior influences parent-child conflict, (3) parent-child conflict and adolescent risk behavior influence each other,

(4) parent-child conflict and adolescent risk behavior do not influence each other, and (5) the relationship between parent-child conflict and adolescent risk behavior is spurious. Therefore, studies with longitudinal designs are indispensable if we assess the direction of influences between parent-child conflict and adolescent risk behavior. It would be exciting if more time points over a longer period of time can be included in the future studies.

Lastly, there is a paucity of studies incorporating multiple positive and negative personal well-being measures in a single study. For instance, Sun and Shek (2011) investigated the relationships among positive youth development, life satisfaction, and problem behavior simultaneously in a single study. The results showed that positive youth development inversely predicted adolescent risk behavior, with life satisfaction as a mediating factor. These results shed light on the importance of promoting psychosocial competencies in adolescents to reduce adolescent risk behavior. Therefore, it is pertinent to include multiple positive and negative personal well-being measures in a single study in order to obtain a clear picture of adolescent risk behavior.

The Way Forward

Recognizing the importance of family to social harmony, in his address at the Legislative Council meeting on October 14, 2009, the former Chief Executive of the Special Administrative Region of Hong Kong, Mr. Donald Tsang said that "many social problems, including juvenile drug abuse, prostitution…, could be traced back to the family. Better family relationships meant fewer social problems" (Family Council, 2011, p. 1).

There are several observations pertaining to family development in Hong Kong. First, the number of non-intact families in Hong Kong is soaring. According to the Census and Statistics Department (2007), the number of divorces in 2006 was eight times that in 1981, suggesting that more children are affected. Second, employees in Hong Kong have longer working hours than many other cities and countries, such as London and the United States (Wharton & Blair-Loy, 2006). As a result, fathers in Hong Kong spent an average of 6 min a day with their children (Bracey, Montie, Xiang, and Schweinhart 2007). Obviously, the long working hours hamper parent-adolescent communication which has adverse effects on adolescent psychological health (e.g., Stivers, 1988). Third, the number of families with economic disadvantage in Hong Kong is increasing, with about one-quarter of children and adolescents experiencing economic disadvantage (Shek, 2006). The Commission on Poverty reported that the poor population in Hong Kong was about 1.02 million (403,000 households), representing a poverty rate of 15.2 %. Among the 1.02 million people below the poverty line, about 209,000 were people under 18 years old, suggesting that one in five Hong Kong children is living below the poverty line (Commission on Poverty, 2013). Finally, the Hong Kong Council of Social Service (2012) found that the Social Development Index showed a drop of family solidarity, from −215 in

2004 to −309 in 2010, suggesting a gradual disintegration of families in Hong Kong (Hong Kong Council of Social Service, 2012). It is obvious that these issues would influence family processes which would eventually affect adolescent development. It is therefore important to explore those topics individually in more detail to reach a clear understanding of how family works and how the family context may influence early adolescent development and the occurrence of risk behaviors, which will be the main focus of the chapters in this book.

Apart from issues on the family levels, there are also findings suggesting that adolescents in Hong Kong are egocentric and immature growing up in a "greenhouse." Hence, how positive youth development attributes may protect adolescents from risk behavior is an important question to be answered. As it is a neglected research gap in the Chinese literature, this issue is also covered in the relevant chapters of this book. It is our modest wish that through further understanding of how family processes and positive youth development attributes may contribute to adolescent developmental outcomes, some insights into the promotion of adolescent development will be crystallized.

Acknowledgments The preparation for this work and the Project P.A.T.H.S. were financially supported by The Hong Kong Jockey Club Charities Trust.

References

Bandura, A. (1997). *Self-efficacy: The exercise of control*. New York: Freeman.

Barber, B. K. (1996). Parental psychological control: Revisiting a neglected construct. *Child Development, 67*(6), 3296–3319.

Baumrind, D. (1991). The influence of parenting style on adolescent competence and substance use. *Journal of Early Adolescence, 11*(1), 56–95.

Bean, R. A., Barber, B. K., & Crane, D. R. (2006). Parental support, behavioral control, and psychological control among African American youth: The relationships to academic grades, delinquency, and depression. *Journal of Family Issues, 27*(10), 1335–1355.

Beveridge, R. M., & Berg, C. A. (2007). Parent-adolescent collaboration: An interpersonal model for understanding optimal interactions. *Clinical Child and Family Psychology, 10*(1), 25–52.

Boughton, K. L., & Lumley, M. N. (2011). Parent prediction of child mood and emotional resilience: The role of parental responsiveness and psychological control. *Depression Research and Treatment*. Retrieved from http://www.hindawi.com/journals/drt/2011/375398/

Bracey, G., Montie, J. E., Xiang, Z. P., & Schweinhart, L. J. (2007). *The IEA preliminary study: Findings and policy implications*. Ypsilanti, MI: High/Scope Educational Research Foundation.

Bronfenbrenner, U. (1979). *The ecology of human development*. Cambridge, MA: Harvard University Press.

Catalano, R. F., Berglund, M. L., Ryan, J. A. M., Lonczak, H. S., & Hawkins, J. D. (2004). Positive youth development in the United States: Research findings on evaluations of positive youth development programs. *The Annals of the American Academy of Political and Social Science, 591*(1), 98–124.

Catalano, R. F., Hawkins, J. D., Berglund, M. L., Pollard, J. A., & Arthur, M. W. (2002). Prevention science and positive youth development: Competitive or cooperative frameworks? *Journal of Adolescent Health, 31*, 230–239.

Census and Statistics Department. (2007, November). *Hong Kong monthly digest of statistics: Marriage and divorce trends in Hong Kong, 1981–2006*. Hong Kong: Census and Statistics Department.
Census and Statistics Department. (2012). *Hong Kong annual digest of statistics*. Hong Kong: Census and Statistics Department.
Chang, L., Mcbride-Chang, C., Stewart, S. M., & Au, E. (2003). Life satisfaction, self-concept, and family relations in Chinese adolescents and children. *International Journal of Behavioural Development, 27*, 182–189.
Cheung, P. C., & Lau, S. (1985). Self-esteem: Its relationship to the family and school social environments among Chinese adolescents. *Youth and Society, 16*, 438–456.
Children's Council. (2006). *Motion 4: The government should set up a task force to improve parent-child relationships*. Retrieved from http://www.childrencouncil.org.hk/app/webroot/files/cms/4th_Motion4.pdf
Ciarrochi, J., Scott, G., Deane, F. P., & Heaven, P. C. L. (2003). Relations between social and emotional competence and mental health: A construct validation study. *Personality and Individual Differences, 35*, 1947–1963.
Commission on Poverty. (2013, September 13). *Hong Kong's first official poverty line – Purpose and value*. Retrieved from: http://www.povertyrelief.gov.hk/eng/pdf/20130930_article.pdf
Conger, R. D. (2005). *The effects of poverty and economic hardship across generations*. Davis, CA: Centre for Public Policy Research, University of California, Davis.
Conger, R. D., & Conger, K. J. (2002). Resilience in Midwestern families: Selected findings from the first decade of a prospective, longitudinal study. *Journal of Marriage and Family, 64*, 361–373.
Department of Child and Adolescent Health and Development. (2001). *Broadening the horizon: Balancing protection and risk for adolescents*. Geneva, Switzerland: World Health Organization.
Family Council. (2011, July 4). *Policy recommendations arising from the four researches on child neglect, elderly neglect, youth drug abuse and youth prostitution*. Retrieved from https://www.google.com.hk/#q=Donald+tsang+October+14+2009+legislative+council+meeting
Feldman, S. S., Wentzel, K. R., Weinberger, D. A., & Munson, J. A. (1990). Marital satisfaction of parents of preadolescent boys and its relationship to family and child functioning. *Journal of Family Psychology, 4*(2), 213–234.
Fok, H. K., & Shek, D. T. L. (2011). A conceptual critique of parenting research in Hong Kong. *International Journal of Adolescent Medicine and Health, 23*(2), 101–107.
Gao, Y., Yu, Y., & Ng, T. K. (2013). A study on the moderating effect of family functioning on the relationship between deviant peer affiliation and delinquency among Chinese adolescents. *Advances in Applied Sociology, 3*(3), 178–185.
Gebauer, J. E., Riketta, M., Broemer, P., & Maio, G. R. (2008). Pleasure and pressure based prosocial motivation: Divergent relations to subjective well-being. *Journal of Research in Personality, 42*, 399–420.
Ho, D. Y. F. (1981). Traditional patterns of socialization in Chinese society. *Acta Psychologica Taiwanica, 23*, 81–95.
Hoffman, L., Marquis, J., Poston, D., Summers, J. A., & Turnbull, A. (2006). Assessing family outcomes: Psychometric evaluation of the Beach Center Family Quality of Life Scale. *Journal of Marriage and Family, 68*(4), 1069–1083.
Hong Kong Council of Social Service. (2012). *Family and community services in Hong Kong*. Retrieved from: https://www.google.com.hk/#q=increase+in+families+with+economic+disadvantage+in+Hong+Kong
Jessor, R., Turbin, M. S., Costa, F. M., Dong, Q., Zhang, H., & Wang, C. (2003). Adolescent problem behavior in China and the United States: A cross-national study of psychosocial protective factors. *Journal of Research on Adolescence, 13*(3), 329–360.
Kang, Y., & Moore, J. (2011). Parenting style and adolescents' school performance in Mainland China. *US-China Education Review, B1*, 133–138.
Korkeila, K., Kivela, S. L., Suominen, S., Vahtera, J., Kivmaki, M., Sundell, J., et al. (2004). Childhood adversities, parent-child relationships and dispositional optimism in adulthood. *Social Psychiatry and Psychiatric Epidemiology, 39*(4), 286–292.

Kraemer, H. C., & Thiemann, S. (1987). *How many subjects? Statistical power analysis in research*. Newbury Park, CA: Sage.

Lai, Y. C. (2007). Personal and family correlates of suicidal ideation in Chinese adolescents in Hong Kong. *Unpublished doctoral thesis. Hong Kong: The Chinese University of Hong Kong*.

Lai Kwok, S. Y. C., & Shek, D. T. L. (2010). Personal and family correlates of suicidal ideation among Chinese adolescents in Hong Kong. *Social Indicators Research, 95*, 407–419. doi:10.1007/s11205-009-9528-4.

Lamborn, S. D., Mounts, N. S., Steinberg, L., & Dornbusch, S. M. (1991). Patterns of competence and adjustment among adolescents from authoritative, authoritarian, indulgent, and neglectful families. *Child Development, 62*, 1049–1065.

Laudet, A. B., & White, W. L. (2008). Recovery capital as prospective predictor of sustained recovery, life satisfaction, and stress among former poly-substance users. *Substance Use and Misuse, 43*, 27–54.

Law, B. M. F., & Shek, D. T. L. (2013). Self-harm and suicide attempts among young Chinese adolescents in Hong Kong: Prevalence, correlates, and changes. *Journal of Pediatric and Adolescent Gynecology, 26*, S26–S32.

Lee, T. Y., & Shek, D. T. L. (2013). Compensated dating in Hong Kong: Prevalence, psychosocial correlates, and relationships with other risky behaviours. *Journal of Pediatric and Adolescent Gynecology, 26*, S42–S48.

Lee, A., & Tsang, C. K. K. (2004). Youth risk behavior in a Chinese population: A territory-wide youth risk behavioral surveillance in Hong Kong. *Public Health, 118*, 88–95.

Lee, M. T. Y., Wong, B. P., Chow, B. W. Y., & McBride-Chang, C. (2006). Predictors of suicide ideation and depression in Hong Kong adolescents: Perceptions of academic and family climates. *Suicide and Life-Threatening Behaviour, 36*(1), 82–96.

Lent, R. W. (2004). Toward a unifying theoretical and practical perspective on well-being and psychosocial adjustment. *Journal of Consulting Psychology, 51*, 482–509.

Leung, K., & Lau, S. (1989). Effects of self-concept and perceived disapproval on delinquent behavior in school children. *Journal of Youth and Adolescence, 18*, 345–359.

Luk, L. (2010). A review of the positive youth development and prevention programs for adolescents in Macau. *Macau Journal of Nursing, 9*(1), 21–25.

Luk, L. (2011). Adopting a positive youth development program in Macau: Difficulties and challenges. *Macau Journal of Nursing, 10*(1), 35–39.

McLoyd, V. C. (1990). The impact of economic hardship on black families and children: Psychological distress, parenting, and socioemotional development. *Child Development, 61*, 311–346.

Mechanic, D., & Hansell, S. (1989). Divorce, family conflict, and adolescents' well-being. *Journal of Health and Social Behaviour, 30*(1), 105–116.

Olson, D. H., Russell, C. S., & Sprenkle, D. H. (1983). Circumplex model of marital and family systems: VI. Theoretical update. *Family Process, 22*(1), 69–83.

Olson, D. H., Sprenkle, D. H., & Russell, C. S. (1979). Circumplex model of marital and family systems: I. Cohesion and adaptability dimensions, family types, and clinical applications. *Family Process, 18*(1), 3–28.

Parker, H. S. (2000). *Parent structure and support and adolescent problems: Delinquency, substance abuse, and peer and self-esteem deficits*. Dissertation, Virginia Polytechnic Institute and State University, Blacksburg, VA.

Putnam, R. D. (1995). Bowling alone: America's declining social capital. *Journal of Democracy, 6*(1), 64–78.

Ruth, J. L., & Brooks-Gunn, J. (2003). What exactly is a youth development program? Answers from research and practice. *Applied Developmental Science, 7*(2), 94–111.

Rutter, M. (1987). Psychosocial resilience and protective mechanisms. *American Journal of Orthopsychiatry, 57*(3), 316–331.

Shek, D. T. L. (1993). Perceptions of parental treatment styles and psychological well-being in Chinese college students. *Psychologia, 36*, 159–166.

Shek, D. T. L. (1997). The relation of family functioning to adolescent psychological well-being, school adjustment, and problem behavior. *The Journal of Genetic Psychology, 158*(4), 467–479.

Shek, D. T. L. (2001a). Chinese adolescents and their parents' views on a happy family: Implications for family therapy. *Family Therapy, 28*(2), 73–104.

Shek, D. T. L. (2001b). Paternal and maternal influences on family functioning among Hong Kong Chinese families. *The Journal of Genetic Psychology, 162*(1), 56–74.

Shek, D. T. L. (2002). Assessment of family functioning in Chinese adolescents: The Chinese version of the Family Assessment Device. *Research on Social Work Practice, 12*, 504–524.

Shek, D. T. L. (2003). Economic stress, psychological well-being and problem behavior in Chinese adolescents with economic disadvantage. *Journal of Youth and Adolescence, 32*(4), 259–266.

Shek, D. T. L. (2005a). A longitudinal study of perceived family functioning and adolescent adjustment in Chinese adolescents with economic disadvantage. *Journal of Family Issues, 26*, 518–543. doi:10.1177/0192513X04272618.

Shek, D. T. L. (2005b). Perceived parental control processes, parent-child relational qualities, and psychological well-being in Chinese adolescents with and without economic disadvantage. *Journal of Genetic Psychology, 166*, 171–188.

Shek, D. T. L. (2006). Assessment of perceived parental psychological control in Chinese adolescents in Hong Kong. *Research on Social Work Practice, 16*, 382–391.

Shek, D. T. L. (2007). Intact and non-intact families in Hong Kong: Differences in perceived parental control processes, parent-child relational qualities, and adolescent psychological well-being. *Journal of Divorce & Remarriage, 47*(1–2), 157–172.

Shek, D. T. L. (2008a). Economic disadvantage, perceived family life quality, and emotional well-being in Chinese adolescents: A longitudinal study. *Social Indicators Research, 85*(2), 169–189.

Shek, D. T. L. (2008b). Perceived parental control processes, parent-child relational qualities, and adolescent psychological well-being in intact and non-intact families: Longitudinal findings in the Chinese culture. *Journal of Divorce & Remarriage, 49*(1–2), 171–189.

Shek, D. T. L. (2013). Sexual behaviour and intention to engage in sexual behaviour in junior secondary school students in Hong Kong. *Journal of Pediatric and Adolescent Gynecology, 26*, S33–S41.

Shek, D. T. L., & Lee, T. Y. (2005). Hopelessness and Chinese adolescents in Hong Kong: Demographic and family correlates. *International Journal of Adolescent Medicine and Health, 17*, 279–290.

Shek, D. T. L., & Lee, T. Y. (2007). Perceived parental control processes, parent-child relational qualities and psychological well-being of Chinese adolescents in intact and non-intact families in Hong Kong. *International Journal of Adolescent Medicine and Health, 19*, 167–175.

Shek, D. T. L., & Ma, C. M. S. (2011). Impact of the Project P.A.T.H.S. in the junior secondary school years: Individual growth curve analyses. *The Scientific World Journal, 11*, 253–266.

Shek, D. T. L., & Ma, C. M. S. (2012). Impact of the Project P.A.T.H.S. in the junior secondary school years: Objective outcome evaluation based on eight waves of longitudinal data. *The Scientific World Journal, 2012*, Article ID 170345, 12 pp. doi:10.1100/2012/170345.

Shek, D. T. L., & Sun, R. C. F. (2010). Effectiveness of the Tier 1 program of Project P.A.T.H.S.: Findings based on three years of program implementation. *The Scientific World Journal, 10*, 1509–1519.

Shek, D. T. L., & Sun, R. C. F. (2013). Development of a positive youth development program in Hong Kong. In D. T. L. Shek & R. C. F. Sun (Eds.), *Development and evaluation of positive adolescent training through holistic social programs (P.A.T.H.S.)*. Singapore/New York: Springer.

Shek, D. T. L., & Tsui, P. F. (2012). Family and personal adjustment of economically disadvantaged Chinese adolescents in Hong Kong. *The Scientific World Journal*. Available at: http://www.ncbi.nlm.nih.gov/pmc/articles/PMC3415177/. doi:10.1100/2012/142689.

Shek, D. T. L., & Yu, L. (2011a). Prevention of adolescent problem behavior: Longitudinal impact of the Project P.A.T.H.S. in Hong Kong. *The Scientific World Journal, 11*, 546–567.

Shek, D. T. L., & Yu, L. (2011b). A review of validated youth prevention and positive youth development programs in Asia. *International Journal of Adolescent Medicine and Health, 23*(4), 317–324.

Shek, D. T. L., & Yu, L. (2012). Longitudinal impact of the Project P.A.T.H.S. on adolescent risk behavior: What happened after five years. *The Scientific World Journal, 2012*, Article ID 316029, 13 pages. doi:10.1100/2012/316029.

Steinberg, L. (2001). *The role of the family in adolescent development: Preventing risk, promoting resilience*. Children, Youth and Families Education and Research Network. Retrieved from: http://www1.cyfernet.org/conffav/05-01-Steinberg.html

Steinberg, L., Lamborn, S. D., Dornbusch, S. M., & Darling, N. (1992). Impact of parenting practices on adolescent achievement: Authoritative parenting, school involvement, and encouragement to succeed. *Child Development, 63*, 1266–1281.

Steinberg, L., Mounts, N. S., Lamborn, S. D., & Dornbusch, S. M. (1991). Authoritative parenting and adolescent adjustment across varied ecological niches. *Journal of Research on Adolescence, 1*, 19–36.

Stivers, C. (1988). Parent-adolescent communication and its relationship to adolescent depression and suicide proneness. *Adolescence, 23*(90), 291–295.

Sun, R. C. F., & Shek, D. T. L. (2010). Life satisfaction, positive youth development, and problem behavior among Chinese adolescents in Hong Kong. *Social Indicators Research, 95*, 455–474.

Sun, R. C. F., & Shek, D. T. L. (2011). Positive youth development, life satisfaction and problem behavior among Chinese adolescents in Hong Kong: A replication. *Social Indicators Research*. Retrieved from: http://link.springer.com/article/10.1007/s11205-011-9786-9/fulltext.html

Sun, R. C. F., & Shek, D. T. L. (2012). Positive youth development, life satisfaction and problem behavior among Chinese adolescents in Hong Kong: A replication. *Social Indicators Research, 105*(3), 541–559.

Sun, R. C. F., & Shek, D. T. L. (2013). Longitudinal influences of positive youth development and life satisfaction on problem behavior among adolescents in Hong Kong. *Social Indicators Research, 114*, 1171–1197. doi:10.1007/s11205-012-0196-4.

Tabachnick, B. G., & Fidell, L. S. (1989). *Using multivariate statistics*. New York: Harper and Row.

Tremblay, R. E., Pagani-Kurtz, L., Masse, L. C., Vitaro, F., & Pihi, R. O. (1995). A bimodal preventive intervention for disruptive kindergarten boys: Its impact through mid-adolescence. *Journal of Counselling and Clinical Psychology, 63*(4), 560–568.

Vecchio, G. M., Gerbino, M., Pastorelli, C., Del Bove, G., & Caprara, G. V. (2007). Multi-faceted self-efficacy beliefs as predictors of life satisfaction in late adolescence. *Personality and Individual Differences, 43*, 1807–1818.

Wharton, A. S., & Blair-Loy, M. (2006). Long work hours and family life. *Journal of Family Issues, 27*(3), 415–436.

Yip, P., Cheung, S. L. K., Tsang, S., Tse, S., Wong, O. L., Laidler, K., et al. (2011). *A study on drug abuse among youths and family relationships*. Hong Kong: University of Hong Kong.

Yu, L., & Shek, D. T. L. (2013). Internet addiction in Hong Kong adolescents: A three-year longitudinal study. *Journal of Pediatric and Adolescent Gynecology, 26*, S10–S17.

A Longitudinal Study of the Personal Well-Being and Family Quality of Life Among Chinese Adolescents in Hong Kong

Daniel T.L. Shek and Cecilia M.S. Ma

Abstract While cross-sectional studies have been commonly employed to examine personal well-being and family quality of life among Chinese adolescents, comparatively fewer efforts were put in longitudinal studies in different Chinese societies. To examine the personal well-being and quality of family life in Chinese adolescents in Hong Kong, a groundbreaking 6-year longitudinal study was launched within the Project P.A.T.H.S. in Hong Kong. After comparing and contrasting the strengths and weaknesses of cross-sectional and longitudinal studies in adolescent development research, this chapter outlines the methodology of this longitudinal study, including the sample, instruments on personal well-being and family quality of life, and procedures. Moreover, the methodological unique features of the study are highlighted, and the demographic characteristics of the sample in the junior secondary school years are presented.

Keywords Adolescent development • Longitudinal research • Chinese adolescents • Personal well-being • Family quality of life

Introduction

For an individual, adolescence is a transitional period between childhood and adulthood in which many physical, emotional, cognitive, and behavioral changes take place. To fully understand the nature of such transition, researchers argued that there is a need to keep track the development of adolescents over time (Moore, 1997). Besides understanding the nature of changes in different areas, such knowledge also informs us what key resources and needs are vital during adolescence, which can further help shaping and improving public policies and welfare programs for adolescents and their families.

D.T.L. Shek, Ph.D., B.B.S., S.B.S., J.P. (✉) • C.M.S. Ma, Ph.D.
Department of Applied Social Sciences, The Hong Kong Polytechnic University, Hunghom, Hong Kong
e-mail: daniel.shek@polyu.edu.hk

D.T.L. Shek et al. (eds.), *Chinese Adolescents in Hong Kong*, Quality of Life in Asia 5, DOI 10.1007/978-981-287-143-5_2

Cross-Sectional Versus Longitudinal Studies

In the field of adolescent research, two approaches are commonly used – cross-sectional and longitudinal designs. Both methods have their own strengths and weaknesses. For cross-sectional research designs, the first strength is its convenience because it is basically a social survey at single point of time. Second, compared to experimental studies, the sample in a cross-sectional survey may be more representative because it involves subjects of different ages in a single study. Third, if a representative sample is selected, cross-sectional surveys can generate findings on the prevalence and profiles of certain behavior (e.g., Internet addiction) in the population under study. Fourth, in terms of resources, the cost of a cross-sectional study is comparatively lower than that of a longitudinal study. Finally, in contrast to longitudinal design, adolescent development at different ages can be understood within a short period of time. Probably because of these strengths, cross-sectional research design is widely used to understand adolescent development (e.g., Escobar-Chaves et al., 2005; Kanuga & Rosenfeld, 2004; Kwan, 2010; Shek, 2005a; Shek, Ma, & Tang, 2012).

Regarding the weaknesses of cross-sectional design, cohort effect may contaminate the effect of age on the developmental outcomes as participants of different ages are involved. Second, it is difficult to determine the causal relationships among different variables because they are assessed at the same time point. Although some statistical techniques such as structural equation modeling may be used to determine the relationships among different variables statistically, simultaneous collection of data on the predictor and criterion variables cannot give a definitive answer on the causal relationships among the variables. In fact, the abuse in using such sophisticated statistical technique may create pseudoscientific knowledge only.

In contrast, longitudinal studies make it possible to understand changes in adolescent behavior across time without the confounding of cohort effect. Besides, as predictors and criterion variables are assessed at different time points, the dynamic relationships among the predictor and criterion variables and the causal relationships can be assessed better. In particular, through the use of structural equation modeling, different models such as reversed causation models can be adequately tested in longitudinal studies (Ma & Shek, 2013; Shuster, Li, & Shi, 2012; Sun & Shek, 2012).

In spite of the aforesaid strengths, several weaknesses of longitudinal studies should be realized. First, compared with cross-sectional studies, longitudinal studies are more expensive. Second, to adequately assess the cause-effect relationships between the predictor and criterion variables, researchers have to wait for the completion of data collection at different waves of data collection. This may be a problem for new researchers who desperately need publications for tenure. Third, subject attrition over time is a challenge faced by researchers using longitudinal studies. If subject attrition is high, the data integrity of longitudinal studies would be compromised. In order to reduce subject attrition, resources must be used to maintain contact with the participants. Fourth, as sophisticated statistical analyses are employed in longitudinal data analyses, researchers must be well-versed in statistical analyses such as individual growth curve modeling.

Over the past decade, one noticeable change in adolescent research is observed. More longitudinal studies with different antecedents and/or correlates of adolescents' developmental outcomes have been carried out (e.g., Shek & Ma, 2012a; Shek & Yu, 2012). These studies demonstrate how the potential impact of early experience interacts with later experience and helps us understand the consequences of children's exposure to an accumulation of risk and protective factors that lead to developmental outcomes (Sroufe, Coffino, & Carlson, 2010). Researchers noted that "understanding developmental processes underlying continuity and change are more important than simply understanding that early experience often predicts later behavior" (Sroufe et al., 2010, p. 44). In particular, studies showed that the use of multiple ecological factors is more effective than focusing on individual factors when understanding adolescent problem behavior (Adalbjarnardottir & Hafsteinsson, 2001). Therefore, it would be interesting to ask whether intrapersonal developmental attributes and interpersonal factors (e.g., family characteristics, parenting style) in early years predict healthy youth development and academic performance at later stages. In order to answer this question, longitudinal research designs are indispensable.

Besides the call for more longitudinal studies, another limitation in the field is over-emphasis of the negative outcomes of adolescents and under-emphasis on positive youth development. As pointed out by Moore, Lippman, and Brown (2004), "from the youth development perspective, a focus on the negatives has another critical shortcoming, in that it fails to serve and inspire youth development programs... having positive outcomes incorporated into the national indicator system would provide a specific vision that includes not just what we do not want but what we do want for children and adolescents" (p. 126). To better monitor changes in adolescent development, a broad array of outcome variables, including both positive and negative well-being, is suggested in order to capture a more balanced picture when studying the trend of adolescent development.

Another limitation in the field is the lack of longitudinal studies in non-Western contexts. When reviewing the literature over the past decade, most of the studies were conducted in the West and comparatively fewer studies were conducted in different Chinese communities. This is further supported by searching in the database PsyINFO in October 2013. Using the key words "longitudinal" and "adolescent," a total of 19,403 articles were found. However, together with "Chinese," only 168 articles were found. Moreover, as shown in Table 1, among those longitudinal studies in different Chinese societies, the duration involved was not long. Given the dearth of studies examining the longitudinal development of adolescents in different Chinese contexts, more research in this area is warranted.

Extension Phase of the Project P.A.T.H.S. in Hong Kong

The Project P.A.T.H.S. is a positive youth development program which attempts to promote the holistic development of junior secondary school students in Hong Kong. In the initial phase of the project, the Research Team developed a positive

Table 1 Examples of longitudinal studies conducted in the past decade

Authors	Year	Age	Context	Duration	Variables
Adalbjarnardottir and Hafsteinsson	2001	14–17	Iceland	3 years	Parenting style, substance use behavior (parents' and adolescents')
Boislard and Poulin	2011	14–16	Canada	2 years	Family structure, parent-child relationship, sexual behavior
Booker et al.	2007	13–14	China	1 year	Smoking behavior, stressful life event
Bowers et al.	2011	10–11	United States	7 years	Positive youth development, delinquency, parental education, socioeconomic status, and after-school activity
Brook, Brook, and Whiteman	2007	12–17	United States	3 years	Violent and substance use behavior (parents', adolescents', and siblings')
Denault and Pouline	2012	12–13	Canada	5 years	Academic performance, after-school activity, depression, problem behaviors, parental involvement and beliefs
Elkington, Bauermeister, and Zimmerman	2011	14–15	United States	4 years	Substance use (adolescents' and parents'), parental support, and family involvement
Farrell, Sullivan, Esposito, Meyer, and Valois	2005	10–12	United States	5 years	Substance use and delinquency
Heard	2007	14–15	United States	1 year	Family structure, academic school performance
Hennessy, Bleakley, Fishbein, and Jordan	2009	14–16	United States	3 years	Sexual behavior and consumption of pornography materials
Keijsers, Branje, VanderValk, and Meeus	2010	13–16	Netherlands	1 year	Delinquency, parental control, parental knowledge, parental solicitation
Kerr, Stattin, and Burk	2010	12–15	Sweden	3 years	Parental control, parental knowledge, parent-child relationship, delinquency

(continued)

Table 1 (continued)

Authors	Year	Age	Context	Duration	Variables
Laird, Bridges, and Marsee	2013	12–13	United States	3 years	Depression, antisocial behavior, and parent-child relationship
Law and Shek	2013	11–13	Hong Kong	2 years	Self-harm and suicide attempts
Leung, Mc-Bride-Chang, and Lai	2004	11–14	Hong Kong	8 months	Parenting style
					Life satisfaction
					Perceived academic performance and academic self-concept
Liljeberg, Eklund, Fritz, and Klinteberg	2011	14–18	Sweden	18 months	Delinquent behavior and school bonding
Ma and Shek	2013	11–13	Hong Kong	3 years	Family functioning, positive youth development, consumption of pornography materials
Metzger, Dawes, Mermelstein, and Wakschlag	2011	15–16	United States	2 years	Smoking (adolescents' and peers') and after-school time activity
Nocentini, Menesini, and Salmivalli	2013	13–15	Italy	3 years	Aggressive behavior, depression
Odgers et al.	2009	5–10	United Kingdom	2 years	Delinquency (adolescents' and parents') and family socioeconomic status
Ostaszewski and Zimmerman	2006	14–16	United States	4 years	Substance use, parental education level, resilience, and parent support
Rueter and Kwon	2005	12–13	United States	7 years	Suicide-related thoughts and behavior (adolescents', parents', siblings', and peers')
Scales, Benson, Roehlkepartain, Sesma, and van Dulmen	2006	13–15	United States	3 years	Positive youth development and academic performance
Shek	2005b	12–16	Hong Kong	2 years	Perceived family functioning, psychological well-being, and problem behavior

(continued)

Table 1 (continued)

Authors	Year	Age	Context	Duration	Variables
Shek	2007a	11–19	Hong Kong	2 years	Parental psychological control, hopelessness, mastery, life satisfaction, and self-esteem
Shek	2007b	11–13	Hong Kong	1 year	Parental behavioral control
					Parental psychological
					control
					Parent-child relational qualities
Shek	2008	11–13	Hong Kong	3 years	Parental control
					Parent-child relational quality
Shuster et al.	2012	12–14	China	3 years	Cultural values
					Parenting practices
					Adolescent aggression
Sun and Shek	2012	12–14	Hong Kong	1 year	Life satisfaction, positive youth development, problem behavior
van den Eijnden, Meerkerk, Vermulst, Spijkerman, and Engels	2008	12–15	Netherlands	6 months	Compulsive Internet use, depression, and loneliness
Wang, Pomerantz, and Chen	2007	12–13	China	6 months	Parents' psychological control, autonomy support, behavioral control, and academic functioning
Wight, Williamson, and Henderson	2006	13–14	Scotland	2 years	Parental monitoring and sexual behavior
Yu and Shek	2013	11–13	Hong Kong	3 years	Internet addiction, positive youth development, and family functioning

youth development program, trained the implementers, implemented the program, and evaluated the program (Shek & Ma, 2012a; Shek & Sun, 2013; Shek & Yu, 2012). The project was financially supported by The Hong Kong Jockey Club Charities Trust, with an earmarked grant of HK$400 million. In the extension phase of the project, the developed program was implemented for another cycle from 2009/2010 to 2011/2012 school years with an addition earmarked grant of HK$350 million. In the extension phase, a 6-year longitudinal study has been implemented since the 2009/2010 school year.

The purpose of this chapter is to outline the research design of this 6-year longitudinal study, including the instruments employed, sample recruited, and procedures involved in data collection. The demographic characteristics of the sample successfully matched across the first three waves, and the unique features of the longitudinal study are highlighted at the end of this chapter.

Overview of the Study

Participants and Procedures

In the academic year 2009/2010, a total of 3,328 Secondary 1 students (Grade 7) from 28 schools randomly selected from schools in Hong Kong participated in this 6-year longitudinal study of adolescent development and their families in Hong Kong. Among the participants, 1,719 (52 %) were boys and 1,572 (48 %) were girls, with 37 of them did not give any response. In the school years of 2010/2011 and 2011/2012, 3,638 Grade 8 students and 4,106 Grade 9 students participated in the study, respectively. A total of 2,667 participants completed the questionnaires in all three waves. The demographic characteristics of the participants matched across three waves are shown in Table 2.

Written consent was obtained from the schools, the parents, and the students. During data collection, the purpose of the study was mentioned and confidentiality of the collected data was ensured. A research assistant was present throughout the administration process. Participants completed a battery of questionnaires in 20–30 min and received a souvenir in return for completion of the questionnaires. The study was approved by The Hong Kong Polytechnic University Institutional Review Board.

Instruments

Respondents were asked to complete a battery of questionnaires containing questions regarding their demographic characteristics (e.g., age, gender, and immigrant status), family background (e.g., parental education level, parental employment and marital status, family economic status), personal well-being, academic performance and adjustment, family quality of life, and after-school activities (see Table 3). Different scales used in the study are described below.

Measures of Personal Well-Being

1. *Positive youth development*
   A total of 45 items of the Chinese Positive Youth Development Scale (CPYDS) were used to assess 15 dimensions of positive youth development, including

Table 2 Demographic information of the respondents matched across all three waves

	Wave 1 (N=3,328)		Wave 2[a] (N=3,638)		Wave 3[b] (N=4,106)	
Gender						
Male	1,306 (50 %)		1,309 (50 %)		1,317 (50 %)	
Female	1,333 (50 %)		1,321 (50 %)		1,332 (50 %)	
Place of birth						
Hong Kong	2,093 (79 %)		2,099 (80 %)		2,128 (80 %)	
Mainland China	515 (19 %)		479 (18 %)		446 (17 %)	
Others	47 (2 %)		50 (2 %)		43 (2 %)	
Parents' marital status						
Married	2,256 (85 %)		2,228 (84 %)		2,238 (84 %)	
Divorced/separated	216 (8 %)		237 (9 %)		255 (10 %)	
Remarried	96 (4 %)		101 (4 %)		112 (4 %)	
Others	78 (3 %)		82 (3 %)		55 (2 %)	
Receiving financial aids						
Yes	169 (6 %)		146 (6 %)		139 (5 %)	
No	2,143 (81 %)		2,202 (83 %)		2,185 (83 %)	
Others	331 (13 %)		305 (12 %)		322 (12 %)	
Parental education level	*Father*	*Mother*	*Father*	*Mother*	*Father*	*Mother*
Elementary education level or less	334 (13 %)	342 (13 %)	342 (13 %)	329 (13 %)	311 (12 %)	298 (11 %)
Secondary educational level	1,003 (39 %)	1,171 (45 %)	981 (27 %)	1,135 (43 %)	951 (36 %)	1,113 (42 %)
Tertiary education level	366 (14 %)	314 (12 %)	677 (26 %)	341 (13 %)	407 (15 %)	334 (13 %)
Others	879 (34 %)	810 (31 %)	908 (34 %)	837 (31 %)	970 (37 %)	885 (34 %)

Note: A total of 2,667 participants completed the questionnaires in all three waves
[a]317 students voluntarily joined in Wave 2 as repeaters (n=249) and newcomers (n=68)
[b]567 students voluntarily joined in Wave 3 as repeaters (n=132), newcomers (n=66) and those who did not participate in Waves 1–2 (n=369)

bonding, resilience, social competence, recognition for positive behavior, emotional competence, cognitive competence, behavioral competence, moral competence, self-determination, self-efficacy, clear and positive identity, beliefs in the future, prosocial involvement, prosocial norms, and spirituality. The details of the items can be seen in Shek, Siu, and Lee (2007). Based on multigroup confirmatory factor analysis, these 15 primary factors could be represented by four secondary factors, including cognitive-behavioral competencies (CBC), prosocial attributes (PA), positive identity (PI), and general positive youth development qualities (GPYDQ). The internal consistency of these measures can be seen in Table 2. A 6-point Likert scale was used to gauge the responses of the participants. A higher total score indicates a higher level of positive youth development qualities. The reliability and validity of the scale have been supported (Shek & Ma, 2010a).

Table 3 Summary of the measures used in the study

Area	Measure	Used in previous studies
(A) Personal well-being (positive and negative mental health)	Positive youth development	Law and Shek (2013), Lee and Shek (2013), Ma and Shek (2013), Shek (2005a, 2005b, 2006, 2007b, 2008), Shek and Ma (2012b), Shek et al. (2012), Shek and Yu (2012), Sun and Shek (2012), and Yu and Shek (2013)
	Life satisfaction	
	Hopelessness	
(B) Personal well-being (risk behavior)	Delinquency	
	Substance use	
	Problem behavior intention	
	Internet addiction	
	Pornography consumption	
	Self-harm	
	Suicidal behavior	
	Compensated dating	
(C) Academic adjustment	Perceived academic and school performance	
	Views on the new secondary school curriculum	
(D) Family quality of life	Paternal knowledge and maternal knowledge	
	Paternal expectation and maternal expectation	
	Paternal monitoring and maternal monitoring	
	Paternal psychological control and maternal psychological control	
	Paternal-child relational qualities and maternal-child relational qualities	
	Satisfaction with paternal control and maternal control	
	Systemic family functioning	
(E) After-school activities	After-school activities	
	After-school tutorial programs	
(F) Demographic and family characteristics	Age	
	Gender	
	Immigrant status	
	Parental education level	
	Parental employment status	
	Parents' marital status	
	Family socioeconomic status	
	Amount of time parents spent with their child	

2. *Life satisfaction*
   The translated version of the five-item Life Satisfaction Scale (Diener, Emmons, Larsen, & Griffin, 1985) with 6-point scale was used to assess the respondents' level of life satisfaction. A higher composite score reflects a higher sense of life satisfaction. The reliability and validity of the scale have been supported (Shek, 1998).
   Apart from measuring the positive aspects of participants' personal well-being, their personal well-being was also assessed in the negative sides as follows:

3. *Hopelessness*
   Based on the work of Beck and colleagues (Beck, Weissman, Lester, & Trexler, 1974), a five-item modified scale was used to assess the respondents' level of hopelessness. A 6-point scale was used with a higher score reflecting a higher sense of hopelessness. The reliability and validity of the scale have been supported (Shek, 1993).

4. *Risk behavior*
   Eight categories of risk behaviors were covered in the study as follows:

(a) *Delinquency*
   A total of 12 items were developed to assess the frequency of adolescent delinquent behavior in the past year, including stealing, cheating, truancy, running away from home, damaging others' properties, assault, having sexual intercourse with others, gang fighting, speaking foul language, staying outside the home overnight without parental consent, bullying or harassing others, and trespassing. A 6-point Likert scale was used with a higher composite score indicating a higher level of delinquent behavior. The reliability of the scale has been supported (Shek et al., 2012).

(b) *Substance use*
   Eight items were used to assess the participants' frequency of using different types of substances in the past half year, including alcohol, tobacco, ketamine, cannabis, cough mixture, organic solvent, pills (including ecstasy and methaqualone), and heroin. A 6-point scale was used with a higher composite score indicating a higher level of substance use. The reliability of the scale has been supported (Shek & Ma, 2012b).

(c) *Problem behavior intention*
   Five items were used to assess the participants' intention to engage in problem behaviors, including drinking alcohol, smoking, using illegal drugs (ketamine, cannabis, or ecstasy), gambling, and having sexual intercourse. A 4-point scale was used with a higher composite score indicating a higher level of intention to engage in problem behavior in the next 2 years. The reliability of the scale has been supported (Shek et al., 2012).

(d) *Internet addiction*
   Based on Young's work (1998), ten dichotomous items (yes/no) were used to assess participants' Internet addictive behavior. Respondents were asked to report whether they had the stated Internet addictive behaviors in the past 12 months. The Chinese translated version of the scale was used. A higher composite score

shows a higher level of Internet addictive behavior in the past year. The reliability of the scale has been supported (Yu & Shek, 2013).

(e) *Pornography consumption*
Twelve items were used to assess participants' consumption of two types of pornographic materials in the past 12 months, including online (e.g., pornographic stories, pictures, videos, and websites) and traditional pornography (e.g., pornographic movies, rental films, movies on cable TV, magazines, books, and comics). A 6-point scale was used with a higher composite score indicating a higher level of pornography use in the past 12 months. The reliability of the scale has been supported (Ma & Shek, 2013).

(f) *Self-harm*
A total of 17 dichotomous items (yes/no) were used to assess whether the participants had engaged in self-harm behaviors (e.g., wrist cutting, burning with cigarette or fire, carving words or marks on the body, self-scratching, self-biting, rubbing sandpaper against the body, acid dripping, bleach scrubbing, putting sharp objects into the body, rubbing glass against the body, breaking bones, head banging, self-punching, and preventing wounds from healing) in the past 12 months. A higher composite score indicates a higher level of self-harm behavior. The reliability of the scale has been supported (Law & Shek, 2013).

(g) *Suicidal behavior*
Four items were used to assess whether the participants had suicidal thoughts, plans, and attempts in the past 12 months. A higher composite score indicates a higher level of suicidal behavior. The reliability of the scale has been supported (Law & Shek, 2013).

(h) *Compensated dating*
Four dichotomous items (yes/no) were used to assess participants' engagement in compensated dating behaviors in the past 12 months. A higher composite score indicates a higher level of engaging in compensated dating. The reliability of the scale has been supported (Lee & Shek, 2013).

Measures of Academic Performance and Adjustment

Two measures were used to assess students' perceived academic performance and adjustment as follows:

1. *Perceived academic and school performance*
Three items were employed to examine how participants perceived their academic and school performance. A 5-point scale was used with a higher composite score reflecting a higher perceived competence on academic and school performance. The reliability of the scale has been supported (Shek & Yu, 2012).
2. *Views on new secondary school curriculum*
Four items were used to assess participants' views on the new school curriculum implemented in Hong Kong. A 4-point scale was used to assess students' confidence, perceived stress, and received support when facing the new school curriculum.

Measures of Family Quality of Life

Several measures were used to assess participants' perceived quality of the parent-child subsystem and systemic family functioning. For the parent-child system, two sets of identical items were used to measure the father-child subsystem and mother-child subsystem. Each set of measure has 17 items and they were divided into six subscales:

1. Parent-child subsystem
   (a) *Paternal knowledge and maternal knowledge about the child*
   Two identical items with a 4-point scale were developed to assess paternal and maternal knowledge about the child. A higher total score on the subscale indicated a higher level of parental knowledge of the child's behavior. The reliability of the scale has been supported (Shek, 2006).
   (b) *Paternal expectation and maternal expectation*
   Two identical items with a 4-point scale were developed to assess paternal and maternal expectation on the child. A higher total score on the subscale indicated a higher level of parental expectation of the child's behavior. The reliability of the scale has been supported (Shek, 2008).
   (c) *Paternal monitoring and maternal monitoring*
   Three identical items with a 4-point scale were developed to assess paternal and maternal monitoring. A higher score on the subscale indicate a higher level of parental monitoring of the child's behavior. The reliability of the scale has been supported (Shek, 2008).
   (d) *Paternal psychological control and maternal psychological control*
   Four identical items with a 4-point scale were developed to assess of paternal and maternal psychological control. A higher score on the subscale indicates a higher level of parental psychological control of the child's behavior. The reliability of the scale has been supported (Shek, 2005b).
   (e) *Paternal-child relational qualities and maternal-child relational qualities*
   Three identical items with a 4-point scale were developed to assess paternal parent-child and maternal parent-child relational qualities. A higher score on the subscale indicates a more positive quality of parent-child relationship. The reliability of the scale has been supported (Shek, 2005b).
   (f) *Satisfaction with paternal and maternal control*
   Three items with a 4-point scale were developed to assess satisfaction with paternal and maternal control. A higher score on the subscale indicates a higher level of satisfaction with parental control. The reliability of the scale has been supported (Shek, 2006).
2. *Family functioning*
   The Chinese Family Assessment Instrument (CFAI) scale was used to assess family functioning, including mutuality, communication, conflicts, and harmony in three subscales (Shek, 2002). These subscales were assessed using a 5-point

scale. A higher total score indicates a higher level of positive family functioning. The hierarchal structure and factorial invariance of the CFAI have been supported in a previous study (Shek & Ma, 2010b).

Measures of After-School Activities

Two measures were used to assess adolescent after-school activities as follows:

1. *After-school activities*
   Participants were asked to report how they usually spend their time after school by using a single-item indicator (i.e., 1 = returned home with the presence of adult, 2 = returned home without the presence of adult, 3 = returned home with the presence of siblings only, 4 = extra-curricular activity, 5 = socializing with friends without the presence of adults, 6 = wandering the streets alone).
2. *After-school tutoring programs*
   Four items were asked whether participants joined any after-school tutorial programs (yes/no), types of tutorial programs (i.e., organized by school, private tutorial center, a private tutoring service), amount of time spent per week to attend tutorial programs, and monthly cost of tutorial services.

Uniqueness of the Present Research Design

With reference to the suggestions by Moore (1997), former executive director of Child Trends, several unique features of the study are highlighted. First, a wide array of multiple ecological factors (e.g., developmental assets, behavioral control, and family functioning) and outcomes (e.g., adolescent risk behavior) were included in this study. The inclusion of such factors can give a comprehensive picture on the antecedents and changes in adolescent developmental outcomes. Second, both positive indicators (such as positive youth development qualities, thriving, and life satisfaction) and negative indicators (such as adolescent risk behavior) of personal well-being were assessed. Third, psychometrically sound instruments were used to measure the pattern and changes of adolescent development and their family characteristics. Fourth, a large and representative sample was employed in this study. Finally, as there are few studies examining personal well-being and family quality of life in the Chinese context in a single study, this study is a pioneer attempt. In fact, this is the first known longitudinal study exploring personal well-being, family quality of life, and developmental outcomes in Chinese adolescents.

Acknowledgment The preparation for this work and the Project P.A.T.H.S. were financially supported by The Hong Kong Jockey Club Charities Trust. The authorship is equally shared by the authors.

References

Adalbjarnardottir, S., & Hafsteinsson, L. G. (2001). Adolescents' perceived parenting styles and their substance use: Concurrent and longitudinal analyses. *Journal of Research on Adolescence, 11*(4), 401–423.

Beck, A. T., Weissman, A., Lester, D., & Trexler, L. (1974). The measurement of pessimism: The hopelessness scale. *Journal of Consulting and Clinical Psychology, 42*(6), 861–865.

Boislard, P. M.-A., & Poulin, F. (2011). Individual, familial, friends-related and contextual predictors of early sexual intercourse. *Journal of Adolescence, 34*(2), 289–300. doi:10.1016/j.adolescence.2010.05.002.

Booker, C. L., Unger, J. B., Azen, S. P., Baezconde-Garbanati, L., Lickel, B., & Johnson, A. (2007). Stressful life events and smoking behaviors in Chinese adolescents: A longitudinal analysis. *Nicotine & Tobacco Research, 9*(11), 1085–1094.

Bowers, E. P., von Eye, A., Lerner, J. V., Arbeit, M. R., Weiner, M. B., Chase, P., et al. (2011). The role of ecological assets in positive and problematic developmental trajectories. *Journal of Adolescence, 34*(6), 1151–1165.

Brook, J. S., Brook, D. W., & Whiteman, M. (2007). Growing up in a violent society: Longitudinal predictors of violence in Colombian adolescents. *American Journal of Community Psychology, 40*(1–2), 82–95.

Denault, A. S., & Poulin, F. (2012). Peer group deviancy in organized activities and youths' problem behaviours. *Canadian Journal of Behavioural Science, 44*(2), 83–92.

Diener, E. D., Emmons, R. A., Larsen, R. J., & Griffin, S. (1985). The satisfaction with life scale. *Journal of Personality Assessment, 49*(1), 71–75.

Elkington, K. S., Bauermeister, J. A., & Zimmerman, M. A. (2011). Do parents and peers matter? A prospective socio-ecological examination of substance use and sexual risk among African American youth. *Journal of Adolescence, 34*(5), 1035–1047.

Escobar-Chaves, S. L., Tortolero, S. R., Markham, C. M., Low, B. J., Eitel, P., & Thickstun, P. (2005). Impact of the media on adolescent sexual attitudes and behaviors. *Pediatrics, 116*(1), 303–326.

Farrell, A. D., Sullivan, T. N., Esposito, L. E., Meyer, A. L., & Valois, R. (2005). A latent growth curve analysis of the structure of aggression, drug use, and delinquent behaviors and their interrelations over time in urban and rural adolescents. *Journal of Research on Adolescence, 15*(2), 179–204.

Heard, H. E. (2007). Fathers, mothers, and family structure: Family trajectories, parent gender, and adolescent schooling. *Journal of Marriage and Family, 69*(2), 435–450.

Hennessy, M., Bleakley, A., Fishbein, M., & Jordan, A. (2009). Estimating the longitudinal association between adolescent sexual behavior and exposure to sexual media content. *Journal of Sex Research, 46*, 586–596.

Kanuga, M., & Rosenfeld, W. D. (2004). Adolescent sexuality and the internet: The good, the bad, and the URL. *Journal of Pediatric and Adolescent Gynecology, 17*(2), 117–124.

Keijsers, L., Branje, S. J. T., VanderValk, I. E., & Meeus, W. (2010). Reciprocal effects between parental solicitation, parental control, adolescent disclosure, and adolescent delinquency. *Journal of Research on Adolescence, 20*(1), 88–113.

Kerr, M., Stattin, H., & Burk, W. J. (2010). A reinterpretation of parental monitoring in longitudinal perspective. *Journal of Research on Adolescence, 20*(1), 39–64.

Kwan, Y. K. (2010). Life satisfaction and self-assessed health among adolescents in Hong Kong. *Journal of Happiness Studies, 11*(3), 383–393.

Laird, R. D., Bridges, B. J., & Marsee, M. A. (2013). Secrets from friends and parents: Longitudinal links with depression and antisocial behavior. *Journal of Adolescence, 36*(4), 685–693.

Law, B. M. F., & Shek, D. T. L. (2013). Self-harm and suicide attempts among young Chinese adolescents in Hong Kong: Prevalence, correlates, and changes. *Journal of Pediatric and Adolescent Gynecology, 26*, S26–S32.

Lee, T. Y., & Shek, D. T. L. (2013). Compensated dating in Hong Kong: Prevalence, psychological correlates, and relationships with other risky behaviors. *Journal of Pediatric and Adolescent Gynecology, 26*, S42–S48.

Leung, C. Y. W., McBride-Chang, C., & Lai, B. P. Y. (2004). Relations among maternal parenting style, academic competence, and life satisfaction in Chinese early adolescents. *Journal of Early Adolescence, 24*(2), 113–142.

Liljeberg, J., Eklund, J., Fritz, M., & Klinteberg, B. (2011). Poor school bonding and delinquency over time: Bidirectional effects and sex differences. *Journal of Adolescence, 34*(1), 1–9.

Ma, C. M. S., & Shek, D. T. L. (2013). Consumption of pornographic materials in early adolescents in Hong Kong. *Journal of Pediatric and Adolescent Gynecology, 26*, S18–S25.

Metzger, A., Dawes, N., Mermelstein, R., & Wakschlag, L. (2011). Longitudinal modeling of adolescents' activity involvement, problem peer associations, and youth smoking. *Journal of Applied Developmental Psychology, 32*(1), 1–9.

Moore, K. A. (1997). Criteria for indicators of child well-being. In R. M. Hauser, B. V. Brown, & W. R. Prosser (Eds.), *Indicators of children's well-being* (pp. 36–44). New York: Russell Sage Foundation.

Moore, K. A., Lippman, L., & Brown, B. (2004). Indictors of child well-being: The promise for positive youth development. *The Annals of the American Academy of Political and Social Science, 591*(1), 125–145.

Nocentini, A., Menesini, E., & Salmivalli, C. (2013). Level and change of bullying behavior during high school: A multilevel growth curve analysis. *Journal of Adolescence, 36*(3), 495–505.

Odgers, C. L., Moffitt, T. E., Tach, L. M., Sampson, A., Taylor, R. J., Matthews, C. L., et al. (2009). The protective effects of neighborhood collective efficacy on British children growing up in deprivation: A developmental analysis. *Developmental Psychology, 45*(4), 942–957.

Ostaszewski, K., & Zimmerman, M. A. (2006). The effects of cumulative risks and promotive factors on urban adolescent alcohol and other drug use: A longitudinal study of resiliency. *American Journal of Community Psychology, 38*(3–4), 237–249.

Rueter, M. A., & Kwon, H. K. (2005). Developmental trends in adolescent suicidal ideation. *Journal of Research on Adolescence, 15*(2), 205–222.

Scales, P. C., Benson, P. L., Roehlkepartain, E. C., Sesma, A., Jr., & van Dulmen, M. (2006). The role of developmental assets in predicting academic achievement: A longitudinal study. *Journal of Adolescence, 29*(5), 691–708.

Shek, D. T. L. (1993). Measurement of pessimism in Chinese adolescents: The Chinese Hopelessness Scale. *Social Behavior and Personality, 21*(2), 107–119.

Shek, D. T. L. (1998). Adolescent positive mental health and psychological symptoms: A longitudinal study in a Chinese context. *Psychologia, 41*(4), 217–225.

Shek, D. T. L. (2002). Assessment of family functioning Chinese adolescents: The Chinese family assessment instrument. In N. N. Singh, T. Ollen-dick, & A. N. Singh (Eds.), *International perspectives on child and adolescent mental health* (pp. 297–316). Amsterdam: Elsevier.

Shek, D. T. L. (2005a). Perceived parental control and parent-child relational qualities in Chinese adolescents in Hong Kong. *Sex Roles, 53*(9–10), 635–646.

Shek, D. T. L. (2005b). Perceived parental control processes, parent-child relational qualities, and psychological well-being in Chinese adolescents with and without economic disadvantage. *Journal of Genetic Psychology, 166*(2), 171–188.

Shek, D. T. L. (2006). Assessment of perceived parental psychological control in Chinese adolescents in Hong Kong. *Research on Social Work Practice, 166*(4), 382–391.

Shek, D. T. L. (2007a). A longitudinal study of perceived parental psychological control and psychological well-being in Chinese adolescents in Hong Kong. *Journal of Clinical Psychology, 63*(1), 1–22.

Shek, D. T. L. (2007b). Perceived parental control based on indigenous Chinese parental control concepts in adolescents in Hong Kong. *American Journal of Family Therapy, 35*(2), 123–137.

Shek, D. T. L. (2008). Perceived parental psychological control in Chinese adolescents: A three-year longitudinal study in Hong Kong. *The Open Family Studies Journal, 1*, 7–16.

Shek, D. T. L., & Ma, C. M. S. (2010a). Dimensionality of the Chinese positive youth development scale: Confirmatory factor analyses. *Social Indicators Research, 98*(1), 41–59.

Shek, D. T. L., & Ma, C. M. S. (2010b). The Chinese Family Assessment Instrument (C-FAI): Hierarchical confirmatory factor analyses and factorial invariance. *Research on Social Work Practice, 20*(1), 112–123.

Shek, D. T. L., & Ma, C. M. S. (2012a). Impact of the Project P.A.T.H.S. in the junior secondary school years: Objective outcome evaluation based on eight waves of longitudinal data. *The Scientific World Journal, 2012,* 12 pp. doi:10.1100/2012/170345.

Shek, D. T. L., & Ma, C. M. S. (2012b). Substance abuse in junior secondary school students in Hong Kong: Prevalence and psychosocial correlates. *International Journal of Child Health and Human Development, 4*(4), 433–442.

Shek, D. T. L., Ma, C. M. S., & Tang, C. Y. P. (2012). Delinquency and problem behavior intention among early adolescents in Hong Kong: Profiles and psychosocial correlates. *International Journal on Disability and Human Development, 11*(2), 151–158.

Shek, D. T. L., Siu, A. M. H., & Lee, T. Y. (2007). The Chinese positive youth development scale: A validation study. *Research on Social Work Practice, 17*(3), 380–391.

Shek, D. T. L., & Sun, R. C. F. (Eds.). (2013). *Development and evaluation of positive adolescent training through holistic social programs (P.A.T.H.S.).* Heidelberg, Germany: Springer.

Shek, D. T. L., & Yu, L. (2012). Longitudinal impact of the Project P.A.T.H.S. on adolescent risk behavior: What happened after five years? *The Scientific World Journal, 2012,* 12 pp. doi:10.1100/2012/316029.

Shuster, M. M., Li, Y., & Shi, J. (2012). Maternal cultural values and parenting practices: Longitudinal associations with Chinese adolescents' aggression. *Journal of Adolescence, 35*(2), 345–355.

Sroufe, L. A., Coffino, B., & Carlson, E. (2010). Conceptualizing the role of early experience: Lessons from the Minnesota longitudinal study. *Developmental Review, 30*(1), 36–51.

Sun, R. C. F., & Shek, D. T. L. (2012). Positive youth development, life satisfaction and problem behaviour among Chinese adolescents in Hong Kong: A replication. *Social Indicators Research, 105*, 541–559.

van den Eijnden, R. J., Meerkerk, G. J., Vermulst, A. A., Spijkerman, R., & Engels, R. C. (2008). Online communication, compulsive internet use, and psychosocial well-being among adolescents: A longitudinal study. *Developmental Psychology, 44*(3), 635–665.

Wang, Q., Pomerantz, E. M., & Chen, H. (2007). The role of parents' control in early adolescents' psychological functioning: A longitudinal investigation in the United States and China. *Child Development, 28*(5), 1592–1610.

Wight, D., Williamson, L., & Henderson, M. (2006). Parental influences on young people's sexual behaviour: A longitudinal analysis. *Journal of Adolescence, 29*(4), 473–494.

Young, K. S. (1998). Internet addiction: The emergence of a new clinical disorder. *CyberPsychology and Behavior, 1*(3), 237–244.

Yu, L., & Shek, D. T. L. (2013). Internet addiction in Hong Kong adolescents: A three-year longitudinal study. *Journal of Pediatric and Adolescent Gynecology, 26*, S10–S17.

Positive Youth Development in Junior Secondary School Students: Do Gender and Time Matter?

Daniel T.L. Shek and Florence K.Y. Wu

Abstract There is a dearth of studies examining gender and time differences in positive youth development attributes among Chinese adolescents. To fill this research gap, this study examined the direct effects of gender and time and the interaction effect of gender and time on different indicators of positive youth development. Over 3 years, the data were collected from a sample of junior secondary school students randomly drawn from secondary schools in Hong Kong. The results showed that gender effect was significant. While boys scored higher than girls on cognitive-behavioral competence and positive identity, girls were found to score higher than boys on prosocial attributes and general positive youth development qualities. Significant time differences were found for some indicators of positive youth development. No interaction effect of gender and time was found. The theoretical and practical implications of the findings were discussed.

Keywords Gender effect • Time effect • Positive youth development program • Project P.A.T.H.S • Holistic development

Introduction

In the past few decades, many Western scholars in the fields of psychology, education, public health, and human development have searched for a new direction in understanding and promoting holistic development of young people (Benson & Scales, 2009; Ferrer-Wreder, 2014; Seligman & Csikszentmihalyi, 2000; Smith, Osgood, Caldwell, Hynes, & Perkins, 2013). According to Ferrer-Wreder (2014), this paradigm shift is known as the positive youth development (PYD) movement, which is a scholarly and public reaction against the overemphasis on youth

D.T.L. Shek, Ph.D., B.B.S., S.B.S., J.P. (✉) • F.K.Y. Wu, Ed.D.
Department of Applied Social Sciences, The Hong Kong Polytechnic University, Hunghom, Hong Kong
e-mail: daniel.shek@polyu.edu.hk

D.T.L. Shek et al. (eds.), *Chinese Adolescents in Hong Kong*,
Quality of Life in Asia 5, DOI 10.1007/978-981-287-143-5_3

problems in conventional psychology and psychiatry and endorsement of the effort to prevent the problem behaviors of children and adolescents. The perspective of positive youth development raises doubts about the deficit-oriented approaches that might lead to an incomplete and biased understanding of children and adolescents (Catalano, Berglund, Ryan, Lonczak, & Hawkins, 2004); and scholars have urged for a more balanced understanding of adolescent development. Hence, instead of focusing on child pathologies and problems, PYD scholars have suggested that talents, strengths, interests, and future potentials in youth should be the legitimate foci and they see children and adolescents as resources (Damon, 2004; Seligman & Csikszentmihalyi, 2000).

The strength-based perception of youth development also influences youth intervention programs. Numerous research studies have consistently showed that risk factors at different levels (e.g., individual, family, school, and community) contribute to adolescent risk behavior (Pittman, Irby, Tolman, Yohalem, & Ferber, 2003). Therefore, the focus of youth intervention programs in the traditional prevention framework was to prevent adolescent problem behaviors (such as substance abuse, delinquency, or premature sexual behaviors) by reducing risk factors (Catalano et al., 2004). However, with growing awareness of the importance of developing children and adolescents holistically, the focus of the youth intervention programs lies on the strengthening of the psychosocial competence of young people and on their ability to cope with future challenges. It is argued that promotion of protective factors at the individual level (e.g., healthy attribution style, optimism, and faith) and different ecological systems (e.g., supportive adults and environments) would help reduce the likelihood of engaging in risk behavior (Benson & Scales, 2009). During the process of the intervention, young people are "intrinsically energized" (Larson, 2000) by discovering their uniqueness and potentials, and they ignite life energy to overcome life hurdles. The positive youth intervention programs are implemented with the goal of understanding how individual-context interactions lead to optimal development of the adolescents and a better transition to adulthood (Ferrer-Wreder, 2014).

In the Hong Kong context, there are similar concerns about holistic children and adolescent development (e.g., Shek, 2010; Shek, Sun, & Merrick, 2012; Shek & Yu, 2013). For example, Shek and Leung (2013) reviewed several adolescent development issues, including adolescent substance abuse, Internet addiction, materialistic orientation, sexual issues, bullying, adolescent poverty, and unemployment. How are we going to nurture young people in the face of such developmental issues? According to Shek, Siu, and Lee (2007), understanding the competencies and strengths of adolescents in fact has equal importance compared with understanding adolescent pathologies. Besides removing risk factors, it is equally important to build up psychosocial competences in young people in Hong Kong. The basic argument in the positive youth development approach is simple and attractive – when a young person acquires psychosocial competence and inner strengths, he or she will have the strength to resist risk behavior.

Against the above background, programs utilizing positive youth development constructs should be developed to promote adolescent holistic development and to facilitate adolescent well-being. With particular reference to Hong Kong, the Project P.A.T.H.S. ("Positive Adolescent Training through Holistic Social Programs") funded by The Hong Kong Jockey Club Charities Trust is one of the few yet validated positive youth development programs in different Chinese contexts. The focus of the project is the promotion of psychosocial skills or qualities in young people with reference to 15 positive constructs in youth development. The project has two tiers of programs. The Tier 1 Program is a universal positive youth development program with structured curricula. Typically, students in Secondary 1 to Secondary 3 receive 20 h of training in each grade (Shek, 2010). For students with greater psychosocial needs, the Tier 2 program is designed. Based on many evaluation studies of the project, junior secondary school students who participated in the program had significantly better positive outcomes in terms of psychosocial competence, academic and school behaviors, and global positive youth development than did the students in the control group (Shek & Sun, 2013; Shek & Yu, 2013). Longitudinal data were collected in both the experimental and control schools in the initial phase of the project with two limitations. First, the participants were not randomly selected from the student population in Hong Kong. Hence, generalizability of the findings may be limited. Second, as the focus of the evaluation study was to examine the program effects of the Project P.A.T.H.S., gender differences were not examined in depth in the study. To address the limitations of the scientific literature, the present study aims to examine time and gender differences in positive youth development in a randomly selected student sample in Hong Kong.

Empirical studies on gender differences in youth developmental outcomes are numerous across different cultures and contexts (e.g., Bennett, Farrington, & Huesman, 2005; DuBois, Burk-Braxton, Swenson, Tevendale, & Hardesty, 2002; Ohannessian, Lerner, Lerner, & von Eye, 1999; Rojewski, Wicklein, & Schell, 1995). Scholars and researchers are interested in understanding how male and female adolescents respond, react, or develop differently in different aspects of their developmental trajectories. In reviewing this vast literature on gender differences of adolescents, there is no consistent pattern on how male and female adolescents differ in various developmental indicators. For example, it is traditionally believed that males are more prone to crime and violence, yet females are less vulnerable to the development of delinquent behaviors and psychosocial adversities (Bennett et al., 2005). However, Herreraa and McCloskey (2001) discovered that girls were arrested for violent offences more than boys. While little is known about the reasons accounted for this phenomenon, conducting the research with different methodologies and student samples as well as cultural sensitivity might lead to a clearer answer with regard to the gender differences in adolescent development.

While some attempts have been made to examine gender differences in mental health problems (e.g., Ohannessian et al., 1999; Park & Peterson, 2006), there are relatively fewer studies examining gender differences in positive youth development measures in the Western contexts. Bennett et al. (2005) investigated the gender differences in social-cognitive competence, and Larsson and Frisk (1999) explored how age and gender influenced adolescent social-emotional competence. It would be interesting to study this "gap" to understand how male and female adolescents develop differently through positive youth development. In the Chinese context, specifically the local Hong Kong context, although Shek and colleagues have extensively explored how Hong Kong adolescents (with special attention to the junior secondary school students) grow or change according to the positive youth development constructs (Shek, 2010; Shek & Ma, 2010; Shek et al., 2012; Shek & Yu, 2013), empirical evidence on gender differences in positive youth development constructs is still limited.

When one examines gender differences in positive youth development, one basic issue that should be addressed is how positive youth development should be measured. Shek et al. (2007) have identified two problems in the assessment of positive youth development constructs. First, only few measures of positive youth development could be adopted after monitoring individual differences in different cultures especially as there is no valid and available measure for the Chinese context. Second, the conception of positive youth development might vary across cultures, and such wide variations might affect the measurement of the essence and the effectiveness of the positive youth development programs. Hence, they argued for the development of a validated and cultural-specific assessment tool for the Chinese students, and they developed the Chinese Positive Youth Development Scale (CPYDS). The scale was based on the 15 positive youth development constructs identified in the review of Catalano et al. (2004), which consists of 15 subscales, including bonding (BO), resilience (RE), social competence (SC), recognition for positive behavior (PB), emotional competence (EC), cognitive competence (CC), behavioral competence (BC), moral competence (MC), self-determination (SD), self-efficacy (SE), clear and positive identity (CPI), beliefs in future (BF), prosocial involvement (PI), prosocial norms (PN), and spirituality (SP). The CPYDS has good internal consistency reliability, and the scale and the subscale scores are able to discriminate adolescents with and without positive youth development (Shek et al., 2007). Shek and Ma (2010) further examined the dimensionality of the scale and found a strong support for its dimensionality. Hierarchical confirmatory factor analysis (HCFA) has been conducted to test the factor structure of the CPYDS, suggesting that the 15 aspects of positive youth development assessed by the CPYDS can be subsumed under four constructs of "cognitive-behavioral competencies" (CBC), "prosocial attributes" (PA), "positive identity" (PI), and "general positive youth development qualities" (GPYDQ) (Shek & Ma, 2010). In the present study, gender differences and the positive youth development are examined based on the four subsumed higher-order factors.

To address the above issues and the identified research gaps, the present study utilized a large and random sample of Secondary 1 to Secondary 3 students in Hong Kong to investigate gender differences in the four dimensions of positive youth development, including cognitive-behavioral competencies (CBC), prosocial attributes (PA), positive identity (PI), and general positive youth development qualities (GPYDQ) (Shek & Ma, 2010) via a set of 3-wave longitudinal data. Besides, whether positive youth development changes over time is also examined in this study. The 3-wave longitudinal data offers a more dynamic picture of how gender differences interact with time in influencing positive youth development constructs. Three basic questions are addressed in the present study: (1) Are there any gender differences in positive youth development among junior secondary school students in Hong Kong? (2) Are there any time differences in positive youth development among junior secondary school students in Hong Kong? (3) Do gender and time interact to influence positive youth development?

Method

Participants and Procedures

The Project P.A.T.H.S. is a pioneer positive youth development program which attempts to promote holistic youth development in adolescents in Hong Kong. The participants in the current study were recruited from 28 schools randomly selected among all the secondary schools in Hong Kong. The sampling frame of the study was all government and aided schools in Hong Kong. As the questionnaire was administered in Chinese, international schools and non-Chinese speaking schools were excluded from the present investigation. The present study was part of a large-scale longitudinal research project investigating youth development and family environment of early adolescents in Hong Kong. The first wave (Wave 1) of the study was conducted during the 2009–2010 academic year, with 3,325 Secondary 1 (equivalent to Grade 7) students (mean age = 12.59 years, SD = .74). The second wave (Wave 2) and third wave (Wave 3) of data were collected in the 2010–2011 and 2011–2012 academic years, respectively. The third wave of data was collected during the 2011–2012 academic year, with 4,106 Secondary 3 (Grade 9) students (mean age = 14.65 years, SD = .80). Based on the Wave 3 data, the majority of the respondents were Chinese who were born in Hong Kong (79.4 %), while the others were from Mainland China (18.9 %) or other countries (1.7 %). Additional demographic information of the participants is shown in Table 1.

The data were collected at schools in a classroom setting by trained research staff and/or school teachers with briefings in advance. The questionnaire was self-administered by the students. Prior to data collection, ethical approval was obtained from The Hong Kong Polytechnic University. Parental and school consent was sought before the data collection and student consent was also sought during data collection. Anonymity and confidentiality were emphasized during the administration process, and participants were given sufficient time to complete the questionnaire.

Instruments

At each wave of data collection, the participants were invited to respond to the abridged version of the Chinese Positive Youth Development Scale. The details of the items in the original scale are presented in Shek et al.'s (2007) study. A composite

Table 1 Sociodemographic profile of participants (Wave 3)

	N	%
Gender		
Male	2,185	53.7
Female	1,885	46.3
Place of birth		
Hong Kong	3,195	79.4
Mainland	762	18.9
Others	68	1.7
Father's education		
Primary education or below	455	17.6
Secondary education	1,656	63.9
Tertiary education or above	481	18.6
Mother's education		
Primary education or below	497	19.9
Secondary education	1,432	57.2
Tertiary education or above	573	22.9

score was calculated by averaging all item scores in the scale which gives an overall score on positive youth development (CPYDS). Using confirmatory factor analyses, Shek and Ma (2010) showed that the 15 primary factors of the scale are subsumed under four higher-order factors, including cognitive-behavioral competencies (CBC), prosocial attributes (PA), positive identity (PI), and general positive youth development qualities (GPYDQ). Support for different types of factorial invariance was also found. In order not to overburden the students, an abridged version of the CPYDS was used in this study. Previous studies showed that the abridged version of the scale possesses good psychometric properties (Leung & Shek, 2013).

Results

Descriptive statistics of the key variables of the present study are reported in Table 2. Reliability analyses showed that the abridged version of the scale was highly reliable (Table 2). The internal consistency reliability coefficient of the complete scale was .96, and the coefficients for the subscales ranged from .83 to .93 across all waves.

To examine gender effect, time effect, and the interaction effect of gender and time, five two-way mixed ANOVA analyses were conducted with gender (male vs. female) as the between-subject factor, time (Wave 1, Wave 2, Wave 3) as the within-subject factor, and the different indicators of positive youth development as the dependent variables. To examine the effects of gender and time on adolescents' cognitive-behavioral competencies (CBC), a mixed ANOVA analysis was conducted (see Table 3). Results yielded a main effect of gender, $F(1, 2355)=7.55$, $p=.006$, $\eta^2=.003$. Further analyses using Bonferroni test suggested that while CBC levels did not differ between genders at Wave 1, male and female adolescent scores were different at Wave 2 where male adolescents reported higher levels of CBC (M=4.48,

Table 2 Descriptive statistics and internal consistency coefficients of positive youth development constructs (Waves 1–3)

	Mean (SD)									Cronbach's α		
	W1			W2			W3					
	Male	Female	Total	Male	Female	Total	Male	Female	Total	W1	W2	W3
CBC	4.49 (.74)	4.44 (.70)	4.46 (.72)	4.47 (.74)	4.40 (.68)	4.44 (.71)	4.48 (.70)	4.40 (.66)	4.44 (.68)	.87	.87	.89
PA	4.44 (.89)	4.65 (.77)	4.54 (.84)	4.33 (.89)	4.55 (.74)	4.44 (.83)	4.33 (.86)	4.54 (.80)	4.44 (.80)	.83	.84	.83
GPYDQ	4.57 (.70)	4.65 (.65)	4.60 (.68)	4.52 (.71)	4.59 (.63)	4.54 (.67)	4.50 (.71)	4.58 (.61)	4.55 (.65)	.93	.93	.93
PI	4.28 (.97)	4.23 (.92)	4.26 (.94)	4.25 (.98)	4.14 (.90)	4.19 (.94)	4.23 (.95)	4.11 (.88)	4.18 (.92)	.87	.89	.89
PYD	4.51 (.69)	4.57 (.64)	4.53 (.67)	4.46 (.69)	4.50 (.61)	4.46 (.67)	4.45 (.69)	4.49 (.60)	4.47 (.64)	.96	.96	.96

Note. W1 Wave 1, *W2* Wave 2, *W3* Wave 3, *CBC* cognitive-behavioral competencies, *PA* prosocial attributes, *GPYDQ* general positive youth development qualities, *PI* positive identity, *PYD* total score of positive youth development.

Table 3 Mixed ANOVA results on the second-order positive youth development constructs

Variable	Time		Gender		Time × gender	
	df (hypothesis df, error df)	*F*	df (hypothesis df, error df)	*F*	df (hypothesis df, error df)	*F*
CBC	2, 2,354	1.76	1, 2,355	7.55**	2, 2,354	.57
PA	2, 2,507	25.90***	1, 2,508	63.98***	2, 2,507	.06
GPYDQ	2, 2,149	14.27***	1, 2,150	9.91**	2, 2,149	.12
PI	2, 2,491	12.54***	1, 2,492	8.96**	2, 2,491	2.45
PYD	2, 1,829	16.27***	1, 1,830	2.82	2, 1,829	.26

Note. $^{**}p<.01$; $^{***}p<.001$

Table 4 Post hoc pairwise comparisons on second-order positive youth development constructs

	CBC		PA		GPYDQ		PI		PYD	
	Gender		Gender		Gender		Gender		Gender	
	Male	Female	Male	Female	Male	Female	Male	Female	Male	Female
W1	.108		**.000**		**.004**		.181		.071	
W2	**.009**		**.000**		**.012**		**.003**		.193	
W3	**.008**		**.000**		**.006**		**.005**		.205	
W1 versus W2	1.000	.144	**.000**	**.000**	**.021**	**.001**	.434	**.000**	**.016**	**.000**
W1 versus W3	1.000	.254	**.000**	**.000**	**.002**	**.000**	.162	**.000**	**.004**	**.000**
W2 versus W3	1.000	1.000	1.000	1.000	1.000	1.000	1.000	.752	1.000	1.000

Note. Significant results are marked in bold
p-values were adjusted using Bonferroni method
W1 Wave 1, *W2* Wave 2, *W3* Wave 3

SD=.02) than their female counterparts (M=4.40, SD=.02). Similar differences were found in Wave 3 (M=4.48, SD=.02 vs. M=4.40, SD=.02). No significant interaction effects were observed (see Table 4).

Results from mixed ANOVA analysis investigating prosocial attributes (PA) revealed a main effect of both time (Wilks' $\lambda=.98$, $F(2, 2{,}507)=25.90$, $p=.000$, $\eta^2=.020$) and gender ($F(1, 2{,}508)=63.98$, $p=.000$, $\eta^2=.025$). Further analyses showed that positive attributes scores decreased from Wave 1 (M=4.55, SD=.02) to Wave 2 (M=4.44, SD=.02) but remained stable from Wave 2 to Wave 3 (M=4.43, SD=.02). In general, female adolescents reported higher positive attributes scores than males in all waves. However, no significant interaction effect between gender and time was yielded.

Mixed ANOVA examining general positive youth development qualities (GPYDQ) revealed significant main effects of both time (Wilks' $\lambda=.99$, $F(2, 2{,}149)=14.27$, $p=.000$, $\eta^2=.01$) and gender ($F(1, 2{,}150)=9.91$, $p=.002$, $\eta^2=.005$). Additional analyses revealed that GPYDQ scores decreased from Wave 1 (M=4.61, SD=.02) to Wave 2 (M=4.56, SD=.01) but remained the same from Wave 2 to Wave 3 (M=4.54,

SD = .01). Furthermore, female adolescents scored higher than males in their GPYDQ in all 3 waves. No significant interaction effect was yielded.

Mixed ANOVA analysis examining positive identity (PI) yielded a significant main effect of time (Wilks' $\lambda = .99$, $F(2, 2{,}491) = 12.54$, $p = .000$, $\eta^2 = .01$) and gender ($F(1, 2{,}492) = 17.05$, $p = .003$, $\eta^2 = .00$). Pairwise comparisons showed that PI scores decreased from Wave 1 (M = 4.26, SD = .02) to Wave 2 (M = 4.19, SD = 0.2) but remained stable from Wave 2 to Wave 3 (M = 4.13, SD = .02). It is noteworthy that although male adolescents did not differ from females in their reported levels of positive identity at Wave 1, significant differences emerged at Wave 2 and Wave 3, where adolescent males reported higher levels of positive identity than did their female counterparts. No significant interaction effect was yielded.

Finally, regarding positive youth development (PYD), a main effect of time was found (Wilks' $\lambda = .98$, $F(2, 1{,}829) = 16.27$, $p = .000$, $\eta^2 = .02$). Further analyses suggested that PYD scores decreased from Wave 1 (M = 4.54, SD = .02) to Wave 2 (M = 4.48, SD = .02) yet no changes were observed from Wave 2 to Wave 3 (M = 4.47, SD = .02). No significant interaction effect was found.

Discussion

This study attempted to examine the main effects of gender and time and the interaction effect of gender and time on the positive youth development indicators among junior secondary school students in Hong Kong. There are several strengths of this paper. First, a large and representative sample was employed. Second, a validated and indigenous measure of positive youth development scale and other indicators derived from the scale were used. Third, longitudinal data over a period of 3 years were collected. Finally, in response to the lack of data on the positive youth development constructs in different Chinese communities, Chinese adolescents participated in this study.

Gender differences are found on the four higher-order factors. In their review of core constructs of effective positive youth development programs, Catalano et al. (2004) stated that an adolescent with cognitive-behavioral competencies is able to develop and apply cognitive skills in reading and interpreting social cues and in taking effective actions after understanding the behavioral norms. Across different cultures, most researchers and scholars have acknowledged that there are gender differences in the development of cognitive-behavioral competencies. Studies in Western and Asian contexts have consistently showed that female adolescents move toward adult status physically, cognitively, and socially earlier and faster than male adolescents do (Chess & Thomas, 1984; Hughes & Zhang, 2007; Rojewski et al., 1995). Cognitive delays in males are commonly articulated in the literature. From a biological perspective, variations in the functional organization of the brain may contribute to differences in devising information processing strategies (Caplan & Caplan, 1997). Caplan and colleagues stated that as females tend to utilize both right and left brain in completing different tasks, the increased connectedness of the two hemispheres can lead to better cognitive processing (Caplan, MacPherson, & Tobin, 1985). Much evidence has indicated that males perform less well than females do in cognitive processes and behavioral responses.

Surprisingly, the male adolescents in the present study reported a slightly higher score in cognitive-behavioral competencies (CBC) than did their female counterparts. The results of the present study are consistent with the findings of Hyde and Linn's (1988) study that there is almost no gender difference in social-cognitive skills; however, there is a need to understand the reasons behind. One possible explanation of the results might be due to the perception of cognitive competence in the ideal gender roles. Although studies have shown that the patterns of cognitive abilities might not be related to sex-role identification (Keyes, 1984), the normative sex-role expectations, especially in the Chinese culture, might affect one's perception on the values and meanings of their cognitive abilities. For males in the Chinese cultural context, having good cognitive competence is regarded as signs of intelligence and leadership. On the other hand, females may be highly anxious to show the "success" of their cognitive competence, especially the reasoning cognition (Beilock, Gunderson, Ramirez, & Levine, 2010). It is possible for Hong Kong female adolescents to show similar "anxiety," and they might perceive that showing their cognitive competence might appear to be not congruent with the female image in Hong Kong. Hence, female adolescents may regard cognitive competence as relatively undesirable. However, these conjectures should be further investigated in the future research on the gender role expectations on the cognitive abilities.

The observation that females scored higher than males on prosocial attributes is in line with the literature that female adolescents outperform males in involvement of prosocial activities and prosocial behaviors (Bybee, 1998; Hansen, Larson, & Dworking, 2003; Rutten et al., 2007). The gender differences in the prosocial involvement and related attributes might be related to adaptive sex-role specialization (Bennett et al., 2005). Males, especially during adolescence, are prone to competitive and performance-oriented environment, such as the expectation for them to win the game or outperform their male counterparts (Rutten et al., 2007). Such environment facilitates the negative effects on prosocial behaviors in male adolescents. In addition, weak social-cognitive capabilities may impede male adolescents' ability to communicate effectively with others and might hinder their bonding with their peers or significant others. Thus, males are more likely to develop the antisocial traits and experience negative outcomes such as peer rejection, academic difficulties, or depression (Eme & Kavanaugh, 1995).

Besides, the existing evidence suggested that females, in both of their childhood and adolescence phases, decode nonverbal expressions better than males (Banerjee, 1997). This distinct socialization practice might encourage girls to read facial and bodily expressions more readily than boys, and girls are thus more eager to engage in relationships with their counterparts. In addition, females are more likely to take the empathic role and have a greater degree of ethical sensitivity, which in turn assists females to be better involved in group settings and to interact more positively with their counterparts (Bybee, 1998). The relational support, which is a strong predictor of behavioral adjustment (DuBois, Holloway, Valentine, & Cooper, 2002), and quality relationships with others might protect female adolescents from antisocial behavior and promote prosocial behavior. In their review, Bennett et al. (2005) summarized the research about gender differences in crime proneness. Male adolescents tend to feel guilty about aggressive behaviors but feel less guilty than females during adolescence, while female adolescents are especially more likely to feel guilty about inconsideration or antisocial behaviors than their male counterparts. This gender difference is due to the more mature social-cognitive skills. The maturity may assist females to have empathetic understanding and better moral judgments and thus inhibit females from committing antisocial behaviors.

There is consistent evidence that inadequate parenting interferes with the development of competent prosocial cognitive information processing skills (Bennett et al., 2005; Kelley, Loeber, Keenan, & DeLamatre, 1997). Parental interactions might exert some influences on children's perceptions of the world and may also affect the way in which children are perceived as well as the way people in their environment react to them. As parents provide initial opportunities for learning social cognition for their children, less effective communication or conflicting relationships between parents and children, especially boys, are more likely to lead to the behavioral problems and maladaptation to the prosocial norms. Moreover, during the childhood, boys usually encounter harsher discipline than girls do. This might in turn affect their perception of the world, and as a result, boys are more likely to develop conflictual perception of others and the world as well as develop more aggressive behaviors in their adolescence (Eme & Kavanaugh, 1995).

The present study suggests a slight gender difference on general positive youth development: females scored higher than did males on some positive development constructs. This finding is consistent with the results obtained from the Western and local contexts (Larsson & Frisk, 1999; Park & Peterson, 2006; Shek et al., 2007). The available literature suggests that male and female adolescents perform differently on various constructs. Female adolescents were more prone to spiritual development, higher awareness of the sociomoral reasoning, and better emotional management (Catalano et al., 2004; Furrow, King, & White, 2004; Rutten et al., 2007), whereas male adolescents tend to have higher self-efficacy during their pubertal maturation and are more resilient in adverse situations (Benjet & Hernandez-Guzman, 2001; Catalano et al., 2004).

In this study, male adolescents scored higher on positive identity; the tendency which is not commonly found across different cultures. In the research of DuBois et al. (2002), females, especially white female adolescents, had stronger awareness of their gender identity. The stronger sense of their gender identity was ascribed to their higher consciousness of gender-specific development and social-cognitive maturity (Bennett et al., 2005; Rojewski et al., 1995). However, some researchers argued that the self-image becomes increasingly more negative during pubertal maturation among females (i.e., in the period of junior secondary school years in the local context) but not among males (Tobin-Richards, Boxer, & Petersen, 1983). For Chinese adolescents, similar finding was found that female adolescents are inclined to perceive themselves negatively, especially when it comes to body image, and the relationship between body satisfaction and depression is only significant for females

(Davis & Katzman, 1997). In addition, during the early adolescence, parents tend to exert more control on female adolescents and allow more autonomy for male adolescents (Benjet & Hernandez-Guzman, 2001). The parental control might increase the tendency that female adolescents conform with parental expectations, and thus parental control may hinder the autonomy of female adolescents who are searching for their identity.

In the present study, male adolescents in the Hong Kong context had higher cognitive-behavioral competencies than did their female counterparts. These competencies might help male adolescents to be more aware of their internal dynamic organization of drives and beliefs which in turn help them understand themselves better (Catalano et al., 2004). Scholars have asserted that if male adolescents have wrong perceptions about themselves, they are more at risk in engaging in risk-taking behaviors such as premarital sex and delinquent behaviors (Swanson, Spencer, Dell'Angelo, Harpalani, & Spencer, 2002). Although male adolescents are less prone to prosocial involvement during adolescence, their stronger sense of developing a positive and healthy identity, as found in the present study, may reduce the possibility of male adolescents' risk behaviors.

Regarding time differences in positive youth development, there was a drop in the scores on the dimensions of "prosocial attributes," "general positive youth development qualities," and "positive identity" from Wave 1 to Wave 2, but the scores remained relatively stable from Wave 2 to Wave 3. One possible reason for the declining scores from Wave 1 to Wave 2 is the gap between the expectations and awareness of their identity as "adolescents." In Wave 1, when the adolescents first transited from primary school to secondary school, they might experience the "transition excitement" – having the opportunity to grow and starting to be aware of the new identity as "secondary school students." The transition excitement may remain for 1 year (Nottelmann, 1987). Marcia (1980) asserted that early adolescence is the first moment in life that physical development, cognitive skills, and social expectations coincide. This awareness might be more obvious when adolescents grow and might arouse adolescents' anxieties of changing the identity and the awareness of different social expectations. These anxieties might make adolescents have confused expectations on their growth and at the same time lead them to know their limitations. These confusions and anxieties might contribute to the decrement of the reported scores in the present study. In addition, the findings suggest that the adolescents perceive themselves more negatively in the aspects of their sexual identity, self-image, and competency level in early adolescence (Keefer, Holden, & Parker, 2013; Marcia, 1980). The confusions and uncertainty arisen from the physical and psychological changes might lower their self-confidence (Tobin-Richards et al., 1983).

There was a more stable development in Wave 3 in all the dimensions measured. Similar findings have been observed across the Western contexts (Berry, Phinney, Sam, & Vedder, 2006; Nottelmann, 1987) and Chinese contexts (Chang, 2003; Shek et al., 2005). There are two possible reasons accounted for this "plateau" phenomenon. First, growth happens in a gradual rather than an abrupt manner. Nottelmann (1987) argued that growth in competence and self-esteem still happens even if there is no notable change or transitions found from childhood to adolescence. Second, the junior secondary school students are still developing self-awareness of their changes which might become stabilized in Grade 9.

There are several methodological limitations of the present study. First, the sample of this study was confined in Hong Kong; therefore, further studies are needed to replicate the current findings in other Chinese communities to have a more generalized understanding of the gender differences in youth development in the Chinese cultural context. Second, the data collected on positive youth development are derived from self-reports. The responses from teachers and peers should be obtained to further facilitate the comprehension of the positive youth development issue. Last, qualitative methods such as in-depth interviews or focus group discussions can be adopted to obtain a better understanding of the issue regarding positive youth development.

Acknowledgment The preparation for this work and the Project P.A.T.H.S. were financially supported by The Hong Kong Jockey Club Charities Trust. The authorship is equally shared by the first author and second author.

References

Banerjee, M. (1997). Peeling the onion: A multilayered view of children's emotional development. In S. Hala (Ed.), *The development of social cognition* (pp. 241–272). Hove, England: Psychology Press.

Beilock, S. L., Gunderson, E. A., Ramirez, G., & Levine, S. C. (2010). Female teachers' math anxiety affects girls' math achievement. *Proceedings of the National Academy of Sciences of the United States of America, 107*(5), 1860–1863.

Benjet, C., & Hernandez-Guzman, L. (2001). Gender differences in psychological well-being of Mexican early adolescents. *Adolescence, 36*(141), 47–65.

Bennett, S., Farrington, D. P., & Huesmann, L. R. (2005). Explaining gender differences in crime and violence: The importance of social cognitive skills. *Aggression and Violent Behavior, 10*(3), 263–288.

Benson, P. L., & Scales, P. C. (2009). The definition and preliminary measurement of thriving in adolescence. *The Journal of Positive Psychology, 4*(1), 85–104.

Berry, J. S., Phinney, J. S., Sam, D. L., & Vedder, P. (2006). Immigrant youth: Acculturation, identity, and adaptation. *Applied Psychology: An International Review, 55*(3), 303–332.

Bybee, J. (1998). The emergence of gender differences in guilt during adolescence. In J. Bybee (Ed.), *Guilt and children* (pp. 113–125). San Diego, CA: Academic.

Caplan, P. J., & Caplan, J. B. (1997). Do sex-related cognitive differences exist, and why do people seek them out? In P. J. Caplan, M. Crawford, J. S. Hyde, & J. T. E. Richardson (Eds.), *Gender differences in human cognition* (pp. 52–80). New York: Oxford University Press.

Caplan, P. J., MacPherson, G. M., & Tobin, P. (1985). Do sex-related differences in spatial abilities exist? A multilevel critique with new data. *American Psychologist, 40*(7), 786–799.

Catalano, R. F., Berglund, M. L., Ryan, J. A. M., Lonczak, H. S., & Hawkins, J. D. (2004). Positive youth development in the United States: Research findings on evaluations of positive youth development programs. *Annals of the American Academy of Political and Social Science, 591*, 98–124.

Chang, L. (2003). Variable effects of children's aggression, social withdrawal, and prosocial leadership as functions of teacher beliefs and behaviors. *Child Development, 74*(2), 535–548.

Chess, S., & Thomas, A. (1984). *Origins and evolution of behavior disorders: From infancy to early adult life*. New York: Brunner/Mazel.

Damon, W. (2004). What is positive youth development? *Annals of the American Academy of Political and Social Science, 591*, 13–24.

Davis, C., & Katzman, M. (1997). Charting new territory: Body esteem, weight satisfaction, depression, and self-esteem among Chinese males and females in Hong Kong. *Sex Roles, 36*(7–8), 449–459.

DuBois, D. L., Burk-Braxton, C., Swenson, L. P., Tevendale, H. D., & Hardesty, J. L. (2002). Race and gender influences on adjustment in early adolescence: Investigation of an integrative model. *Child Development, 73*(5), 1573–1592.

DuBois, D. L., Holloway, B. E., Valentine, J. C., & Cooper, H. (2002). Effectiveness of mentoring programs for youth. A meta-analytic review. *American Journal of Community Psychology, 30*(2), 157–197.

Eme, R. F., & Kavanaugh, L. (1995). Sex differences in conduct disorder. *Journal of Clinical Child Psychology, 24*(4), 406–426.

Ferrer-Wreder, L. (2014). Advancing child and adolescent well-being through positive youth development and prevention programs. In *Handbook of child well-being* (pp. 3025–3041). Dordrecht: Springer.

Furrow, J. L., King, P. E., & White, K. (2004). Religion and positive youth development: Identity, meaning, and prosocial concerns. *Applied Developmental Science, 8*(1), 17–26.

Hansen, D. M., Larson, R. W., & Dworking, J. B. (2003). What adolescents learn in organized youth activities: A survey of self-reported developmental experiences. *Journal of Research on Adolescence, 13*(1), 25–55.

Herreraa, V. M., & McCloskey, L. A. (2001). Gender differences in the risk for delinquency among youth exposed to family violence. *Child Abuse & Neglect, 25*(8), 1037–1051.

Hughes, J. N., & Zhang, D. (2007). Effects of the structure of classmates' perceptions of peers' academic abilities on children's perceived cognitive competence, peer acceptance, and engagement. *Contemporary Educational Psychology, 32*(3), 400–419.

Hyde, J. S., & Linn, M. C. (1988). Gender differences in verbal ability: A meta-analysis. *Psychological Bulletin, 104*(1), 53–69.

Keefer, K. V., Holden, R. R., & Parker, J. D. A. (2013). Longitudinal assessment of trait emotional intelligence: Measurement invariance and construct continuity from late childhood to adolescence. *Psychological Assessment, 25*(4), 1255–1272.

Kelley, B. T., Loeber, R., Keenan, K., & DeLamatre, M. (1997). *Developmental pathways in boys' disruptive and delinquent behavior.* US Department of Justice, Office of Justice Programs, Office of Juvenile and Delinquency Prevention. Retrieved from http://www.ncjrs.org/jjbulletins/jjbul2_1297/jjb1297.html

Keyes, S. (1984). Measuring sex-role stereotypes: Attitudes among Hong Kong Chinese adolescents and the development of the Chinese sex-role inventory. *Sex Roles, 10*(1–2), 129–140.

Larson, R. W. (2000). Toward a psychology of positive youth development. *American Psychologist, 55*(1), 170–183.

Larsson, B., & Frisk, M. (1999). Social competence and emotional/behaviour problems in 6-16 year-old Swedish school children. *European Child & Adolescent Psychiatry, 8*(1), 24–33.

Leung, J. T. Y., & Shek, D. T. L. (2013). Parent-adolescent discrepancies in perceived family functioning and developmental outcomes in Chinese adolescents experiencing economic disadvantage. *International Journal on Disability and Human Development, 12*(2), 163–174.

Marcia, J. E. (1980). Identity in adolescence. *Handbook of Adolescent Psychology, 9*, 159–187.

Nottelmann, E. D. (1987). Competence and self-esteem during transition from childhood to adolescence. *Developmental Psychology, 23*(3), 441–450.

Ohannessian, C. M., Lerner, R. M., Lerner, J. V., & von Eye, A. (1999). Does self-competence predict gender differences in adolescent depression and anxiety? *Journal of Adolescence, 22*(3), 397–411.

Park, N., & Peterson, C. (2006). Moral competence and character strengths among adolescents: The development and validation of the Values in Action Inventory of Strengths for Youth. *Journal of Adolescence, 29*(6), 891–909.

Pittman, K. J., Irby, M., Tolman, J., Yohalem, N., & Ferber, T. (2003). *Preventing problems, promoting development, encouraging engagement: Competing priorities or inseparable goals?* Washington, DC: The Forum for Youth Investment, Impact Strategies, Inc. Retrieved from http://forumfyi.org/files/Preventing%20Problems,%20Promoting%20Development,%20Encouraging%20Engagement.pdf

Rojewski, J. W., Wicklein, R. C., & Schell, J. W. (1995). Effects of gender and academic-risk behavior on the career maturity of rural youth. *Journal of Research in Rural Education, 11*(2), 92–104.

Rutten, E. A., Stams, G. J. J. M., Biesta, G. J. J., Schuengel, C., Dirks, E., & Hoeksma, J. B. (2007). The contribution of organized youth sport to antisocial and prosocial behavior in adolescent athletes. *Journal of Youth Adolescence, 36*(3), 255–264.

Seligman, M. E. P., & Csikszentmihalyi, M. (2000). Positive psychology: An introduction. *American Psychologist, 55*(1), 5–14.

Shek, D. T. L. (2010). Using students' weekly diaries to evaluate positive youth development programs: Are findings based on multiple studies consistent? *Social Indicators Research, 95*(3), 475–487.

Shek, D. T. L., & Leung, J. T. Y. (2013). Adolescent development issues in Hong Kong: Phenomena and implications for youth service. In D. T. L. Shek & R. C. F. Sun (Eds.), *Development and Evaluation of Positive Adolescent Training through Holistic Social Programs (P.A.T.H.S.)* (pp. 1–13). New York: Springer Science and Business Media.

Shek, D. T. L., & Ma, C. M. S. (2010). Dimensionality of the Chinese positive youth development scale: Confirmatory factor analyses. *Social Indicators Research, 98*(1), 41–59.

Shek, D. T. L., Siu, A. M. H., & Lee, T. Y. (2007). The Chinese positive youth development scale: A validation study. *Research on Social Work Practice, 17*(3), 380–391.

Shek, D. T. L., & Sun, R. C. F. (2013). Evaluation of project P.A.T.H.S. by the program implementers: Findings based on the extension phase. *International Journal of Adolescent Medicine and Health, 25*(4), 415–423.

Shek, D. T. L., Sun, R. C. F., & Merrick, J. (2012). Positive youth development constructs: Conceptual review and application. *The Scientific World Journal, 2012*, Article ID 152923.

Shek, D. T. L., & Yu, L. (2013). Impact of the Project PA.T.H.S. On adolescent risk behavior: A five-year longitudinal study. In D. T. L. Shek & R. C. F. Sun (Eds.), *Development and evaluation of Positive Adolescent Training through Holistic Social Programs (P.A.T.H.S.)* (pp. 85–106). New York: Springer.

Smith, E. P., Osgood, D. W., Caldwell, L., Hynes, K., & Perkins, D. F. (2013). Measuring collective efficacy among children in community-based afterschool programs: Exploring pathways toward prevention and positive youth development. *American Journal of Community Psychology, 52*(1–2), 27–40.

Swanson, D. P., Spencer, M. B., Dell'Angelo, T., Harpalani, V., & Spencer, T. R. (2002). Identity processes and the positive youth development of African Americans: An explanatory framework. *New Directions for Youth Development, 95*, 73–100.

Tobin-Richards, M. H., Boxer, A. M., & Petersen, A. C. (1983). The psychological significance of pubertal change: Sex differences in perception of self during early adolescence. In J. Brooks-Gunn & A. C. Petersen (Eds.), *Girls at puberty: Biological and psychological perspectives* (pp. 127–154). New York: Plenum Press.

Parental Behavioral Control, Parental Psychological Control and Parent-Child Relational Qualities: Relationships to Chinese Adolescent Risk Behavior

Daniel T.L. Shek and Moon Y.M. Law

Abstract Over three consecutive years, Chinese junior secondary school students responded to the measures of parenting (perceived behavioral control and perceived psychological control), parent-child relational qualities and adolescent risk behavior (substance abuse, delinquency, self-harm behavior, and suicidal behavior). Factor analysis showed that three distinct factors (namely parental behavioral control, parental psychological control, and parent-child relational qualities) were extracted from the father-child and mother-child relational measures, and good internal consistency among the items on the three factors was indicated. In line with the hypotheses, correlation and partial correlation analyses showed that parental behavioral control, parental psychological control, and parent-child relational qualities at Time 1 predicted adolescent risk behavior and their change at Time 3. Regarding the different contributions of fathers and mothers to adolescent risk behavior, results showed that maternal influence predicted changes in adolescent substance abuse and delinquency whereas paternal influence predicted adolescent deliberate self-harm and suicidal behavior over time.

Keywords Chinese adolescents • Parental behavioral control • Parental psychological control • Parent-child relational quality • Adolescent risk behavior

Introduction

Family has been considered to be important in the development of children and youth (Barker & Hunt, 2006). According to the ecological model (Bronfenbrenner, 1988), the development of individuals is influenced by the qualities and interactions between different systems. Among different systems, the dynamic and interaction

D.T.L. Shek, Ph.D., B.B.S., S.B.S., J.P. (✉) • M.Y.M. Law, M.S.W.
Department of Applied Social Sciences, The Hong Kong Polytechnic University, Hunghom, Hong Kong
e-mail: daniel.shek@polyu.edu.hk

D.T.L. Shek et al. (eds.), *Chinese Adolescents in Hong Kong*, Quality of Life in Asia 5, DOI 10.1007/978-981-287-143-5_4

effects arisen from different family processes, such as parenting and parent-child relationship, influence adolescent development deeply (Hepworth, Rooney, Rooney, & Strom-Gottfried, 2013).

In the parent-child dyad, parenting and parent-child relationship have been identified as important factors affecting adolescent development (Shek, 2008). Also, warmth and responsive parental control are important parenting dimensions. Generally speaking, there are two types of parental control (Barber, 1996, 2002; Steinberg, 1990). While parental behavioral control refers to "rules, regulations and restrictions that parents have for their children" (Smetana & Daddis, 2002, p. 563), psychological control refers to "parents attempt to control the child's activities in ways that negatively affect the child's psychological world and thereby undermines the child's psychological development" (Smetana & Daddis, p. 563).

Parental behavioral control has been conceptualized and assessed based on the global dimensions such as demandingness (Maccoby & Martin, 1983), and specific dimensions such as knowledge and monitoring (Smetana & Daddis, 2002). Shek (2005, 2006, 2007) concluded the available research findings and argued that there are at least five different aspects of parental behavioral control. These included (a) how much the parent knows about the child (parental knowledge), (b) rules imposed and expectations of the parent (parental expectations), (c) parental surveillance and tracking (parental monitoring), (d) reward and punishment of the child (parental discipline), and (e) global parental control such as parental demandingness.

The parental psychological control refers to parental behaviors that include constraining verbal expression, invalidating feelings, personal attack, guilt induction, love withdrawal, and erratic emotional behavior. Barber (1996) pointed out that "although psychological control was included in some of the earliest conceptualization of parenting and continues to be implicit in much of the major work, focused attention to the construct has been lacking" (p. 3298) and that "there is little research specifically measuring psychological control and its covariates" (p. 3313). Barber and Harmon (2002) further showed that the relevant scientific literature does not suffice.

Although studies on behavioral control and psychological control have been carried out, few researchers have simultaneously included parent-child relational quality in their studies. In their review of the related studies in this area, Crouter and Head (2002) criticized that "many studies of parental monitoring or knowledge have examined possible antecedents without reference to the quality of the parent-child relationship" (p. 473) and argued that "it is impossible to conceptualize the possible antecedents of parental monitoring or parental knowledge without acknowledging that the quality of the parent-child relationship is the fundamental platform that gives rise to them" (p. 472). Although parent-child relationship is commonly used to reflect parent-child relational quality, different indicators have been proposed (Shek, 2007, 2008). These include parent-child relationship, parental trust of their children, children's trust of their parents, children's satisfaction with parental parenting, and readiness of the child to disclose to parents (Shek, 2007, 2008).

Shek (2005, 2006) suggested that three aspects of parent-child relational qualities are of particular importance. The first aspect is mutual trust between the parents and their children. Shek (2010) found that parental trust of the children and children's trust of their parents were closely related to parental behavioral and psychological controls. However, there is a dearth of research on these two aspects in the existing literature. The second aspect is the readiness of the child to communicate with the parents. It can be inferred that as the child's readiness to communication increases, parental knowledge would also increase. Shek (2007) revealed that readiness of the child to communicate was related to parental behavioral control and psychological control. The third aspect is the child's satisfaction with parental control. For children who are more satisfied with parental control, they are also more willing to be socialized. Shek's (2007) study showed that children's satisfaction with parental control was related to parental behavioral control and psychological control.

Previous research has showed that parenting and parent-child relational qualities influence adolescent externalized behaviors, such as risk behaviors or delinquency (Dishion & Loeber, 1985). For example, Patterson and colleagues (Patterson, Capaldi, & Bank, 1991) disclosed that parental behavioral control may prevent adolescents from committing delinquent behaviors. Family researchers also reported that warm and responsive parental control predicts cooperative and appropriate behaviors, as well as social competence of adolescents (Booth, Rose-Krasnor, McKinnon, & Rubin, 1994; Hart, DeWolf, Wozniak, & Burts, 1992). However, excessive or inadequate behavioral control may lead to externalized problems of children and adolescents (Barber, Olsen, & Shagle, 1994).

Parent-child relational qualities also benefit adolescents' behavior. Good parent-child relationship and interaction provide nurture to children and youth as it gives them a solid emotional foundation based on secure attachment and positive interaction, which may further help them develop appropriate behaviors and competences as they grow up (Coates & Lewis, 1984; Greenberg, Speltz, & DeKlyen, 1993; Kochanska, Murray, & Harlan, 2000). A longitudinal study with the sample of 672 adolescents in 405 adoptive families was conducted to examine the relationship between adolescent behavior problems and parent-child relationship (Klahr, McGue, Iacono, & Burt, 2010). The results showed that poor parent-child relationship predicted adolescent behavior problems. As participants of this study are not genetically influenced by their adoptive parents, this study is likely to suggest that parent-child relational qualities influence adolescent risk behaviors. In contrast, poor parental monitoring and control might encourage adolescents to associate with deviant peers, and expose them to higher level of deviant behaviors (Smith & Krohn, 1995).

While parental behavioral control and good parent-child relational qualities have been identified as protective factors for adolescent risk behavior, parental psychological control might serve as a risk factor which can lead to an increase in adolescent risk behavior (Bean, Bush, McKenry, & Wilson, 2003). For example, results of the study conducted by Pettit and colleagues (Petti, Laird, Dodge, Bates, & Criss, 2001) revealed that a higher level of psychological control was associated with greater deviant behavioral problems of adolescents.

Parental control and parent-child relational quality are strongly related to adolescent substance abuse problem. According to previous studies, parental behavioral control is a protective factor to adolescent drug use (Brody & Forehand, 1993). Researchers found that adolescents under poor parental behavioral control were more vulnerable to abuse drugs (Chassin, Pillow, Curran, Molina, & Barrera, 1993). In addition, researchers also found that parental psychological control was positively related to adolescent substance use. According to the study of Silk and colleagues (Silk, Morris, Kanaya, & Steinberg, 2003), psychological control predicts adolescent drug use and deviant behaviors. Furthermore, except parental control, poor parent-child relational qualities also predict the substance use among adolescents (Windlin & Kuntsche, 2012).

Regarding adolescent internalizing problems, previous studies showed that parent-child relational qualities were strongly associated with adolescent self-harm and suicidal behavior (Borowsky, Ireland, & Resnick, 2001; Tomori, 1999). According to the study of Hsu, Chen, and Lung (2013), parental bonding was a strong predictor of the intention to commit suicide or self-harm among adolescents. Also, a recent study (Consoli et al., 2013) revealed that adolescents with negative relationships with parents were more likely to commit suicide.

Parenting was also found to be related to adolescent suicidal behavior. For example, based on a longitudinal study, Johnson et al. (2002) found that negative parenting might induce the difficulties regarding inter-personal relationships for adolescents, which may result in the possibility of suicidal behavior. Furthermore, some researchers (Harrington et al., 1998; Soenens, Vansteenkiste, Luyten, Duriez, & Goossens, 2005) examined the link between psychological control and adolescent well-being. Results of these studies showed that parental psychological control was one crucial factor of adolescent deliberate self-harm and depression. According to Bowen (1976, 1991), young people have to experience psychological separation from their parents and learn to build up their self-determination and independent thinking during adolescence. Adolescents who have experienced parental psychological control may fail to develop a better sense of self-determination and have difficulties in making appropriate decisions. As a result, these young people are more likely to have higher anxiety level and have different internalized problems.

Although much work has been done to examine the relationship between parenting and adolescent risk behavior (Bean et al., 2003; Huang et al., 2010; Petti et al., 2001), there are several limitations in the existing literature. First, while many studies have been carried out in the Western context, only a few studies are done in Chinese communities. Studies conducted in the Chinese cultural context are important because Chinese people constitute roughly one-fifth of the world's population. Second, there are few longitudinal studies in the field. Longitudinal studies can help researchers and frontline practitioners to understand the causality, stability, and continuity among different variables over time (Fok & Shek, 2011). In other words, more knowledge on the dynamic and reciprocal processes between parenting, parent-child relationship, and adolescent risk behavior are needed, because this can further benefit the service development in future. Third, there are few studies that simultaneously include multiple adolescent risk behaviors. In the present longitudinal study, several adolescent risk behaviors including substance abuse, delinquency, deliberate self-harm, and suicidal behavior are investigated. Finally, few studies have examined the relationship between parental control (behavioral control and psychological control) and parent-child relational quality and adolescent risk behavior in a single study. Inclusion of these areas can give a more dynamic picture about the role of different family processes in adolescent development.

Against the above background, there are several objectives of this study. First, factorial validity and internal consistency of the measures of behavioral control, psychological control and parent-child relational quality for the father-child and mother-child subsystems were examined. Second, the relationships between the parent-child subsystem quality and adolescent risk behavior were examined. It is predicted that (a) paternal and maternal behavioral control would be negatively related to adolescent risk behavior over time (Hypotheses 1a and 1b); (b) paternal and maternal psychological control would be positively related to adolescent risk behavior over time (Hypotheses 2a and 2b), (c) father-child relational quality and mother-child relational quality would be negatively related to adolescent risk behavior overtime (Hypotheses 3a and 3b). Concerning the different contributions from fathers and mothers to adolescent risk behavior, there are two general predictions.

First, based on the theories and findings suggesting that mothers are more important than fathers (see Shek, 1999a), it is predicted that compared with the father-child subsystem quality, the mother-child subsystem quality would exert stronger influence on adolescent risk behavior (Hypothesis 4a). On the other hand, based on theories and research findings highlighting the important role of the fathers (see Shek, 1999b), it is predicted that father-child subsystem quality would exert a stronger influence on adolescent risk behavior than did mother-child subsystem quality (Hypothesis 4b). The findings reported in this article were derived from the Wave 1, Wave 2 and Wave 3 data of a longitudinal study on the psychosocial adjustment of adolescents in their junior secondary school years (Shek & Ma, 2012; Shek & Yu, 2012).

Method

Participants and Procedures

The present study is part of a 6-year longitudinal study on adolescent development and the data was derived from the first three waves of the project. Students from 28 secondary schools in Hong Kong participated in the study, and these schools were randomly selected from all the secondary schools in Hong Kong. For these 28 schools, students from all classes in Secondary 1 were invited to participate in the study in 2009/10 school year. In school year 2011/12, all Secondary 3 students in the selected 28 schools were invited to attend the third wave of survey. A total of 4,106 Secondary 3 students responded to the questionnaire (male = 2,185; female = 1,885; no indication of gender = 36). The mean age of the participants was 14.65 years (SD = 0.80). From Secondary 1 to Secondary 3, the data from 2,667 students was successfully matched, indicating an acceptable attrition rate of 19.8 %. The procedures for collecting the data can be seen in Chap. 2 of the book and other publications of the project (e.g., Ma & Shek, 2013).

Instruments

Assessment of Parental Behavioral Control

Validated measures of parental behavioral control have been developed in previous studies by the first author (Shek, 2005, 2006, 2007). Because of time limitation in administering the questionnaires, items were selected to measure parental behavioral control based on the item-total correlation coefficients. Three aspects of parental behavioral control were covered in this study:

Paternal Knowledge and Maternal Knowledge: Two items were developed to assess paternal knowledge ("My father knows my situation in my school"; "My father clearly knows who my friends are"). Similar items were used to assess maternal knowledge. The total score of these two items was used as an indicator of the level of parental knowledge of the child's behavior, with a higher score indicating a higher level of knowledge.

Paternal Expectation and Maternal Expectation: Two items were developed to assess paternal expectation ("My father expects me to have good behavior in school"; "My father has clear expectations about how I make friends"). Similar items were used to assess maternal expectations. The total score of these two items was used as an indicator of the level of parental expectation of the child's behavior, with a higher score indicating a higher level of expectations.

Paternal Monitoring and Maternal Monitoring: Three items were developed to assess paternal monitoring ("My father actively understands my situation at school"; "My father actively understands my friends", "My father actively understands my afterschool activities"). Similar items were used to assess maternal monitoring. The total score of these three items was used as an indicator of the level of parental monitoring of the child's behavior, with a higher score indicating a higher level of monitoring.

Assessment of Parental Psychological Control

Four items were selected from the Chinese Paternal Psychological Control Scale (CPPCS) (e.g., "My father always wants to change my views and experiences"; "My father wants to control everything I do"). Similar items were used to assess maternal monitoring that formed the Chinese Maternal Psychological Control Scale (CMPCS). The total score of these items was used as an indicator of the level of parental psychological control of the child's behavior, with a higher score indicating a higher level of psychological control. Previous studies showed that the CPPCS and CMPCS possessed good psychometric properties.

Assessment of Parent-Child Relational Qualities

Based on the measures of parent-child relational qualities used in previous studies (Shek, 2005, 2006, 2007), the items that assess the parent-child relation in the following two aspects were selected. First, three items on the respondent's satisfaction with paternal control (e.g., "My father's discipline of me is reasonable") were selected. Similar items were used to assess the respondent's satisfaction with maternal control. Second, two items on the father-child relationship ("I actively tell my father what happens to me"; "I actively share my experience with my father") were used to assess father-child communication. Similar items were used to assess the respondent's satisfaction with mother-child communication.

Assessment of Adolescent Risk Behaviors

- *Substance Use Scale* (*DRUG*): Eight items were used to assess the participants' frequency of using different types of substance (i.e., alcohol, tobacco, ketamine, cannabis, cough mixture organic solvent, heroin, and pills such as ecstasy and methaqualone) during the past year. Participants answered on a 6-point Likert-scale (0 = never; 1 = 1–2 times; 2 = 3–5 times; 3 = more than 5 times; 4 = several times a month; 5 = several times a week; 6 = everyday). A composite score was calculated by averaging all eight item scores in order to obtain the mean score on the overall substance use.
- *Delinquency Scale* (*DELIN*): This scale comprises 12 items that assess the frequency of delinquent behavior of the participants in the past year, including stealing, cheating, truancy, running away from home, damaging others' properties, assault, having sexual relationship with others, gang fighting, speak foul language, staying away from home without parental consent, strong arm others, and break in others' places. Respondents rated the frequency of these behaviors in the past half a year on a six-point Likert-scale (0 = never, 1 = 1–2 times; 2 = 3–4 times; 3 = 5–6 times; 4 = 7–8 times; 5 = 9–10 times; 6 = more than 10 times).
- *Deliberate Self-Harm Behavior Scale* (*DSHS*): This scale comprises 17 items that assess the occurrence of different deliberate self-harming behaviors of the participants in the past year such as cutting wrist and burning oneself. Respondents answered yes (coded as 1) or no (coded as 0) on these 17 items according to their actual behavior in the past year. A composite score of DSHS was calculated for each individual by averaging the 17 item scores, with higher score representing more self-harm behaviors.
- *Suicidal Behavior Scale* (*SBS*): Participants' suicidal behaviors were measured by a four-item SBS in the three aspects: suicidal thought, suicidal plan, and suicidal attempt. A composite score of SBS was computed by averaging scores of item 1, item 2 and the recoded item 3, which represents for a general suicidal tendency of the participants.

Results

To measure the paternal factors (paternal behavioral control, paternal psychological control and father-child relational qualities items), we used a principal components analysis to extract the factors. The results showed that the three factors with eigenvalues exceeding unity explained 64.94 % in the variance of the paternal factors. Scree test showed that the three factors could be meaningfully extracted. Hence, varimax factor rotation was carried out. Factor I included the items on paternal behavioral control (item 1 to item 7). The second factor included the items on father-child relationship (item 8 to item 10, item 15 to item 17). The third factor included the items on paternal psychological control (item 11 to item 14). The factor solution can be seen in Table 1.

To test the maternal factors (maternal behavioral control, maternal psychological control and mother-child relational quality items), similar factor analysis (i.e., principal components analysis followed by varimax rotation) was conducted. The three factors explained 60.3 % in the variance of the maternal factors. Factor I was mother-child relational quality (item 8 to item 10, item 15 to item 17). The second factor included the items on maternal behavioral control (item 1 to item 7). The third factor included items on maternal psychological control (item 11 to item 14). The factor solution can be seen in Table 2. The findings gave support to the factorial validity of the measures of the quality of the father-child and mother-child subsystems.

Table 1 Varimax rotated factor solution based on measures of perceived paternal behavioral control, paternal psychological control and father-child relational quality based on the Time 1 data

		Paternal behavioral control	Father-child relational quality	Paternal psychological control
Item 1	My father knows my situation in school	*.712*	.384	−.003
Item 2	My father clearly knows who my friends are	*.725*	.341	−.009
Item 3	My father expects me to have good behavior in school	*.502*	.333	.230
Item 4	My father has clear expectations about how I make friends	*.642*	.174	.284
Item 5	My father actively understands my situation at school	*.807*	.236	.027
Item 6	My father actively understands my friends	*.850*	.194	.076
Item 7	My father actively understands my afterschool activities	*.737*	.261	.104
Item 8	My father's discipline of me is reasonable	.268	*.811*	−.057
Item 9	I am glad to do what my father expects me to do	.245	*.821*	−.014

(continued)

Table 1 (continued)

		Paternal behavioral control	Father-child relational quality	Paternal psychological control
Item 10	I believe my father's discipline of me is good to me	.278	*.813*	.022
Item 11	My father always wants to change my views and experiences	.167	.265	*.661*
Item 12	My father puts more weight on his views than my views	−.039	−.158	*.814*
Item 13	My father wants to control everything I do	.059	−.208	*.825*
Item 14	My father always attempts to change me to reach his standard	.131	−.035	*.813*
Item 15	I am satisfied with the relationship with my father	.306	*.753*	−.135
Item 16	I actively tell my father what happens to me	.491	*.599*	−.052
Item 17	I actively share my experience with my father	.498	*.586*	−.045

Note: The highest loading obtained by a variable among the factors is in italics. Factor 1=Paternal Behavioral Control. Factor 2=Father-child Relational Quality. Factor 3=Paternal Psychological Control

Table 2 Varimax rotated factor solution based on measures of perceived maternal behavioral control, maternal psychological control and mother-child relational quality based on the Time 1 data

		Mother-child relational quality	Maternal behavioral quality	Maternal psychological control
Item 1	My mother knows my situation in school	.470	*.657*	−.039
Item 2	My mother clearly knows who my friends are	.460	*.664*	−.033
Item 3	My mother expects me to have good behavior in school	.261	*.635*	.142
Item 4	My mother has clear expectations about how I make friends	.166	*.677*	.263
Item 5	My mother actively understands my situation at school	.274	*.814*	−.002
Item 6	My mother actively understands my friends	.248	*.835*	.042
Item 7	My mother actively understands my afterschool activities	.290	*.740*	.031
Item 8	My mother's discipline of me is reasonable	*.771*	.304	−.115
Item 9	I am glad to do what my mother expects me to do	*.805*	.243	−.019

(continued)

Table 2 (continued)

		Mother-child relational quality	Maternal behavioral quality	Maternal psychological control
Item 10	I believe my mother's discipline of me is good to me	*.781*	.298	−.003
Item 11	My mother always wants to change my views and experiences	.147	.142	*.750*
Item 12	My mother puts more weight on her views than my views	−.200	.008	*.843*
Item 13	My mother wants to control everything I do	−.194	.019	*.868*
Item 14	My mother always attempts to change me to reach her standard	−.037	.084	*.828*
Item 15	I am satisfied with the relationship with my mother	*.765*	.266	−.173
Item 16	I actively tell my mother what happens to me	*.755*	.318	−.033
Item 17	I actively share my experience with my mother	*.759*	.298	−.030

Note: The highest loading obtained by a variable among the factors is in italics. Factor 1 = Mother-Child Relational Quality. Factor 2 = Maternal Behavioral Control. Factor 3 = Maternal Psychological Control

Reliability analyses were carried out for the measures on paternal and maternal behavioral control (knowledge, expectations, monitoring and omnibus behavioral control), psychological control, parent-child relational qualities (satisfaction with parental control and readiness to communicate), and positive parent-child subsystem (behavioral control plus parent-child relational qualities items) at Time 1 and Time 3. As shown in Tables 3 and 4, the measures had good internal consistency reliability.

To understand the relationships between quality of the parent-child subsystem (behavioral control, psychological control and parent-child relational qualities) and adolescent risk behavior, two sets of analyses were performed (Table 5). First, bivariate correlations examined the relationship between Time 1 parent-child subsystem quality and Time 3 adolescent risk behavior. Second, partial correlation analyses examined the relationship between Time 1 parent-child subsystem quality and Time 3 adolescent risk behavior, controlling the effect of Time 1 adolescent risk behavior. Two observations can be highlighted from the findings. First, the hypotheses of the study were generally supported (i.e., positive parent-child subsystem quality predicted lowered adolescent risk behavior). Second, the effect size of the related correlation coefficients was not large.

To examine the relative influence of fathers and mothers on risk behavior and the change of risk behavior over time, multiple regression analyses were carried out (Table 6). According to the regression models, while both the paternal and maternal factors predicted substance abuse, delinquency and deliberate self-harm, only paternal factors predicted adolescent suicidal behavior. We also conducted the regression with the changes in risk behavior as the dependent variable. The results showed that

Table 3 Internal consistency reliability of the different measures within the father-child subsystem and mother-child subsystem at Time 1

Measure	Mean inter-item correlation	Mean item-total correlation	Coefficient alpha
Father-child measures			
PK	.713	.713	.832
PE	.516	.516	.680
PM	.676	.739	.862
SPC	.707	.766	.879
PPC	.500	.617	.801
FCR	.657	.729	.853
PBC	.538	.688	.891
PCRQ	.603	.792	.899
PPCS	.493	.674	.926
Mother-child measures			
MK	.754	.754	.859
MEXP	.520	.520	.676
MMON	.687	.749	.868
SMC	.715	.772	.882
MPC	.589	.695	.853
MCR	.687	.758	.870
MBC	.554	.700	.897
MCRQ	.626	.747	.907
PMCS	.508	.686	.930

PK Paternal Knowledge Scale, *PE* Paternal Expectation Scale, *PM* Paternal Monitoring Scale, *SPC* Satisfaction with Paternal Control, *PPC* Paternal Psychological Control, *FCR* Father-child Relationship, *PBC* Paternal Behavioral Control, *PCRQ* Father-Child Relational Quality, *PPCS* Positive Father-Child Subsystem, *MK* Maternal Knowledge Scale, *ME* Maternal Expectation Scale, *MM* Maternal Monitoring Scale, *SMC* Satisfaction with Maternal Control, *MPC* Maternal Psychological Control, *MCR* Mother-Child Relationship, *MBC* Maternal Behavioral Control, *MCRQ* Mother-child Relational Quality, *PMCS* Positive Mother-Child Subsystem

Table 4 Internal consistency of the different measures within the father-child subsystem and mother-child subsystem at Time 3

Measure	Mean inter-item correlation	Mean item-total correlation	Coefficient alpha
Father-child measures			
PK	.746	.746	.854
PE	.491	.491	.658
PM	.720	.776	.884
SPC	.729	.784	.890
PPC	.600	.703	.857
FCR	.682	.753	.868
PBC	.546	.694	.893
PCRQ	.615	.738	.904
PPCS	.500	.618	.928

(continued)

Table 4 (continued)

Measure	Mean inter-item correlation	Mean item-total correlation	Coefficient alpha
Mother-child measures			
MK	.757	.757	.861
MEXP	.552	.552	.707
MMON	.717	.774	.884
SMC	.724	.780	.887
MPC	.671	.762	.892
MCR	.686	.759	.870
MBC	.557	.703	.898
MCRQ	.623	.744	.906
PMCS	.494	.675	.926

PK Paternal Knowledge Scale, *PE* Paternal Expectation Scale, *PM* Paternal Monitoring Scale, *SPC* Satisfaction with Paternal Control, *PPC* Paternal Psychological Control, *FCR* Father-child Relationship, *PBC* Paternal Behavioral Control, *PCRQ* Father-Child Relational Quality, *PPCS* Positive Father-Child Subsystem, *MK* Maternal Knowledge Scale, *ME* Maternal Expectation Scale, *MM* Maternal Monitoring Scale, *SMC* Satisfaction with Maternal Control, *MPC* Maternal Psychological Control, *MCR* Mother-Child Relationship, *MBC* Maternal Behavioral Control, *MCRQ* Mother-child Relational Quality, *PMCS* Positive Mother-Child Subsystem

Table 5 Relationships between parent-child relational qualities measures and adolescent risk behavior

	Substance abuse		Delinquency	
Measure	T3	P3	T3	P3
Father-child measures				
T1 PBC	−.092***	−.040*	−.136***	−.028
T1 PPC	.043*	.025	.029	.012
T1 PCRQ	−.125***	−.071***	−.155***	−.043*
T1 PPCS	−.119***	−.059**	−.158***	−.039*
Mother-child measures				
T1 MBC	.115***	−.072**	−.130**	−.040*
T1 MPC	.064**	.041**	.048*	.010
T1 MCRQ	.156***	−.101***	−.167***	−.050*
T1 PMCS	.147***	−.094**	−.162***	−.049*
	Deliberate self-harm		Suicidal behavior	
Measure	T3	P3	T3	P3
Father-child measures				
T1 PBC	−.079***	−.049*	−.061**	−.023
T1 PPC	.043*	.031	.063**	.047*
T1 PCRQ	−.136***	−.088***	−.123***	−.070***
T1 PPCS	−.115***	−.074***	−.098***	−.050*
Mother-child measures				
T1 MBC	.074***	−.042*	−.038*	−.002

(continued)

Table 5 (continued)

	Deliberate self-harm		Suicidal behavior	
Measure	T3	P3	T3	P3
T1 MPC	.055**	.029	.099***	.072***
T1 MCRQ	.114***	−.056**	−.112***	−.066**
T1 PMCS	.103***	−.054**	−.081***	−.034

Note: *T1* Time 1, *T3* Time 3, *P3* Partial correlation between Time 1 predictor and Time 3 outcome variable controlling for Time 1 measure
PBC Paternal Behavioral Control, *PPC* Paternal Psychological Control, *PCRQ* Father-Child Relational Quality, *PPCS* Positive Father-Child Subsystem, *MBC* Maternal Behavioral Control, *MPC* Maternal Psychological Control, *MCRQ* Mother-child Relational Quality, *PMCS* Positive Mother-Child Subsystem
*** $p<.001$; ** $p<.01$; * $p<.05$

Table 6 Relationships between parent-child subsystem factors at Time 1 (predictor variables) and adolescent risk behavior at Time 3 (criterion variable)

Dependent variable	Predictor variables	Beta	R^2
T3 DRUG	T1 PCS	−.066**	.024
	T1 MCS	−.115***	
T3 DELIN	T1 PCS	−.105***	.035
	T1 MCS	−.115***	
T3 DSH	T1 PCS	−.086***	.016
	T1 MCS	−.063**	
T3 SB	T1 PCS	−.080***	.011
	T1 MCS	−.040	
T3 DRUG	T1 DRUG	.374***	.159
	T1 PCS	−.022	
	T1 MCS	−.074***	
T3 DELIN	T1 DELIN	.450***	.217
	T1 PCS	−.021	
	T1 MCS	−.036a	
T3 DSH	T1 DSH	.360***	.143
	T1 PCS	−.058**	
	T1 MCS	−.025	
T3 SB	T1 SB	.318***	.11
	T1 PCS	−.043*	
	T1 MCS	−.010	

Note: *T1* Time 1, *T3* Time 3, *DRUG* Substance abuse, *DELIN* Delinquency, *DSH* Deliberate self-harm, *SB* Suicidal behavior, *PCS* Father-Child Subsystem, *MCS* Mother-Child Subsystem
*** $p<.001$; ** $p<.01$; * $p<.05$

while the negative mother-child subsystem quality at Time 1 predicted an increase in substance abuse and delinquency in Time 3, negative father-child subsystem quality at Time 1 did not. On the other hand, while negative father-child subsystem quality at Time 1 predicted an increase in deliberate self-harm and suicidal behavior in Time 3, the negative mother-child subsystem quality at Time 1 did not.

Discussion

The first research objective of this study was to examine whether the three aspects of the parent-child subsystem for fathers and mothers could be empirically established. With specific reference to the father-child subsystem, factor analysis clearly showed that three distinct dimensions emerged from the data – paternal behavioral control, father-child relational qualities and paternal psychological control dimensions (Table 1). Similarly, factor analysis revealed that three distinct dimensions emerged from the data also for on the mother-child dyad – maternal behavioral control, mother-child relational quality and maternal psychological control dimensions (Table 2). Reliability analyses showed that the scales that test the quality of the father-child subsystem and mother-child subsystem at Time 1 had good internal consistency reliability. These findings are generally consistent with the full version of the measures reported previously (Shek, 2006). The present study addresses the research problem identified by Shek (2002, 2010) that there is a lack of instruments that measures family and parenting processes in the Chinese cultural context. The findings also suggest that the adapted measures used in this study possess acceptable psychometric properties.

The present findings are consistent with the general parenting literature that positive parenting characteristics are related to better adolescent developmental outcomes (e.g., Shek, 1999b). Consistent with the findings of Rogers, Buchanan, and Winchell (2003), the present study also suggests that the behavioral control and psychological control of parents have different effects on adolescent development. Regarding parental control effects, the present study is consistent with the findings that parental behavioral control and parent-child relational qualities were negatively related to adolescent externalized behavioral problems, such as delinquency and risk behavior (Burt, McGue, Iacono, & Krueger, 2006; Eccles, Early, Frasier, Belansky, & McCarthy, 1997). The present findings are also consistent with the previous findings that parental psychological control contributed to adolescent internalized problems, such as depression and anxiety (Barber & Harmon, 2002) which would result in deliberate self-harm or suicidal behavior.

Regarding the research question on the relationship between parent-child subsystem qualities and adolescent risk behavior over time, the results generally supported the hypotheses (Hypotheses 1a, 1b, 2a, 2b, 3a and 3b). For adolescent substance abuse, different measures of the quality of the parent-child subsystem at Time 1 were related to substance abuse and the changes in it at Time 3. This finding is consistent with the previous research findings. In a recent longitudinal study, Wang et al. (2013) suggested that good parent-child relational qualities could facilitate children's disclosure of information which would eventually reduce the possibility of adolescent substance abuse. Other research also suggested that parental behavior control also has positive impact on preventing adolescent substance use (Fletcher, Steinberg, & Williams-Wheeler, 2004; Windlin & Kuntsche, 2012).

Regarding delinquency, with the exception of psychological control, different measures of the quality of the parent-child subsystem at Time 1 predicted delinquency and the change of it at Time 3. The present findings are consistent with previous studies (Bean, Barber, & Crane, 2006; Laird, Pettit, Bates, & Dodge, 2003) and they further support the argument that parental behavior control and high quality of parent-child relationship can help to reduce adolescent delinquent behavior. The results also further corroborate Bradford et al.'s (2003) findings that maternal psychological control contributes to adolescent externalized behavioral problems.

Except for the parental psychological control, different measures on the quality of the parent-child subsystem at Time 1 predicted deliberate self-harm and the change of it at Time 3. These findings are consistent with the research suggesting that poor parent-child relationship is a risk factor for deliberate self-harm behavior (Crowell et al., 2008). In contrast, family cohesiveness (Webb, 2002) was shown to be a protective factor in adolescent deliberate self-harm. Finally, different measures on the quality of the parent-child subsystem at Time 1 predicted suicidal behavior at Time 3. Besides, psychological control and parent-child relational quality at Time 1 predicted adolescent suicidal behavior at Time 3. These findings are in line with the results of previous research (Soenens, Luyckx, Vansteenkiste, Duriez, & Goossens, 2008), which supports the argument that parental psychological control is positively related to adolescent suicidal attempts and actions, and high quality of parent-child relationship can promote the well-being of adolescent (Kwok-Lai & Shek, 2010).

The findings regarding the different influences of the father-child subsystem and mother-child subsystem support both Hypothesis 4a and Hypothesis 4b. While mothers influenced children's substance abuse and delinquency, fathers did not. It is noteworthy that substance abuse and delinquency are illegal activities (i.e., externalizing behavior). On the other hand, while fathers predicted change in deliberate self-harm and suicidal behavior (i.e., internalizing behavior), mothers did not. These results are consistent with previous findings (Gould, Shaffer, Fisher, & Garfinkel, 1998; Shek, 1998). For example, a longitudinal study revealed that the father-child relationship, rather than mother-child relationship, significantly affected the deliberate self-harm adolescent self-harm (Hilt, Nock, Lloyd-Richardson, & Prinstein, 2008). In short, the present findings suggest that the influence of fathers and mothers on adolescent development is more complicated than we have expected. Shek (1999b) found that compared with mothers, fathers exerted a stronger influence on adolescent development. However, the present study suggests that the relative influences from fathers and mothers vary as a function of different developmental outcomes of children. The present findings suggest that two different pathways may be involved in the differential influence of fathers and mothers on adolescent internalized and externalized behavior.

From a theoretical perspective, the present findings underscore the importance of dyadic family processes in shaping adolescent risk behavior. Two practical implications can be drawn from the present findings. First, as parent-child subsystem attributes (parental control and parent-child relational qualities) influence adolescent risk behavior (Tables 3 and 4), the present findings suggest that there is a need to cultivate healthy parental control and parent-child relational quality processes so that adolescent risk behavior could be reduced. Second, to have a deeper understanding on how parent-child subsystem attributes influence adolescent development, further investigation on different adolescent risk behaviors, such as sexual risk behavior and Internet addiction is needed.

As there are few studies examining all the three parental factors simultaneously to predict of adolescent development (Gamambos, Barker, & Almeida, 2003), this study is innovative, in particular in the Chinese cultural context. Despite the fact that the present study is pioneer in nature, several limitations should be noted. First, since parental control and parent-child relational qualities were only assessed from the child perspective, it would be useful to include data to reflect the point of view of the parents or outsiders to the family. Second, the present longitudinal study was conducted merely among Chinese adolescents in Hong Kong, and more research is needed to replicate the findings in other Chinese contexts. Third, only three time points were involved in this study. If more time points could be included, a more insightful understanding on the psychosocial development of Chinese adolescents would be developed.

Acknowledgement The Project P.A.T.H.S. and preparation for this paper were financially supported by the Hong Kong Jockey Club Charities Trust. The literature review and part of the analyses are based on the doctoral thesis of the second author. The authorship is equally shared between the two authors.

References

Barber, B. K. (1996). Parental psychological control: Revisiting a neglected construct. *Child Development, 67*(6), 3296–3319.
Barber, B. K. (2002). *Intrusive parenting: How psychological control affects children and adolescents.* Washington, DC: American Psychological Association.
Barber, B. K., & Harmon, E. L. (2002). Violating the self: Parental psychological control of early adolescents and adolescents. In B. K. Barber (Ed.), *Intrusive parenting: How psychological control affects children and adolescents* (pp. 15–52). Washington, DC: American Psychological Association Press.
Barber, B. K., Olsen, J. E., & Shagle, S. C. (1994). Associations between parental psychological and behavioral control and youth internalized and externalized behaviors. *Child Development, 65*(4), 1120–1136.
Barker, J. C., & Hunt, G. (2006). Representations of family: A review of the alcohol and drug literature. *International Journal of Drug Policy, 15*(5–6), 347–356.
Bean, R. A., Barber, B. K., & Crane, D. R. (2006). Parental support, behavioral control, and psychological among African American youth: The relationships to academic grades, delinquency, and depression. *Journal of Families Issues, 27*(10), 1335–1355.
Bean, R. A., Bush, K. R., McKenry, P. C., & Wilson, S. M. (2003). The impact of parental support, behavioral control, and psychological control on the academic achievement and self-esteem of African American and European American adolescents. *Journal of Adolescent Research, 18*(5), 523–541.
Booth, C. L., Rose-Krasnor, L., McKinnon, J., & Rubin, K. H. (1994). Predicting social adjustment in middle childhood: The role of preschool attachment security and maternal style. *Social Development, 3*(3), 189–204.
Borowsky, I. W., Ireland, M., & Resnick, M. D. (2001). Adolescent suicide attempts: Risks and protectors. *Pediatrics, 107*(3), 485–493.
Bowen, M. (1976). Theory in the practice of psychotherapy. In P. J. Guerin Jr. (Ed.), *Family therapy: Theory and practice* (pp. 42–90). New York: Gamer Press.
Bowen, M. (1991). Alcoholism as viewed through family systems theory and family psychotherapy. *Family Dynamics Addiction Quarterly, 1*(1), 94–102.
Bradford, K., Barber, B. K., Olsen, J. A., Maughan, S. L., Erickson, L. D., Ward, D., et al. (2003). A multi-national study of interparental conflict, parenting, and adolescent functioning: South

Africa, Bangladesh, China, India, Bosnia, Germany, Palestine, Colombia, and the United States. *Marriage & Family Review, 35*(3–4), 107–137.

Brody, G. H., & Forehand, R. (1993). Prospective associations among family form, family processes, and adolescents' alcohol and drug use. *Behaviour Research and Therapy, 31*(6), 587–593.

Bronfenbrenner, U. (1988). Interacting systems in human development. Research paradigms: Present and future. In N. Bolger, A. Caspi, G. Downey, & M. Morrehouse (Eds.), *Persons in context: Development processes* (pp. 25–49). Cambridge, UK: Cambridge University Press.

Burt, S. A., McGue, M., Iacono, W. G., & Krueger, R. F. (2006). Differential parent-child relationships and adolescent externalizing symptoms: Cross-lagged analyses within a monozygotic twin differences design. *Developmental Psychology, 42*(6), 1289–1298.

Chassin, L., Pillow, D. R., Curran, P. J., Molina, B. S. G., & Barrera, M., Jr. (1993). Relation of parental alcoholism to early adolescent substance abuse use: A test of three mediating mechanisms. *Journal of Abnormal Psychology, 102*(1), 3–19.

Coates, D. L., & Lewis, M. (1984). Early mother-infant interaction and infant cognitive status as predictors of school performance and cognitive behavior in six-year-olds. *Child Development, 55*(4), 1219–1230.

Consoli, A., Peyre, H., Speranza, M., Hassler, C., Falissard, B., Touchette, E., et al. (2013). Suicidal behaviors in depressed adolescents: Role of perceived relationships in the family. *Child and Adolescent Psychiatry and Mental Health, 7*(1), 8–20.

Crouter, A. C., & Head, M. R. (2002). Parental monitoring and knowledge of children. In M. H. Bornstein (Ed.), *Handbook of parenting* (Vol. 3, pp. 461–483). Mahwah, NJ: Erlbaum.

Crowell, S. E., Beauchaine, T. P., McCauley, E., Smith, C. J., Vasilev, C. A., & Stevens, A. L. (2008). Parent-child interactions, peripheral serotonin, and self-inflicted injury in adolescents. *Journal of Consulting and Clinical Psychology, 76*(1), 15–21.

Dishion, T. J., & Loeber, R. (1985). Adolescents marijuana and alcohol use: The role of parents and peers revisited. *American Journal of Drug and Alcohol Abuse, 11*(1–2), 11–25.

Eccles, J. S., Early, D., Frasier, K., Belansky, E., & McCarthy, K. (1997). The relation of connection, regulation, and support for autonomy to adolescents' functioning. *Journal of Adolescent Research, 12*(2), 263–286.

Fletcher, A. C., Steinberg, L., & Williams-Wheeler, M. (2004). Parental influences on adolescent problem behavior: Revisiting Stattin and Kerr. *Child Development, 75*(3), 781–796.

Fok, H. K., & Shek, D. T. L. (2011). A methodological critique of parenting research in Hong Kong. *International Journal of Adolescent Medicine and Health, 23*(2), 93–99.

Gamambos, N. L., Barker, E. T., & Almeida, D. M. (2003). Parents do matter: Trajectories of change in externalizing and internalizing problems in early adolescence. *Child Development, 74*(2), 578–594.

Gould, M. S., Shaffer, D., Fisher, P., & Garfinkel, R. (1998). Separation/divorce and child and adolescent completed suicide. *Journal of the American Academy of Child and Adolescent Psychiatry, 37*(2), 155–162.

Greenberg, M. T., Speltz, M. L., & DeKlyen, M. (1993). The role of attachment in the early development of disruptive behavior problems. *Development and Psychopathology, 5*(1–2), 191–213.

Harrington, R., Kerfoot, M., Dyer, E., McNiven, F., Gill, J., Harrington, V., et al. (1998). Randomized trial of a home-based family intervention for children who have deliberately poisoned themselves. *Journal of the American Academy of Child Adolescent Psychiatry, 37*(5), 512–518.

Hart, C. H., DeWolf, D. M., Wozniak, P., & Burts, D. C. (1992). Maternal and paternal disciplinary styles: Relations with preschoolers' playground behavioral orientations and peer status. *Child Development, 63*(4), 879–892.

Hepworth, D. H., Rooney, R. H., Rooney, G. D., & Strom-Gottfried, K. (2013). *Direct social work practice: Theory and skill* (9th ed.). Belmont, Canada: Brooks/Cole, Cengage Learning.

Hilt, L. M., Nock, M. K., Lloyd-Richardson, E. E., & Prinstein, M. J. (2008). Longitudinal study of nonsuicidal self-injury among young adolescents: Rates, correlates, and preliminary test of an interpersonal model. *Journal of Early Adolescence, 28*(3), 455–469.

Hsu, Y. F., Chen, P. F., & Lung, F. W. (2013). Parental bonding and personality characteristics of first episode intention to suicide or deliberate self-harm without a history of mental disorders. *BMC Public Health, 13*(1), 421–428.

Huang, X., Zhang, H., Li, M., Wang, J., Zhang, Y., & Tao, R. (2010). Mental health, personality, and parental rearing styles of adolescents with internet addiction disorder. *Cyberpsychology, Behavior, and Social Networking, 13*(4), 401–406.

Johnson, J. G., Cohen, P., Gould, M. S., Kasen, S., Brown, J., & Brook, J. S. (2002). Childhood adversities, interpersonal difficulties, and risk for suicide during late adolescent and early adulthood. *Archives of General Psychiatry, 59*(8), 741–749.

Klahr, A. M., McGue, M., Iacono, W. G., & Burt, S. A. (2010). The association between parent-child conflict and adolescent conduct problems over time: Results from a longitudinal adoption study. *Journal of Abnormal Psychology, 120*(1), 46–56.

Kochanska, G., Murray, K. T., & Harlan, E. T. (2000). Effortful control in early childhood: Continuity and change, antecedents, and implications for social development. *Developmental Psychology, 36*(2), 220–232.

Kwok-Lai, S. Y. C., & Shek, D. T. L. (2010). Personal and family correlates of suicidal ideation among Chinese adolescents in Hong Kong. *Social Indicators Research, 95*(3), 407–419.

Laird, R. D., Pettit, G. S., Bates, J. E., & Dodge, K. A. (2003). Parents' monitoring-relevant knowledge and adolescents' delinquent behavior: Evidence of correlated developmental changes and reciprocal influences. *Child Development, 74*(3), 752–768.

Ma, C. M. S., & Shek, D. T. L. (2013). Consumption of pornographic materials in early adolescents in Hong Kong. *Journal of Pediatric and Adolescent Gynecology, 26*, S18–S25.

Maccoby, E. E., & Martin, J. A. (1983). Socialization in the context of the family: Parent-child interaction. In E. Hetheringon (Ed.), *Handbook of child psychology* (Vol. 4, pp. 1–101). New York: Wiley.

Patterson, G. R., Capaldi, D., & Bank, L. (1991). An early starter model for predicting delinquency. In D. J. Pepler & K. H. Rubin (Eds.), *The development and treatment of childhood aggression* (pp. 139–168). Hillsdale, NJ: Erlbaum.

Petti, G. S., Laird, R. D., Dodge, K. A., Bates, J. E., & Criss, M. M. (2001). Antecedents and behavior-problem outcomes of parental monitoring and psychological control in early adolescence. *Child Development, 72*(2), 583–598.

Rogers, K. N., Buchanan, C. M., & Winchell, M. E. (2003). Psychological control during early adolescence: Links to adjustment in differing parent/adolescent dyads. *Journal of Early Adolescence, 23*(4), 349–383.

Shek, D. T. L. (1998). Adolescents' perceptions of paternal and maternal parenting styles in a Chinese context. *Journal of Psychology, 132*, 527–537.

Shek, D. T. L. (1999a). Parenting characteristics and adolescent psychological well-being: A longitudinal study in a Chinese context. *Genetic, Social, and General Psychology Monographs, 125*(1), 27–44.

Shek, D. T. L. (1999b). Perceptions of family functioning among Chinese parents and their adolescent children. *American Journal of Family Therapy, 27*(4), 303–314.

Shek, D. T. L. (2002). The relation of parental qualities to psychological well-being, school adjustment, and problem behavior in Chinese adolescents with economic disadvantage. *American Journal of Family Therapy, 30*(3), 215–230.

Shek, D. T. L. (2005). Perceived parental control processes, parent-child relational qualities, and psychological well-being in Chinese adolescents with and without economic disadvantage. *Journal of Genetic Psychology, 166*(2), 171–188.

Shek, D. T. L. (2006). Perceived parental behavioral control and psychological control in Chinese adolescents in Hong Kong. *American Journal of Family Therapy, 34*(2), 163–176.

Shek, D. T. L. (2007). Perceived parental control based on indigenous Chinese parental control concepts in adolescents in Hong Kong. *American Journal of Family Therapy, 35*(2), 123–137.

Shek, D. T. L. (2008). Perceived parental control processes, parent-child relational qualities, and adolescents psychological well-being in intact and nonintact families: Longitudinal findings in the Chinese culture. *Journal of Divorce & Remarriage, 49*(1/2), 171–189.

Shek, D. T. L. (2010). Parent-adolescent trust and parent-adolescent relationships in Chinese families in Hong Kong: Implications for parent education and family therapy. *American Journal of Family Therapy, 38*(3), 251–265.

Shek, D. T. L., & Ma, C. M. S. (2012). Program implementers' evaluation of the Project P.A.T.H.S.: Findings based on different datasets over time. *The Scientific World Journal.* Article ID 918437, 10 pages. doi:10.1100/2012/918437.

Shek, D. T. L., & Yu, L. (2012). Interim evaluation of the Project P.A.T.H.S.: Findings based on different datasets: *The Scientific World Journal*, Article ID 132826, 8 pages. doi:10.1100/2012/132826.

Silk, J. S., Morris, A. S., Kanaya, T., & Steinberg, L. (2003). Psychological control and autonomy granting: Opposite ends of a continuum or distinct constructs? *Journal of Research on Adolescence, 13*(1), 113–128.

Smetana, J. G., & Daddis, C. (2002). Domain-specific antecedents of parental psychological control and monitoring: The role of parenting beliefs and practices. *Child Development, 73*(2), 563–580.

Smith, C., & Krohn, M. D. (1995). Delinquency and family life among male adolescents: The role of ethnicity. *Journal of Youth and Adolescence, 24*(1), 69–93.

Soenens, B., Luyckx, K., Vansteenkiste, M., Duriez, B., & Goossens, L. (2008). Clarifying the link between perceived parental psychological control and adolescents' depressive feelings: A test of reciprocal versus unidirectional models of influence. *Merrill-Palmer Quarterly, 54*, 411–444.

Soenens, B., Vansteenkiste, M., Luyten, P., Duriez, B., & Goossens, L. (2005). Maladaptive perfectionistic self-representations: The meditational link between psychological control and adjustment. *Personality and Individual Differences, 38*(2), 487–498.

Steinberg, L. (1990). Autonomy, conflict, and harmony in the parent-adolescent relationship. In S. S. Feldman & G. R. Elliott (Eds.), *At the threshold: The developing adolescent* (pp. 255–276). Cambridge, MA: Harvard University Press.

Tomori, M. (1999). Suicide risk in high school students in Slovenia. *Crisis, 20*(1), 23–27.

Wang, B., Stanton, B., Li, X., Cottrell, L., Deveaux, L., & Kaljee, L. (2013). The influence of parental monitoring and parent-adolescent communication on Bahamian adolescent risk involvement: A three-year longitudinal examination. *Social Science & Medicine, 97*, 161–196.

Webb, L. (2002). Deliberate self-harm in adolescence: A systematic review of psychological and psychosocial factors. *Journal of Advanced Nursing, 38*(3), 235–244.

Windlin, B., & Kuntsche, E. (2012). Differences in the impact of the frequency and enjoyment of joint family activities on adolescent substance use and violence. *Journal of Health Psychology, 17*(4), 509–519.

Perceived Family Quality of Life, School Competence, and Academic Adjustment Among Early Adolescents in Hong Kong

Daniel T.L. Shek and Hildie Leung

Abstract Based on the responses of secondary school students recruited from 28 randomly selected schools in Hong Kong over 3 years, the relationships between perceived family functioning (i.e., family mutuality, harmony, and communication) and school competence as well as academic adjustment of young adolescents are examined in this chapter. Correlation analyses showed that family functioning dimensions at Time 1 were correlated with school competence and academic adjustment at Time 1 and Time 3. Multiple regression analyses showed that different dimensions of family functioning at Time 1 predicted different measures of school competence at Time 3. Similarly, family functioning measures at Time 1 predicted academic adjustment over time, but the perceived family functioning measures at Time 1 were unable to predict students' perceived stress regarding the new secondary school curriculum at Time 3. The theoretical and practical implications of the findings are discussed.

Keywords Family functioning • Family quality of life • School competence • Academic adjustment • Adolescents

Introduction

Ecological models on human development theorize how systems in the environment shape adaptive outcomes (Bronfenbrenner, 1986), with the family identified as a microsystem of the proximal process that impacts on adolescent development (Bronfenbrenner & Morris, 1998). The exploration of possible systemic influences of family has lead researchers to the following question, "do parents matter?" There are two views on this issue in the scientific literature. More than a decade ago, Harris (1998) introduced the provocative notion that regarding influences of children and adolescent behavior, parents in fact matter far less than other factors such as peers. On the other hand, both researchers and the general public are skeptical about her

D.T.L. Shek, Ph.D., B.B.S., S.B.S., J.P. (✉) • H. Leung, Ph.D.
Department of Applied Social Sciences, The Hong Kong Polytechnic University, Hunghom, Hong Kong
e-mail: daniel.shek@polyu.edu.hk

D.T.L. Shek et al. (eds.), *Chinese Adolescents in Hong Kong*, Quality of Life in Asia 5, DOI 10.1007/978-981-287-143-5_5

claim, given repeated evidence that suggests how family quality of life impact on adolescent psychological well-being and behavior (Kwan, 2008).

In family theories, family quality of life indexed by both systemic and dyadic family processes has been proposed to influence adolescent development. In particular, family functioning is an important factor shaping adolescent development. Family functioning refers to "the quality of family life at the systemic and dyadic levels and concerns wellness, competence, strengths, and weaknesses of a family" (Shek, 2002a, p. 497). To systematically investigate the impact of family functioning on developmental outcomes, various conceptual models have been proposed as organizational frameworks to assess family functioning. For instance, Barnhill (1979) isolated eight bipolar dimensions of family functioning; individuation-enmeshment, mutuality-isolation, flexibility-rigidity, stability-disorganization, clear-unclear/distorted perception, clear-unclear/distorted communication, role reciprocity-unclear roles/role conflict, and clear-diffuse/breached generational boundaries. Beavers and Hampson (1990) proposed the Beavers Systems Model which posited that families vary on the dimensions of competence and style. A competent family is characterized by the presence of egalitarian leadership, strong parental coalitions, clear boundaries, autonomy, intimacy and trust, and the capacity to accept and overcome differences. The style dimension is related to the degree of closeness in a family which includes attributes such as the meeting of dependency needs, openness to conflicts, physical closeness, expression of emotions, appearance to outsiders, and the management of assertion. The Circumplex Model (Olson, Russell, & Sprenkle, 1989) delineates family cohesion, adaptability, and communication as elements crucial to healthy family functioning. Lastly, the McMaster Family Functioning Model posits that healthy families should be able to successfully deal with maintenance, hazardous, and developmental tasks, with the use of effective problem-solving strategies, communication, clearly defined rules, affective involvement, and behavioral control (Epstein, Bishop, Ryan, Miller, & Keitner, 1993). While each model provides a unique perspective to understand family functioning and outlines different attributes essential for a healthy family, notions such as communication, cohesiveness, and the maintenance of a positive emotional environment are shared across different models.

Despite their important theoretical contributions to family literature, the aforementioned models have all been developed and empirically tested predominantly in Western contexts. Obviously, such investigations can be criticized as merely reflecting "Western investigators' assumptions and interpretations (i.e., the lens through which behavior is viewed) as well as Western ways of functioning (i.e., the incidence and pattern of behavior per se)" (Rothbaum, Rosen, Ujiie, & Uchida, 2002, p. 329), which may result in Western bias. This criticism is valid because studies showed that family functioning differed across cultures (e.g., Hohashi, Honda, & Kong, 2008; Shek, 2001b) and there are warnings that researchers and practitioners should be conscious of cultural variations in the application of family models and assessment tools (Shek, 1998).

Taking into consideration the influence of Chinese cultural values on family, the Chinese Family Assessment Instrument (C-FAI) was developed by Shek (2002b) as an indigenous Chinese family functioning measure to enable researchers and practitioners to perform objective assessment of family functioning in Chinese populations. Five basic dimensions of family functioning were proposed, with communication, mutuality, and harmony as dimensions related to the concept of "family interaction" and parental concern and parental control pertaining to "parenting." The validity and reliability of the C-FAI have been consistently demonstrated across studies (e.g., Shek, 2002b; Shek & Ma, 2010). Using the C-FAI, the aim of the present study is to investigate the influence of the three systemic family functioning dimensions as indicators of family quality of life on school competence and academic adjustment of early adolescents in Hong Kong.

Family Functioning, School Competence, and Academic Adjustment

Many studies have been conducted to identify school and classroom factors affecting student learning and academic outcomes. With the influence of the ecological approach, the scope of the related studies has broadened to encompass family as a contextual variable influencing educational adjustment and achievement of students (Marchant, Paulson, & Rothlisberg, 2001).

Family mutuality refers to a sense of emotional closeness or bonding between family members which is made possible when members have clearly defined identities (Barnhill, 1979). Families with high levels of mutuality are characterized with mutual support and the presence of love and concern among family members (Shek, 2002b). The importance of family mutuality to a child's development has been postulated based on the premise of Bowlby's attachment theory (1979) which asserts that children's self-esteem and sense of competence are influenced by their caregivers' responsiveness, availability, and accepting behaviors. With particular relevance to research on learning, it has been found that the degree of secure attachment in a parent-child relationship is positively correlated to students' academic learning (Kenny, Gallagher, Alvarez-Salvat, & Silsby, 2002). Secure children demonstrated better school adjustment in terms of scholastic, emotional, social, and behavioral adjustment (Granot & Mayseless, 2001). Adolescents who reported higher levels of family closeness experienced fewer academic problems. In addition, college students who reported higher levels of family closeness demonstrated more effective use of self-regulating learning where they were more motivated toward the attainment of learning goals and took more initiative in their learning process. Besides, students experiencing better family functioning were also better adjusted in school, such as having a sense of control over their life and future and feeling comfortable with other students (Lee, Hamman, & Lee, 2007).

The climate within one's family has also been proposed as an underlying mechanism through which attachment impacts on school adjustment, implicating on the importance of family harmony. Family harmony refers to how smoothly a family functions without friction. Harmonious family environments are those in which family members are able to get along well with each other, and parents are perceived to be caring toward the child (Trinidad, Chou, Unger, Johnson, & Li, 2003). Family climate has been operationalized differently across studies. For instance, Kurdek, Fine, and Sinclair (1995) used dimensions of parental supervision (levels of control and monitoring), acceptance (levels of warmth and support), autonomy granting (degree to which children are allowed to make decisions), and conflict (fighting and discord), which were found to be associated with higher levels of academic performance and lower instances of disruptive behaviors at school. Similarly, in a longitudinal study investigating the effects of family environment on early adolescents' school adjustment, Dubois, Eitel, and Felner (1994) found family climate (including dimensions such as expressiveness, conflict, active-recreational orientation, and control) related to reduced absences and higher grades at school, as well as higher levels of academic self-concept. By the same token, family disharmony characterized by high levels of parental and parent-child conflicts had negative outcomes on children's development (Zhou, King, & Chassin, 2006). Specifically, parent-child conflict was shown to have negative impact on adolescent mental health, problem behavior, and school adjustment (Shek, 1997a).

Communication is a dimension that has been included in most systems models as essential to healthy family functioning. Parent-child communication becomes increasingly important during adolescence. Communication has been identified as a protective factor in the family context for healthy adolescent development. Adolescents from families with better communication had higher self-esteem, were more socially competent, more likely to engage in health-promoting behaviors, and experienced less internalizing and externalizing problems (Youngblade et al., 2007). Adolescents with parents who had more discussions with them about their career plans and were more willing to listen to their thoughts had higher academic achievement (Hsu, Zhang, Kwok, Li, & Ju, 2011). Research has also shown that parents who communicated their expectations for academic performance and behavior in schools and inspired their children through reflection-enhancing communication have children who were more adaptive to transitions to school (Taylor, Clayton, & Rowley, 2004).

A survey of the literature on family functioning, school competence, and academic adjustment in adolescents shows that while the majority of studies have been conducted in the West, few studies have been conducted in an Asian context. This is surprising given the collectivistic orientations and value for harmony as well as absence of conflicts in the Chinese culture (Shek, 2001b). Furthermore, most studies investigating the link between family functioning and academic adjustment have operationalized academic adjustment in terms of academic performance (i.e., grades obtained in different subjects, scores on nationwide examinations) or social adjustment (e.g., relationships with peers, disruptive behaviors). Very few research studies have examined how family functioning affects both scholastic performance and academic adjustment of adolescents.

The New Senior Secondary School Curriculum in Hong Kong

As a result of globalization, educational reforms have been initiated in many countries to nurture students to better suit the changing needs of the economy and improve competitiveness. Hong Kong is of no exception. The traditional 9-year (primary 1–6, secondary 1–3) compulsory education system in Hong Kong has been criticized for its over-selectivity and outdated pedagogical orientations. Therefore, starting from 2009/2010 school year, the Hong Kong Government implemented a new senior secondary education system, coined as the "334" academic structure, which represents 3 years of junior secondary education (secondary 1–3), 3 years of senior secondary education (secondary 4–6), and 4 years of university education. It is believed that the reform will enable better alignment with the education systems in China, North America, and Australia to allow graduates to have more vocational or occupational mobility. In addition, the old education system has also been criticized for the fact that only a third of students are able to successfully proceed to pursue the two final years of secondary school education and that students have to take two public examinations – the Hong Kong Certificate of Education Examination (HKCEE) after secondary 5 and the Hong Kong Advanced Level Examination (HKALE) after secondary 7 prior to entering a university.

Under the new secondary school system, students will only have to sit for one public examination – the Hong Kong Diploma of Secondary Education (HKDSE) – with the primary purpose to reduce the stress of the students to sit for two public examinations. In addition, under the "334" curriculum, all students will be given the opportunity to progress to senior secondary education (i.e., students are no longer required to sit for a junior secondary school examination). Furthermore, the subjects that students are required to take under the new curriculum are carefully designed with the objectives of enhancing students' awareness of contemporary issues, broadening their knowledge base, and to strengthen their critical thinking skills, as fundamentals for lifelong learning (Chan & Luk, 2013).

The new curriculum, however, is not without criticisms. Some critics assert that with the abolishment of the first public examination as a filter, there is the danger of "putting all eggs in one basket" and that students may lack experience in taking public examinations. In addition, under the new curriculum, students are required to take Liberal Studies as a core subject, which was previously an elective subject. This new arrangement poses difficulties for students "who have not been previously taught or assessed by this method (inquiry-based learning and teaching approach) … to adapt… This is not something they can get accustomed to easily, it may take years to learn and adapt, from the traditional spoon-fed learning approach" (Chan & Luk, 2013, p. 59). Given these observations, it is important to understand the factors that would impact on the implementation of the education reform or how students adapt and adjust to the changes, so as to better inform the government and practitioners of areas to deploy their resources to. In Cheung and Wong's (2012) recent investigation of the key factors impacting on the effectiveness of the implementation of the new education system, five levels of factors were identified, including external, school, teacher, students, parent, and other factors. Particularly, students' attitude, family background, and parents' understanding and attitude were found critical to implementation. While Cheung and Wong's study provides an encompassing list of factors on different levels that impact on the implementation of the "334" curriculum, the underlying processes have not been examined. Therefore, the focus of the present study lies on the family and parental level and attempted to examine how family quality of life (family mutuality, harmony, and communication) influences young adolescents' adjustment to the new secondary school curriculum in Hong Kong.

The Present Study

Several gaps have been identified in existing research on family functioning and academic adjustment in adolescents. Based on a comprehensive review of studies on family functioning, Bronfenbrenner (1986) concluded that "the body of research reviewed in these pages is curiously one-sided, for its predominant focus on the ecologies of family disorganization and developmental disarray" (p. 738). This trend seems to have persisted over the years as reviewed in the observation of Rask, Âstedt-Kurki, Paavilainen, and Laippala (2003) that "…research about the relationship between adolescent well-being and family functioning have mostly focused on ill-being in the family, …(and) youth problems, conflicts, low self-esteem, and child abuse or substance abuse of parents or adolescents" (p. 129). Hence, there is a call for the need to investigate how healthy family functioning can serve as a protective factor to enable positive youth development, especially in terms of school competence and academic adjustment. With particular reference to the new "334" curriculum in Hong Kong, most standing studies have been conducted to investigate the challenges faced by teachers in the implementation of the new curriculum and their impact on teaching effectiveness (e.g., Cheung & Wong, 2012). To date, no systematic studies have been conducted to investigate the impact of family functioning on students' adjustment to the new academic structure. Against the reformative background of the education system in Hong Kong and the dynamic flux of the Hong Kong family, the present study was conducted with a large representative sample of junior secondary school students in Hong Kong to investigate whether perceived family functioning as a measure of family quality of life (i.e., family mutuality, family harmony, and family communication) predicted adolescents' perceived levels of school competence and academic adjustment. Besides, the profiles of school competence and academic adjustment at different time points were examined.

Method

Participants

Project P.A.T.H.S. (Positive Adolescent Training through Holistic Social Programs) is a pioneering positive youth development program attempting to promote holistic development among adolescents in Hong Kong. Participants in the current study

Table 1 Socio-demographic profiles of respondents at Time 3

Gender	*N*	%
Male	2,185	53.7
Female	1,885	46.3
Place of Birth		
Hong Kong	3,195	79.4
Mainland	762	18.9
Others	68	1.7
Father education		
Primary education or below	455	17.6
Secondary education	1,656	63.9
Tertiary education or above	481	18.6
Mother education		
Primary education or below	497	19.9
Secondary education	1,432	57.2
Tertiary education or above	573	22.9

were recruited from 28 participating schools randomly selected from all secondary schools in Hong Kong to join a longitudinal study. The sampling frame of the study was all government and aided schools in Hong Kong. As the questionnaire was administered in Chinese, international schools and non-Chinese speaking schools were excluded from the present investigation. The present study was part of a large-scale longitudinal research project investigating youth development and family functioning of early adolescents in Hong Kong. The first wave (Time 1) of the study was conducted during the 2009–2010 academic year, with 3,325 secondary 1 (equivalent to Grade 7) students (mean age = 12.59, SD = .74 years). The second wave (Time 2) and third wave (Time 3) of data were collected in 2010–2011 and 2011–2012 academic years, respectively. The present chapter reports data from both Time 1 and Time 3 of the longitudinal study. The third wave of data was collected during the 2011–2012 academic year, with 4,106 secondary 3 (Grade 9) students (mean age = 14.65, SD = .80 years). Based on Time 3 data, majority of the respondents were locals born in Hong Kong (79.4 %), while the others were from Mainland China (18.9 %) or other countries (1.7 %). Particularly, students from Mainland China have resided in Hong Kong for a mean of 8.74 years (SD = 3.90 years). Regarding the duration of parents' stay in Hong Kong, in the past 30 days, students reported a mean of 24.6 days (SD = 10.4 days) for their fathers' stay and a mean of 28.1 days (SD = 6.7 days) for their mothers' stay. Additional demographic information of the participants is shown in Table 1.

Procedures

Data were collected at schools in a classroom setting by trained research staff and/or school teachers with advance briefings. All participants responded en masse to the instrument scales in the questionnaire in a self-administration format. Prior to data collection, ethical approval was obtained from the Hong Kong Polytechnic University, as well as parental and school consent. At the time of data collection, student consent was also sought. Anonymity and confidentiality were emphasized during the administration process, and participants were given sufficient time to complete the questionnaire.

Instruments

The questionnaire distributed comprises items assessing adolescents' demographic information, family environment (e.g., parental control and family functioning), life satisfaction, positive youth development, as well as problem behaviors. The details of the instruments employed can be seen in Yu and Shek (2013) and Ma and Shek (2013). Instruments related to the variables of investigation in the current study are detailed below.

Assessment of Family Functioning

Adolescents' perceived family functioning was assessed by a simplified version of the Chinese Family Assessment Instrument (C-FAI) developed by the first author. The scale includes nine items from three subscales assessing family mutuality, i.e., the presence of support, love, and concern among family members (CFAIM, 3 items; α=.89); family harmony, i.e., the absence of conflicting behaviors in the family (CFAIC, 3 items; α=.79); and family communication, i.e., the frequency and nature of communication within an individual's family (CFAICOM, 3 items; α=.81). Respondents were asked to indicate on a 5-point Likert scale, ranging from 1 (very dissimilar) to 5 (very similar) the extent to which the items resembled their current family situation. A higher score for each subscale indicated a higher level of positive family functioning. A detailed description of the scale and its psychometric properties including validity and reliability analyses is reported in Shek and Ma's (2010) study.

School Competence

Students' school competence was measured using three items. The first item assessed students' perception of his/her academic performance in comparison with his/her fellow schoolmates. Respondents were asked to indicate on a 5-point Likert scale, ranging from 1 (very bad) to 5 (very good) in terms of their relative academic performance. The second item assessed students' satisfaction with his/her academic performance using a 5-point Likert scale ranging from 1 (very dissatisfied) to 5 (very satisfied). The third item assessed students' perceived level of conduct at school using a 5-point Likert scale ranging from 1 (very bad) to 5 (very good). For each of the items, a lower-scale score indicates a lower level of school competence.

Academic Adjustment

Students' academic adjustment was assessed using 3 items. The first item assessed students confidence in coping with the demands of the new curriculum. Respondents were asked to indicate on a 4-point Likert scale, ranging from 1 (not confident at all) to 4 (very confident) the extent that best represented their confidence level. A higher score indicates a higher level of school adjustment. The second item assessed students level of stress when facing the new curriculum. The final item assessed students level of stress regarding their studies in general, both using a 4-point Likert scale, ranging from 1 (not at all) to 4 (very). A lower-scale score on the two items indicated higher school adjustment in this study.

Results

Students' responses to the school competence and academic adjustment items are presented in Table 2. Several observations can be drawn from data reported in Table 2. Concerning school competence, majority of students reported their academic performance to be average as compared with their fellow classmates (53.4 % at Time 1; 50.8 % at Time 3), were generally satisfied with their own academic performance (40.3 % at Time 1; 37.9 % at Time 3), and perceived their school conduct to be average as well (46.0 % at Time 1; 48.8 % at Time 3). A worrying phenomenon, however, was observed as evidenced by the decreasing trend from Time 1 to Time 3 in positive responses reported for both relative academic performance and level of satisfaction with one's academic performance. Fortunately, more students reported better school conduct across time. With regard to academic adjustment, generally speaking, more than half of the students (59.8 %) were confident in adjusting to the new curriculum. However, many of them experienced stress from the new curriculum (50.3 %) and their studies in general (45.0 %). Descriptive statistics on the key variables of the present study are reported in Table 3.

The Effect of Perceived Family Functioning on School Competence

Correlation analyses were conducted among perceived family functioning levels at Time 1 and perceived levels of school competence variables in Time 1 and Time 3, as reported in Table 4. Pearson correlations revealed that family functioning variables were positively correlated with all perceived school competence variables (ranging

Table 2 Frequencies and percentages of responses to school competence and academic adjustment items at Time 1 and Time 3

	Time 1							Time 3						
	1	2	3	4	5	Negative responses (1–2)	Positive responses (3–5)	1	2	3	4	5	Negative responses (1–2)	Positive responses (3–4)
School competence														
1. Academic performance compared with schoolmates	89 (3.3 %)	342 (12.8 %)	1,423 (53.4 %)	705 (26.4 %)	69 (2.6 %)	431 (16.2 %)	2,197 (82.4 %)	130 (4.9 %)	414 (15.5 %)	1,354 (50.8 %)	681 (25.5 %)	75 (2.8 %)	544 (20.4 %)	2,110 (79.1 %)
2. Level of satisfaction with own academic performance	206 (7.7 %)	672 (25.5 %)	1,076 (40.3 %)	594 (22.3 %)	72 (2.7 %)	878 (32.9 %)	1,742 (65.3 %)	326 (12.2 %)	848 (31.8 %)	1,011 (37.9 %)	404 (15.1 %)	64 (2.4 %)	1,174 (44.0 %)	1,479 (55.0 %)
3. Perceived levels of school conduct	32 (1.2 %)	133 (5.0 %)	1,227 (46.0 %)	989 (37.1 %)	227 (8.5 %)	165 (6.2 %)	2,443 (91.6 %)	33 (1.2 %)	131 (4.9 %)	1,302 (48.8 %)	990 (37.1 %)	190 (7.1 %)	164 (6.1 %)	2,482 (93.1 %)
Academic adjustment														
4. Confidence in adjusting to the new curriculum								126 (4.7 %)	938 (35.2 %)	1,465 (54.9 %)	129 (4.8 %)	–	1,064 (39.9 %)	1,594 (59.8 %)
5. Stress regarding the new curriculum								139 (5.2 %)	1,177 (44.1 %)	977 (36.6 %)	364 (13.6 %)	–	1,316 (49.3 %)	1,341 (50.3 %)
6. Stress regarding studies in general								126 (4.7 %)	1,329 (49.8 %)	915 (34.3 %)	285 (10.7 %)	–	1,455 (54.6 %)	1,200 (45.0 %)

Note: For items 1 and 3: *1* very bad, *2* worse than average, *3* average, *4* better than average, *5* very good; Item 2: *1* very dissatisfied, *2* dissatisfied, *3* average, *4* satisfied, *5* very satisfied; Item 4: *1* not confident at all, *2* not confident, *3* confident, *4* very confident; Item 5 and 6; *1* not at all, *2* slightly, *3* quite, *4* very

Table 3 Descriptive statistics of key variables at Time 1 and Time 3

	Mean (SD)	
	Time 1	Time 3
Family functioning		
Family mutuality	3.91 (.88)	3.88 (.84)
Family harmony	3.86 (.89)	3.77 (.90)
Family communication	3.52 (.99)	3.47 (.91)
School competence		
Academic performance compared with schoolmates	3.12 (.79)	3.06 (.85)
Level of satisfaction with own academic performance	2.87 (.94)	2.64 (.96)
Perceived levels of school conduct	3.48 (.77)	3.44 (.75)
Academic adjustment		
Confidence in adjusting to the new curriculum	–	2.60 (.66)
Stress regarding the new curriculum	–	2.59 (.79)
Stress regarding studies in general	–	2.51 (.75)

Table 4 Correlations among family functioning at Time 1 and perceived levels of school competence and academic adjustment variables at Time 1 and Time 3

	Time 1		
	Family mutuality	Family harmony	Family communication
Time 1			
School competence			
Academic performance compared with schoolmates	.17**	.14**	.17**
Level of satisfaction with own academic performance	.18**	.16**	.20**
Perceived levels of school conduct	.21**	.17**	.19**
Time 3			
School competence			
Academic performance compared with schoolmates	.13**	.11**	.14**
Level of satisfaction with own academic performance	.15**	.12**	.16**
Perceived levels of school conduct	.17**	.15**	.15**
Academic adjustment			
Confidence in adjusting to the new curriculum	.19**	.13**	.20**
Stress regarding the new curriculum	–.03	–.01	–.03
Stress regarding studies in general	–.06*	–.06*	–.08**

$^{**}P<.001$; $^{*}P<.01$

Table 5 Multiple regression analyses predicting students' perceived levels of school competence at Time 3 by family functioning at Time 1

	Predictors				
	Family mutuality	Family harmony	Family communication	Model	
	β^a	β^a	β^a	R	R^2
Academic performance compared with schoolmates	.06	.04	.07*	.15	.02
Level of satisfaction with own academic performance	.04	.06*	.10**	.17	.03
Perceived levels of school conduct	.10**	.07*	.03	.18	.03

[a]Standardized coefficients
$^{**}P<.001$; $^{*}P<.01$

from .11 to .20). In general, higher levels of perceived family functioning were associated with higher levels of perceived school competence among adolescents. In order to examine the relative impact that family mutuality, harmony, and communication have on adolescents' perceived school competence, multiple regression analyses were conducted with the three family functioning measures as predictor variables and the different measures of perceived school competence as criterion variables. Findings of the multiple regression analyses are presented in Table 5. The linear combination of perceived family mutuality, harmony, and communication significantly predicted students' perceived levels of academic performance as compared with their schoolmates ($F(3, 2509)=19.18$, $p<.001$), their levels of satisfaction with their own academic performance ($F(3, 2507)=23.92$, $p<.001$), as well as their perceived levels of school conduct ($F(3, 2500)=27.41$, $p<.001$). However, only family communication emerged as a significant predictor of students' perceptions of their own academic performance when compared with their fellow classmates. Family harmony and communication significantly predicted students' levels of prediction with their own school performance. Lastly, family mutuality and harmony significantly predicted students' perceived level of school conduct. Overall speaking, results across analyses suggest that favorable family functioning has positive impact on adolescents' perceived levels of school competence in terms of academic performance and conduct.

The Effect of Perceived Family Functioning on Academic Adjustment

Correlation analyses were conducted among family functioning and academic adjustment measures as presented in Table 4. All family functioning variables were significantly associated with the school adjustment variables, with the exception of students' reported levels of stress regarding the new curriculum. In order to investigate

Table 6 Multiple regression analyses predicting students' perceived levels of academic adjustment at Time 3 by family functioning at Time 1

	Predictors				
	Family mutuality	Family harmony	Family communication	Model	
	β^a	β^a	β^a	R	R^2
Confidence in adjusting to the new curriculum	.09**	.00	.13***	.21	.04
Stress regarding the new curriculum	−.03	.01	−.02	.04	.00
Stress regarding studies in general	.00	−.03	−.07*	.08	.01

[a]Standardized coefficients
****P*<.001; ***P*<.01; **P*<.05

the differential impact of perceived family functioning factors on early adolescents' school adjustment in Hong Kong, three multiple regression analyses were subsequently conducted, using perceived family mutuality, family harmony, and family communication as the predictor variables and students' confidence in adjusting to the new curriculum, students' level of stress regarding the new curriculum, and their stress regarding their studies in general as three dependent variables, respectively. Table 6 presents multiple regression analyses results. The linear combination of perceived family mutuality, harmony, and communication significantly predicted students' confidence levels in adjusting to the new curriculum ($F(3, 2512) = 37.49$, $p < .001$) and their stress levels toward their studies in general ($F(3, 2510) = 5.91$, $p < .01$). Particularly, family mutuality and communication significantly predicted students' confidence in adjusting to the new curriculum. Family communication was also predictive of students' stress regarding their studies. These findings are consistent with previous studies showing the positive impact of healthy family functioning on students' academic adjustment. However, all three of the perceived family functioning variables were unable to predict students' stress regarding the new curriculum ($F(3, 2511) = 1.18$, nonsignificant).

Discussion

The aims of the study are to investigate the influence of perceived levels of family functioning on school competence and academic adjustment among young adolescents in Hong Kong and examine patterns of school competence and academic adjustment at different time points. Several observations can be drawn from the findings. Regarding students' school competence, the profiles showed that most of them were average in terms of academic performance when compared with their classmates and were also relatively satisfied with their academic performances. However, when examining the changes across time, a worrying situation was observed, where there was a declining trend in students' perceived relative academic performance, as well as their levels of satisfaction toward their scholastic performance.

Many studies have been conducted to investigate factors that influence Hong Kong adolescents' academic performance. For instance, recently, Mak, Lee, Ho, Lo, and Lam (2012) found that only 27.4 % of adolescents have more than 8 h of sleep on school-day nights and 21.5 % of students reported symptoms of insomnia. Poor academic performance was associated with sleep debt and insomnia (Mak et al., 2012). Furthermore, Shek, Ma, and Sun (2011) also reported on adolescent developmental problems in Hong Kong, such as Internet addiction and materialistic orientations; both of which have been previously identified as factors that adversely impact on students' academic outcomes and learning motivation (Ku, Dittmar, & Banerjee, 2012; Kubey, Lavin, & Barrows, 2001). Our results call for more research to further explore factors contributing to this phenomenon and for teachers and parents to pay closer attention to problems that students may be facing and to consider their psychological well-being, particularly in the academic domain. On a positive note, across time, students reported higher levels of school conduct.

Regarding academic adjustment, responses to the items reveal that majority of the students were confident in adjusting to the new secondary school curriculum. However, a large proportion of them remained quite stressed about the new curriculum and their studies. This is not surprising given Chinese's emphasis on attaining high academic achievements. The stress patterns reported by students in the present study should not be overlooked, since test anxiety, academic self-concept, and adolescents' perceived parental dissatisfaction with their academic performance have been found to be associated with suicide ideation among adolescents in Hong Kong, underscoring the important role of both academic and family climate in adolescents' well-being (Lee, Wong, Chow, & McBride-Chang, 2006).

Concerning the impact of family functioning on school competence and academic adjustment, family mutuality was predictive of adolescents' perceived levels of school conduct and their confidence in adjusting to the new secondary school curriculum. Results are consistent with studies conducted in the West which found family closeness to be fundamental to the well-being of children and college students' ability to adjust to their schools (Lee, Hamman, & Lee, 2007). Adolescents who reported warm relationships with their parents exhibited fewer behavioral problems and were less likely to be adversely influenced by deviant peers (Crosnoe, Erickson, & Dornbusch, 2002). In addition, family closeness was also related to fewer academic problems and higher levels of self-esteem in adolescents (Youngblade et al., 2007). Students from families with parents who were more accepting and involving had improved academic self-conceptions and declined school misconduct over time (Steinberg, Lamborn, Darling, Mounts, & Dornbusch, 1994). The impact of family closeness on adolescent development is well documented and supported in the current study. Unfortunately, however, researchers report declines in perceived feelings of family support, closeness, and intimacy by adolescents and in observed assessments of family warmth and cohesion during adolescence (Conger & Ge, 1999; Shek, Leung, & Lu, 2013). The findings suggest that family quality of life as a protective factor may decline in the adolescent years.

Family harmony also had positive impact on both adolescents' levels of satisfaction with their academic performance and their school conduct. In general, our findings echo previous research suggesting a positive linkage between family harmony and school competence and conduct in adolescents (Shek, 1997b, 2002b). Family conflicts were predictive of child adjustment and problem behaviors (David, Steele, Forehand, & Armistead, 1996); children from conflictual homes experience a sense of disrupted family relationships which results in higher levels of conduct problems, aggression, and antisocial behaviors (Formoso, Gonzales, & Aiken, 2000). Surprisingly, however, family harmony did not affect adolescents' perceived level of academic achievement relative to their fellow classmates. At this point, one must be cautioned that students' satisfaction with their academic performance and their actual academic achievement are in essence, two distinct concepts. Educational satisfaction is defined as the enjoyment of one's role or experiences as a student. It takes on an affective nature and includes personal appraisals in relation to motivation, achievement goals, and aspirations (Lent, Singley, Sheu, Schmidt, & Schmidt, 2007). On the other hand, academic outcomes are more objective and often operationalized in terms of actual scores obtained in formal assessments within the classroom setting. Thus, the present findings suggest that family harmony functions on an affective and cognitive level where positive emotions derived from a harmonious family impact on students' appraisals in relation to the school context. Indeed, studies have shown that students from harmonious families with parents who provide encouragement and provide appropriate levels of autonomy and support to their children were more likely to seek challenging tasks, demonstrate persistence when confronted with challenges at school, experience more satisfaction with their schoolwork, and reported more favorable attitudes toward school (Gonzalez-DeHass, Willems, & Holbein, 2005). Other external factors such as teachers, peers, school, or classroom environment may play a relatively greater role in determining adolescents' actual academic achievement as opposed to family functioning, which warrants more examination. Future studies should investigate the relations between family harmony, students' satisfaction toward their academic performances, and their academic outcomes to shed light on the inter-level intricacies. Theoretically, the present findings underscore the additive value of relationship harmony to the development of self-esteem and life satisfaction for individuals in collectivistic cultures like Hong Kong (Kwan, Bond, & Singelis, 1997) with empirical evidence from adolescents. This adds also to the greater picture given that students' perceptions of their academic abilities and overall satisfaction with school contribute greatly to their global life satisfaction (Suldo, Riley, & Shaffer, 2006).

Another interesting finding yielded from the present study is the positive impact of family communication on both school competence and academic adjustment. Students from families with better communication reported higher levels of academic performance, levels of satisfaction with their schoolwork, confidence in adjusting to the new curriculum, as well as lower levels of stress regarding their studies in general. There are also findings suggesting that parent-adolescent communication is positively related to the psychological well-being of adolescents (e.g., Raja, McGee, & Stanton, 1992; Schrodt, Ledbetter, & Ohrt, 2007).

The above findings may seem to be counterintuitive in an Asian context given that individuals from collectivistic cultures often engage in behaviors aimed at enhancing and saving "face" (*mianzi*) (Bond & Hwang, 1986). It is not uncommon for Asians to avoid disclosing distressful information or emotional problems that may potentially embarrass oneself or evoke feelings of shame or negative emotions (Ow & Katz, 1999), which suggest that more family communication may not necessarily be associated with positive developmental or psychological outcomes in a collectivistic culture like Hong Kong. However, our findings are consistent with studies from the West in demonstrating the importance of family communication in improving academic outcomes in adolescents. As Hong Kong is relatively westernized, it is not surprising to find that there is a positive relationship between family communication and adolescent developmental outcomes.

Nevertheless, family communication was not associated with students' perceived level of school conduct or their stress toward the new secondary school curriculum in the present study. Several reasons may account for these findings. First, the nature of the communication itself determines its influence on adolescents' behaviors. For instance, studies on the impact of family communication on adolescents' smoking and drinking behaviors show that communication can be categorized as being "hard" (i.e., directive, including sanctions for substance use or explicitly instructing adolescents not to engage in tobacco or drug use), "soft" (i.e., communicating about the harms and consequences of substance use), or "cautionary" (i.e., discussion about media portrayals). Research shows that not all contents of family communication exert positive influences on adolescents' behaviors: parents who engaged in directive and demanding conversations on substance use actually escalated adolescents' substance use. Some adolescents deliberately engage in behaviors that they were told not to do so (Ennett, Bauman, Foshee, Pemberton, & Hicks, 2001). Furthermore, parents in Hong Kong place great value on conduct in their child's behaviors. Parents described an "ideal child" to be one who possesses good character, obeys the law, is not acquainted with undesirable peers, and is not naughty (Shek & Chan, 1999). This is in line with the traditional Chinese family where children are to stay out of trouble and avoid engaging in behaviors that may bring shame and dishonor to the family (Lim & Lim, 2004). Given the sensitivity of the issue, respondents may have refrained from discussing about their school conduct with their parents explaining the nonsignificant associations.

The present findings have implications to future research on family studies. Regarding the relation between family communication and school competence and academic adjustment, the yielded results suggest a complex relation, where family communication may not necessarily be positively related to all aspects of adolescent academic outcomes. Hence, it is more important to have knowledge on what and how information should be communicated between the parent-child dyad in order to gain the expected protective effects of family functioning. As such, future studies should investigate the specific factors underlying the parent-child communication process, the content of discourses, as well as their psychological mediators. This is in line with the comments of Ennett et al. (2001) that "more attention to the nature and measurement of communication is warranted … It is important to conceptualize communication as a multidimensional process and to measure other aspects of communication in addition to occurrence" (p. 49).

Against the educational reformation background of the Hong Kong secondary school curriculum, one of the goals of the present study was to investigate the impact of perceived family functioning on adolescents' adjustment to the new "334" curriculum. Results suggest that perceived family functioning have little impact on adolescents' adjustment. Particularly, neither family mutuality, harmony, nor communication predicted adolescents' stress regarding the new curriculum. Some explanations may account for the phenomenon. In order for family functioning to exert positive influences on adolescents' academic outcomes, it is crucial that parents have sufficient information or knowledge of their children's academic progress, curriculum rationales, learning goals, etc. It may well be the fact that parents, alike with their children, are also adjusting to and unsure of the challenges accompanied with the transition. Repeated studies have shown the importance of parent-school partnership and communication for student learning (Eccles & Harold, 1993). The second explanation is that the outcome variable was measured at secondary 3, the last year of the junior secondary school years. As students still had not entered the senior secondary school years, they might not really feel the stress involved. The third explanation is that as academic excellence is strongly emphasized in the Chinese culture, academic stress might still be high even when a family functions well, hence leading to the nonsignificant findings observed. Obviously, future studies are needed to further explore these possibilities.

Theoretically, the present study underscores the importance of family quality of life in shaping adolescent development. Besides the findings that family processes influence individual well-being in Chinese adolescents (e.g., Shek, 2001a, 2005), the present findings show that the influence extends to the academic domain. In future, research work should be conducted to clarify the processes mediating or moderating the impact of the family on adolescent development. As the development of evidence-based family life education programs in Hong Kong is still at its infancy (Shek, 2014), there is a need to develop evidence-based family life education programs that can promote the quality of family life in Hong Kong.

Although the present study is pioneer in nature, the present investigation has several methodological limitations. First, although the patterns of data yielded in this study are generally consistent with those in the West demonstrating the importance of a healthy family functioning to adolescent development, the sample of this study was confined to Hong Kong adolescents. As such, further replications in other Chinese communities are needed before generalizations can be made to the entire Asian population. Second, as the data collected on family functioning, school competence, and academic adjustment were derived from self-reports, the inclusion of more diverse sources of information from parents, teachers, and peers would create a fuller picture about the problem area. Lastly, as the current study adopted a quantitative approach, it would be interesting for future studies to include qualitative methodologies such as focus groups, in-depth interviews, and discourse analyses to gain a more comprehensive understanding of the issue.

Despite the above limitations, the present study contributes to family functioning literature by elucidating the impact of family functioning on adolescent academic outcomes from an Asian context, which is infrequent in existing research. This is especially important given the traditional Confucian teachings' emphasis on family relations, harmony, and communication which differs from that of the West. In addition, findings with regard to adolescents' adjustment to the new secondary school curriculum in Hong Kong also shed light on the issue worldwide, as many countries are also undergoing educational reforms in meeting the needs of globalization. Evidence reported in the current chapter offers an affirmative answer to the question "do parents matter?" and provides meaningful directions for future research and practice in the family and adolescent development arena.

Acknowledgment The preparation for this paper and the Project P.A.T.H.S. were financially supported by The Hong Kong Jockey Club Charities Trust.

References

Barnhill, L. R. (1979). Healthy family systems. *Family Coordinator, 28*(1), 94–100.
Beavers, W. R., & Hampson, R. B. (1990). *Successful families: Assessment and intervention.* New York: Norton.
Bond, M. H., & Hwang, K. K. (1986). The social psychology of Chinese people. In M. H. Bond (Ed.), *The psychology of the Chinese people* (pp. 213–266). Hong Kong: Oxford University Press.
Bowlby, J. (1979). *The making and breaking of affectional bonds.* London: Tavistock.
Bronfenbrenner, U. (1986). Ecology of the family as a context for human development: Research perspectives. *Developmental Psychology, 22*(6), 723–742.
Bronfenbrenner, U., & Morris, P. A. (1998). The ecology of developmental processes. In W. Damon & R. M. Lerner (Eds.), *Handbook of child psychology: Vol. 1: Theoretical models of human development* (5th ed., pp. 993–1028). Hoboken, NJ: Wiley.
Chan, C. K., & Luk, L. Y. (2013). Faculty Perspectives on the "3+3+4" Curriculum reform in Hong Kong: A case study. *International Education Studies, 6*(4), 56–66.
Cheung, A. C. K., & Wong, P. M. (2012). Factors affecting the implementation of curriculum reform in Hong Kong: Key findings from a large-scale survey study. *International Journal of Education Management, 26*(1), 39–54.
Conger, R. D., & Ge, X. (1999). Conflict and cohesion in parent–adolescent relations: Changes in emotional expression from early to midadolescence. In M. J. Cox & J. Brooks-Gunn (Eds.), *Conflict and cohesion in families: Causes and consequences* (The advances in family research series, pp. 181–206). Mahwah, NJ: Lawrence Erlbaum Associates.
Crosnoe, R., Erickson, K. G., & Dornbusch, S. M. (2002). Protective functions of family relationships and school factors on the deviant behavior of adolescent boys and girls reducing the impact of risky friendships. *Youth & Society, 33*(4), 515–544.
David, C., Steele, R., Forehand, R., & Armistead, L. (1996). The role of family conflict and marital conflict in adolescent functioning. *Journal of Family Violence, 11*(1), 81–91.
DuBois, D. L., Eitel, S. K., & Felner, R. D. (1994). Effects of family environment and parent-child relationships on school adjustment during the transition to early adolescence. *Journal of Marriage and the Family, 56*(2), 405–414.
Eccles, J., & Harold, R. (1993). Parent-school involvement during the early adolescent years. *The Teachers College Record, 94*(3), 568–587.
Ennett, S. T., Bauman, K. E., Foshee, V. A., Pemberton, M., & Hicks, K. A. (2001). Parent-child communication about adolescent tobacco and alcohol use: What do parents say and does it affect youth behavior? *Journal of Marriage and Family, 63*(1), 48–62.
Epstein, N. B., Bishop, D., Ryan, C., Miller, I., & Keitner, G. (1993). The McMaster model: View of healthy family functioning. In F. Walsh (Ed.), *Normal family processes* (pp. 138–160). New York: Guilford Press.

Formoso, D., Gonzales, N. A., & Aiken, L. S. (2000). Family conflict and children's internalizing and externalizing behavior: Protective factors. *American Journal of Community Psychology, 28*(2), 175–199.

Gonzalez-DeHass, A. R., Willems, P. P., & Holbein, M. F. D. (2005). Examining the relationship between parental involvement and student motivation. *Educational Psychology Review, 17*(2), 99–123.

Granot, D., & Mayseless, O. (2001). Attachment security and adjustment to school in middle childhood. *International Journal of Behavioral Development, 25*(6), 530–541.

Harris, J. R. (1998). *The nurture assumption: Why children turn out the way that they do*. New York: Free Press.

Hohashi, N., Honda, J., & Kong, S. K. (2008). Validity and reliability of the Chinese version of the Feetham Family Functioning Survey (FFFS). *Journal of Family Nursing, 14*(2), 201–223.

Hsu, H. Y., Zhang, D., Kwok, O. M., Li, Y., & Ju, S. (2011). Distinguishing the influences of father's and mother's involvement on adolescent academic achievement analyses of Taiwan education panel survey data. *The Journal of Early Adolescence, 31*(5), 694–713.

Kenny, M. E., Gallagher, L. A., Alvarez-Salvat, R., & Silsby, J. (2002). Sources of support and psychological distress among academically successful inner-city youth. *Adolescence, 37*(145), 161–182.

Ku, L., Dittmar, H., & Banerjee, R. (2012). Are materialistic teenagers less motivated to learn? Cross-sectional and longitudinal evidence from the United Kingdom and Hong Kong. *Journal of Educational Psychology, 104*(1), 74–86.

Kubey, R. W., Lavin, M. J., & Barrows, J. R. (2001). Internet use and collegiate academic performance decrements: Early findings. *Journal of Communication, 51*(2), 366–382.

Kurdek, L. A., Fine, M. A., & Sinclair, R. J. (1995). School adjustment in sixth graders: Parenting transitions, family climate, and peer norm effects. *Child Development, 66*(2), 430–445.

Kwan, V. S., Bond, M. H., & Singelis, T. M. (1997). Pancultural explanations for life satisfaction: Adding relationship harmony to self-esteem. *Journal of Personality and Social Psychology, 73*(5), 1038–1051.

Kwan, Y. K. (2008). Life satisfaction and family structure among adolescents in Hong Kong. *Social Indicators Research, 86*(1), 59–67.

Lee, M. T., Wong, B. P., Chow, B. W. Y., & McBride-Chang, C. (2006). Predictors of suicide ideation and depression in Hong Kong adolescents: Perceptions of academic and family climates. *Suicide and Life-threatening Behavior, 36*(1), 82–96.

Lee, P. L., Hamman, D., & Lee, C. C. (2007). The relationship of family closeness with college students' self-regulated learning and school adjustment. *College Student Journal, 41*(4), 779–788.

Lent, R. W., Singley, D., Sheu, H. B., Schmidt, J. A., & Schmidt, L. C. (2007). Relation of social-cognitive factors to academic satisfaction in engineering students. *Journal of Career Assessment, 15*(1), 87–97.

Lim, S. L., & Lim, B. K. (2004). Parenting style and child outcomes in Chinese and immigrant Chinese families-current findings and cross-cultural considerations in conceptualization and research. *Marriage & Family Review, 35*(3–4), 21–43.

Ma, C. M. S., & Shek, D. T. L. (2013). Consumption of pornographic materials in early adolescents in Hong Kong. *Journal of Pediatric and Adolescent Gynecology, 26*(3S), S18–S25.

Mak, K. K., Lee, S. L., Ho, S. Y., Lo, W. S., & Lam, T. H. (2012). Sleep and academic performance in Hong Kong adolescents. *Journal of School Health, 82*(11), 522–527.

Marchant, G. J., Paulson, S. E., & Rothlisberg, B. A. (2001). Relations of middle school students' perceptions of family and school contexts with academic achievement. *Psychology in the Schools, 38*(6), 505–519.

Olson, D., Russell, C. S., & Sprenkle, D. H. (1989). *Circumplex model: Systemic assessment and treatment of families*. New York: Routledge Press.

Ow, R., & Katz, D. (1999). Family secrets and the disclosure of distressful information in Chinese families. *Families in Society: The Journal of Contemporary Social Services, 80*(6), 620–628.

Raja, S. N., McGee, R., & Stanton, W. R. (1992). Perceived attachments to parents and peers and psychological well-being in adolescence. *Journal of Youth and Adolescence, 21*(4), 471–485.

Rask, K., Âstedt-Kurki, P., Paavilainen, E., & Laippala, P. (2003). Adolescent subjective well-being and family dynamics. *Scandinavian Journal of Caring Sciences, 17*(2), 129–138.
Rothbaum, F., Rosen, K., Ujiie, T., & Uchida, N. (2002). Family systems theory, attachment theory, and culture. *Family Process, 41*(3), 328–350.
Schrodt, P., Ledbetter, A. M., & Ohrt, J. K. (2007). Parental confirmation and affection as mediators of family communication patterns and children's mental well-being. *The Journal of Family Communication, 7*(1), 23–46.
Shek, D. T. L. (1997a). Family environment and adolescent psychological well-being, school adjustment, and problem behavior: A pioneer study in a Chinese context. *The Journal of Genetic Psychology, 158*(1), 113–128.
Shek, D. T. L. (1997b). The relation of parent-adolescent conflict to adolescent psychological well-being, school adjustment, and problem behavior. *Social Behavior and Personality: An International Journal, 25*(3), 277–290.
Shek, D. T. L. (1998). The Chinese version of the self-report family inventory: Does culture make a difference? *Research on Social Work Practice, 8*(2), 315–329.
Shek, D. T. L. (2001a). Chinese adolescents and their parents' views on a happy family: Implications for family therapy. *Family Therapy, 28*(2), 73–103.
Shek, D. T. L. (2001b). Family functioning and psychological well-being, school adjustment, and substance abuse in Chinese adolescents: Are findings based on multiple studies consistent? In F. Columbus (Ed.), *Advances in psychology research* (Vol. 7, pp. 63–86). New York: Nova Science.
Shek, D. T. L. (2002a). Family functioning and psychological well-being, school adjustment, and problem behavior in Chinese adolescents with and without economic disadvantage. *The Journal of Genetic Psychology, 163*(4), 497–502.
Shek, D. T. L. (2002b). Assessment of family functioning Chinese adolescents: The Chinese Family Assessment Instrument. In N. N. Singh, T. Ollen-dick, & A. N. Singh (Eds.), *International perspectives on child and adolescent mental health* (pp. 297–316). Amsterdam: Elsevier.
Shek, D. T. L. (2005). A longitudinal study of perceived family functioning and adolescent adjustment in Chinese adolescents with economic disadvantage. *Journal of Family Issues, 26*(4), 518–543.
Shek, D. T. L. (2014). Chinese family quality of life. In A. C. Michalos (Ed.), *Encyclopedia of quality of life and well-being research.* Berlin, Germany: Springer.
Shek, D. T. L., & Chan, L. K. (1999). Hong Kong Chinese parents' perceptions of the ideal child. *The Journal of Psychology, 133*(3), 291–302.
Shek, D. T. L., Leung, H., & Lu, S. (2013). Perceived family life quality in junior secondary school students. *Social Indicators Research.* doi:10.1007/s11205-013-0397-5.
Shek, D. T. L., & Ma, C. M. S. (2010). The Chinese Family Assessment Instrument (C-FAI) Hierarchical confirmatory factor analyses and factorial invariance. *Research on Social Work Practice, 20*(1), 112–123.
Shek, D. T. L., Ma, H. K., & Sun, R. C. F. (2011). A brief overview of adolescent developmental problems in Hong Kong. *The Scientific World Journal, 11*, 2243–2256.
Steinberg, L., Lamborn, S. D., Darling, N., Mounts, N. S., & Dornbusch, S. M. (1994). Over-time changes in adjustment and competence among adolescents from authoritative, authoritarian, indulgent, and neglectful families. *Child Development, 65*(3), 754–770.
Suldo, S. M., Riley, K. N., & Shaffer, E. J. (2006). Academic correlates of children and adolescents' life satisfaction. *School Psychology International, 27*(5), 567–582.
Taylor, L. C., Clayton, J. D., & Rowley, S. J. (2004). Academic socialization: Understanding parental influences on Children's school-related development in the early years. *Review of General Psychology, 8*(3), 163–178.
Trinidad, D. R., Chou, C. P., Unger, J. B., Johnson, C. A., & Li, Y. (2003). Family harmony as a protective factor against adolescent tobacco and alcohol use in Wuhan, China. *Substance Use & Misuse, 38*(8), 1159–1171.

Youngblade, L. M., Theokas, C., Schulenberg, J., Curry, L., Huang, I. C., & Novak, M. (2007). Risk and promotive factors in families, schools, and communities: A contextual model of positive youth development in adolescence. *Pediatrics, 119*(Supplement 1), 47–53.

Yu, L., & Shek, D. T. L. (2013). Internet addiction in Hong Kong adolescents: A three-year longitudinal study. *Journal of Pediatric and Adolescent Gynecology, 26*(3S), S10–S17.

Zhou, Q., King, K. M., & Chassin, L. (2006). The roles of familial alcoholism and adolescent family harmony in young adults' substance dependence disorders: Mediated and moderated relations. *Journal of Abnormal Psychology, 115*(2), 320–331.

Subjective Well-Being of Early Adolescents in Hong Kong

Daniel T.L. Shek and Xiang Li

Abstract There is a pressing need to learn more about the subjective well-being of adolescents because it is an important indicator of the quality of life in adolescence. Utilizing a three-wave longitudinal study with 1-year time interval, the subjective well-being of adolescents in the junior secondary school years in Hong Kong was examined. Measures of subjective well-being (life satisfaction and hopelessness) and school adjustment indicators (academic and school competence, perceptions of the new school curriculum, and participation in tutoring activities) were explored in this study. Six major observations were highlighted from the findings. First, factor analysis showed that life satisfaction and hopelessness were two separable dimensions of subjective well-being. Second, life satisfaction was negatively related to hopelessness concurrently and longitudinally. Third, the negative correlation between life satisfaction and hopelessness was stronger for adolescent girls than for adolescent boys. Fourth, while academic and school competence positively predicted life satisfaction, it negatively predicted hopelessness. Fifth, life satisfaction, hopelessness, and academic and school competence influenced students' perceptions of the new school curriculum, with academic and school competence to be the strongest predictor. Finally, time spent in tutoring was positively related to the hopelessness of the participants.

Keywords Subjective well-being • School adjustment • Early adolescents • Longitudinal study

Introduction

In the past decades, much attention has been paid to the topic "subjective well-being" (Huebner, 2004; Proctor, Linley, & Maltby, 2009). Subjective well-being is commonly regarded as people's evaluation of their lives at the moment and for

D.T.L. Shek, Ph.D., B.B.S., S.B.S., J.P. (✉) • X. Li, Ph.D.
Department of Applied Social Sciences, The Hong Kong Polytechnic University, Hunghom, Hong Kong
e-mail: daniel.shek@polyu.edu.hk

D.T.L. Shek et al. (eds.), *Chinese Adolescents in Hong Kong*, Quality of Life in Asia 5, DOI 10.1007/978-981-287-143-5_6

longer periods (Diener, Oishi, & Lucas, 2003). It is referred to as individuals' own assessment rather than experts' judgments on their own life, and it is typically conceptualized as a higher-order construct including individuals' life satisfaction, positive affect, and negative affect (Ma & Huebner, 2008). While life satisfaction was defined as a "global evaluation by the person of his or her life" (Pavot, Diener, Colvin, & Sandvik, 1991), positive affect refers to the frequency of positive emotion, and negative affect refers to the frequency of negative emotion (Ma & Huebner, 2008). Accordingly, subjective well-being can be assessed by life satisfaction and affect (Suh, Diener, Oishi, & Triandis, 1998). Although life satisfaction and affect are interrelated, life satisfaction is different from affect (Lucas, Diener, & Suh, 1996). Life satisfaction is generally regarded as a cognitive appraisal of one's satisfaction arising from a judgment by the person of his or her life (Diener, 2009), whereas affect is the summed emotional experience of one's reactions to ongoing events in life (Suh et al., 1998) arising from cognitive appraisals (Diener, 2009).

Long, Huebner, Wedell, and Hills (2012) suggested that life satisfaction was negatively related to negative affect. Abramson, Metalsky, and Alloy (1989) also proposed that negative affect could be implied by hopelessness, which was an important indicator of emotional well-being and a measure of psychological symptom that was intrinsic to many forms of mental problems (Shek, 2008). The essence of hopelessness is that individuals become pessimistic and they hold negative expectations about the self and future (Bolland, 2003).

Subjective well-being is highly volatile in early adolescence because it is a developmental period with many changes and shifts in different domains, such as educational and psychological aspects (Eccles, 1999). Some studies (e.g., Kwan, 2010; Leung, McBride-Chang, & Lai, 2004) showed that adolescent life satisfaction significantly declined with age, while adolescent hopelessness increased with age (Han & Shek, 2012). Some scholars (e.g., Suh et al., 1998) postulated that for people who were not satisfied with their life, they might still experience much pleasant emotion. However, more recent studies (e.g., Gilman & Huebner, 2006; Kolarcik, Geckova, Reijneveld, & van Dijk, 2012; Proctor et al., 2009; Shek, 2005) revealed a negative correlation between life satisfaction and hopelessness. As life satisfaction is a potential protective factor against hopelessness (Heisel & Flett, 2004), it can be regarded as a positive indicator, while hopelessness can be regarded as a negative indicator of subjective well-being (Shek, 2005, 2007).

Are there any gender differences in subjective well-being in adolescents? A survey of the literature showed that it was not conclusive. While some studies (e.g., Valois, Zullig, Huebner, & Drane, 2004) showed that boys displayed a higher level of life satisfaction, some studies (e.g., Long et al., 2012) showed that girls had a higher level of life satisfaction or there were no differences between adolescent boys and girls (e.g., Huebner, 2004; Leung et al., 2004; Vecchio, Gerbino, Pastorelli, Del Bove, & Caprara, 2007). Regarding hopelessness, both Bolland (2003) and Park, Morash, and Stevens (2010) reported that boys showed a lower sense of hope than did girls. However, girls tended to react more strongly with depressive symptoms than did boys in response to the same stressful events (Hankin, Mermelstein, & Roesch, 2007), suggesting that when girls are dissatisfied with life or encounter some negative events, they are more likely to display emotional vulnerability such as hopelessness. Telzer and Fuligni (2013) also indicated that girls were more vulnerable to the effects of stressors (e.g., dissatisfying life) than did boys.

As life satisfaction was positively related to positive youth development (Sun & Shek, 2012), adolescents with a higher level of life satisfaction usually showed better adaptive adjustment and positive psychosocial functioning (Suldo & Huebner, 2006), while adolescents with a lower level of life satisfaction displayed more maladaptive outcomes and problem behaviors (McKnight, Huebner, & Suldo, 2002; Shek & Liu, 2014; Sun & Shek, 2012). Besides, higher life satisfaction was found to be related to adolescent school engagement (Gilman & Huebner, 2006; Lewis, Huebner, Malone, & Valois, 2011), and academic competence was significantly related to life satisfaction concurrently and longitudinally (Chow, 2008; Gilman & Huebner, 2006; Huebner, Antaramian, Hills, Lewis, & Saha, 2011; Leung & Leung, 1992; Vecchio et al., 2007). Furthermore, academic achievement was positively related to hope (Gilman & Huebner, 2006) but negatively associated with internalizing problems (Roeser, Eccles, & Freedman-Doan, 1999). For example, academic competence was negatively related to depression (Vecchio et al., 2007) and hopelessness (Sun & Shek, 2012).

With specific reference to Hong Kong, academic excellence is strongly emphasized. Under the influence of the traditional Chinese culture, children and adolescents are expected to have good academic performance in order to climb up the social ladder. Due to the high level of competition in Chinese schools, Chinese students only spent much less time in playing outside and had much heavier study burden than did their Western counterparts (Xu et al., 2012). Research also showed that academic engagement (e.g., classroom conduct, time expenditure) influenced students' academic achievement (Chen, 2005).

To climb up the social ladder, students usually hire private tutors or join classes in tutoring schools to "consolidate" their academic performance. Although tutoring is an international phenomenon, it is especially pervasive in Asia such as Hong Kong (de Castro & de Guzman, 2014). Typically, tutoring is a popular alternative for parents who are unavailable or incompetent to supervise children's study (Tam & Chan, 2010). Since students' academic achievement is the top priority for students themselves, parents, and teachers, many students desire to reach a high level of academic performance by participating in different kinds of tutoring after class. De Castro and de Guzman (2014) consider tutoring to be an effective approach since private tutors are able to tailor their teaching to the needs of students. However, some parents are worried that tutoring services might not be helpful because it may mask children's learning problems (Tam & Chan, 2010). Interestingly, despite the popularity of tutoring schools in Hong Kong, there is very little systematic research in this area.

In recent years, the new senior secondary school curriculum reform (i.e., the "3-3-4 academic structure reform") is a revolution of the education system in Hong Kong.

In this reform, secondary school education is reduced to 6 years, and an additional year is added in the university education (Pun, 2013). Although the goal of the school reform is to help young people get good jobs and succeed in the fast-changing society in the long run (Chan, 2006), secondary school students have to face more difficulties and challenges because of the reformed curriculum. As it is a new initiative in Hong Kong, not much scientific data are available. Hence, it is important to examine this issue with particular reference to the Hong Kong context.

Although the topic of subjective well-being is quite well researched in the Western context, there are very few longitudinal studies on subjective well-being of adolescents, and the research data on Chinese adolescents are slim (Shek & Liu, 2014). As early adolescence is a turbulent and transitional stage that forces youngsters to face a variety of physical and social changes (Lewis et al., 2011), it is of great importance to understand subjective well-being in the transition from childhood to adolescence. Therefore, early adolescents were recruited in this study. Given that longitudinal design is a superior approach to chart changes over time than do cross-sectional studies, longitudinal design was adopted in this study.

Although subjective well-being includes people's cognitive appraisal and emotional evaluation of their lives (Diener et al., 2003; Lucas et al., 1996; Pavot et al., 1991), most researchers only employ life satisfaction as the sole indicator to measure subjective well-being (Diener et al., 2003; Suldo & Huebner, 2006). Nevertheless, although life satisfaction can be viewed as a good indicator of subjective well-being, life satisfaction and affect are independent constructs (Lucas et al., 1996; Suh et al., 1998). Hence, it can be argued that life satisfaction as a single indicator is not sufficient to measure subjective well-being and it would be more illuminating to assess life satisfaction and other related emotional indicators such as hopelessness.

Several research questions were addressed in the present study. The first research question addressed in this study was whether measures of life satisfaction and hopelessness could be differentiated. Based on the existing theories and research findings (e.g., Lucas et al., 1996), it was expected that these two measures were distinct constructs (Hypothesis 1). The second research question was whether there was any relationship between life satisfaction and hopelessness as measures of adolescent well-being. Based on the existing theories and findings (e.g., Gilman & Huebner, 2006; Shek, 2005), it was expected that these two measures would be negatively correlated (Hypothesis 2). As there were research findings showing gender differences in the relationship between life satisfaction and hopelessness (e.g., Yeo, Ang, Chong, & Huan, 2007), this formed the third research question. It was expected that the relationship would be stronger in adolescent girls than in adolescent boys (Hypothesis 3).

In this study, school adjustment was assessed by three measures, including academic and school competence, perceptions of the new school curriculum, and tutoring activities. While happiness is an important goal of schooling (Noddings, 2003), school competence influences the life satisfaction of students (Leung et al., 2004). Hence, the fourth research question was whether there would be a relationship between school competence and subjective well-being in early adolescents. It was hypothesized that there would be a positive relationship between school competence and subjective well-being (Hypothesis 4).

As academic pressure becomes higher as students approach the Hong Kong Diploma of Secondary Education Examination (HKDSEE), it is important to understand the views of young people on the related topics. Hence, students' perceptions of the new secondary school curriculum were explored as the fifth research question. It was expected that both subjective well-being and school competence would be positively related to the perceptions of the new secondary school curriculum (Hypothesis 5). Finally, as tutoring plays an important role in student life in Hong Kong, the sixth research question examined the influence of time spent in tutoring on the subjective well-being of students. It was expected that students who spent more time in tutoring had less life satisfaction and more hopelessness than did those who spent less time in tutoring (Hypothesis 6).

Methods

Participants

The data for the present study were derived from an ongoing longitudinal study aiming at exploring the psychosocial development of secondary school students over six consecutive years in Hong Kong. A total of 28 secondary schools were randomly selected and involved in this large-scale investigation. There were 3,325 Secondary 1 students (1,718 boys and 1,570 girls; $M_{age}=12.59$ years old) participating in the first measurement at the 2009/2010 school year; 3,638 Secondary 2 students (1,864 boys and 1,716 girls; $M_{age}=13.64$ years old) participated in the second measurement at the 2010/2011 school year; and 4,106 Secondary 3 students (2,185 boys and 1,885 girls; $M_{age}=14.65$ years old) participated in the third measurement at the 2011/2012 school year. Totally, 2,667 students (80.21 %) completed all three measurements, and the attrition rate could be regarded as satisfactory according to the criteria of Taris (2000) that a nonresponse rate between 30 and 40 % was quite common (Taris, 2000).

Procedures

The procedures were the same at each wave of data collection. Given that all participating students were under 18 years old, written informed consent was obtained from students themselves, parents, and schools before data collection. The same set of self-report questionnaire was employed at each wave. Students were required to complete the questionnaire independently in their classrooms under the guidance and administration of a research assistant who had received training before data collection. Before filling in the questionnaires at each time, standardized instructions including the research purpose, confidentiality of the data, willingness of the participation, and other related information about this study were introduced to the students. During the data collection process of around 30–35 min, students were discouraged to share their personal answers with each other. If students have questions about the questionnaire, they were encouraged to discuss them with the research assistants. All information collected from the students was kept strictly confidential, and the individual data would not be disclosed to the third party.

Instruments

Besides the basic demographic information, several measures were included in the questionnaire as follows:

Satisfaction with Life Scale (SWLS): The SWLS measures individuals' own global judgment of their quality of life, and it was developed by Diener, Emmons, Larsen, and Griffin (1985). It comprises five items (e.g., I am satisfied with my life) rated on a 6-point Likert scale (1 = *strongly disagree* and 6 = *strongly agree*), and a higher score indicates a higher level of life satisfaction. In the original validation study, the Cronbach's alpha was .87. Shek (1992) translated this scale into Chinese, and good psychometric properties were found for the modified scale (e.g., Shek, 1997; Shek & Lee, 2007).

Hopelessness Scale (HOPEL): The HOPEL (Beck, Weissman, Lester, & Trexler, 1974) was developed to measure the extent to which individuals possess hopeless and unfavorable expectations regarding future life outcomes (Lucas et al., 1996). Shek (1993) translated this scale into Chinese with modifications and validated its applicability in Hong Kong. The high reliability of HOPEL was then confirmed in many studies (e.g., Shek, 1997; Shek & Lee, 2007). The HOPEL, an abridged version based on Shek's earlier studies, consists of five items (e.g., my future seems dark to me) with the highest item-total correlation. It is a 6-point Likert scale ranging from 1 (*strongly disagree*) to 6 (*strongly agree*), with a higher score suggesting a lower sense of hope.

Academic and School Competence Scale (ASC): The ASC, measuring individuals' school performance, is a 5-point Likert scale (1 = *very poor* and 5 = *very good*) with three items including perceived academic performance compared to schoolmates, satisfaction with academic performance, and conduct in school. The high reliability was reported (Shek & Yu, 2012), and a higher score represents a higher level of academic and school competence.

Perceptions of the New School Curriculum (PNSC): Four items were used to assess respondents' perceptions of the new school curriculum implemented in Hong Kong. The first item was constructed to assess students' confidence in adapting to the new school curriculum, and students were asked to rate from 1 (*totally no confidence*) to 4 (*full confidence*). Two items, also ranging from 1 (*totally not*) to 4 (*very much*), were used to measure students' perceived stress on the new school curriculum and current study, respectively. These two items were reverse-scored. The last item was used to assess respondents' perceptions of the learning support provided by schools, and the rating ranges from 1 (*very little*) to 4 (*very enough*).

Tutoring Questions: Three questions were used to understand students' tutoring participation. Students were first asked whether they participated in tutoring. If yes, they were then asked which kinds of tutoring (i.e., in-school tutorial classes, outside-of-school tutorial classes, and private tutoring) they participated in. Finally, students were asked how much time they spent on tutoring each week and how much money they spent on tutoring each month.

Results

To test the hypothesis that life satisfaction and hopelessness represent the two dimensions of subjective well-being (Shek, 2005), exploratory factor analyses were performed to examine the factor structure. At each time point, principal component analysis (PCA) with varimax rotation was used to assess the dimensionality of the measures. Results showed that only the eigenvalues of the first two components were over 1 and they explained a substantial amount of variance across the three waves (65.48 %, 68.10 %, and 68.79 %, respectively). Results of the varimax rotated factor loadings at the three time points consistently showed that the two-factor solution (i.e., life satisfaction and hopelessness) was stable across time (see Table 1). The reliability values of the related measures of subjective well-being were from .620 to .648 across the three time points. Therefore, Hypothesis 1 was supported.

Regarding the reliability values of all measures employed in this study (including SWLS, HOPEL, ASC, and PNSC), results showed that they had high internal consistency at the three waves (see Table 2). While PNSC was only tested at the third time point, its reliability was acceptable. Life satisfaction and academic and school competence showed a significant decreasing trend from Time 1 to Time 3, while adolescent hopelessness significantly increased during this period. The related findings were summarized in Table 3.

For the interrelationships among life satisfaction, hopelessness, academic and school competence, and perceptions of the new school curriculum, the correlation coefficients at each time point were moderately correlated and very stable over time (see Table 4). Several interesting observations deserve our attention. First, consistent with Hypothesis 2, there was significantly negative correlation between life satisfaction and hopelessness at each time point. To further explore the predictive link from life satisfaction to hopelessness, multiple regression analyses were conducted. After controlling for hopelessness at Time 1 and Time 2, life satisfaction at Time 1 still significantly predicted hopelessness at Time 3 ($\beta = -.058$, $t = -3.278$, $p < .002$), suggesting that life satisfaction has a negative impact on hopelessness over time.

To test gender differences, independent *t*-tests were conducted to compare the differences between boys and girls in terms of life satisfaction, hopelessness, academic and school competence, and perceptions of the new school curriculum (see Table 5).

Table 1 Rotated varimax factor loadings for the items of measures of life satisfaction and hopelessness at the three time points

	Time 1		Time 2		Time 3	
	LS	HL	LS	HL	LS	HL
Item 1 In most ways my life is close to my ideal	**.799**	−.231	**.824**	−.248	**.829**	−.235
Item 2 The conditions of my life are excellent	**.809**	−.232	**.823**	−.253	**.835**	−.223
Item 3 I am satisfied with my life	**.830**	−.264	**.834**	−.282	**.845**	−.271
Item 4 So far I have gotten the important things I want in my life	**.782**	−.003	**.802**	−.004	**.783**	.016
Item 5 If I could live my life over, I would change almost nothing	**.728**	.100	**.748**	.063	**.746**	.073
Item 6 I might as well give up because I cannot make things better for myself	−.048	**.796**	−.048	**.816**	−.010	**.815**
Item 7 My future seems dark to me	−.146	**.867**	−.158	**.870**	−.145	**.880**
Item 8 All I can see ahead of me is unpleasantness rather than pleasantness	−.156	**.872**	−.160	**.873**	−.125	**.892**
Item 9 I do not expect to get what I really want	.035	**.748**	−.025	**.762**	−.029	**.781**
Item 10 Things just will not work out the way I want them to	−.253	**.649**	−.227	**.689**	−.259	**.692**

LS life satisfaction, *HL* hopelessness

Table 2 Reliabilities of all scales at the three time points

Variables (no. of items)	Time 1 α	Time 2 α	Time 3 α
LS (5 items)	.851	.870	.868
HL (5 items)	.854	.872	.879
ASC (3 items)	.665	.690	.674
PNSC (4 items)			.601

LS life satisfaction, *HL* hopelessness, *ASC* academic and school competence, *PNSC* perceptions of the new school curriculum

Table 3 Change trends of all variables across the three time points

	Time 1		Time 2		Time 3		Comparisons		
Variables	Mean	SD	Mean	SD	Mean	SD	T1–T2	T2–T3	T1–T3
LS (n=2,503)	19.78	5.39	19.13	5.46	18.83	5.28	↓***	↓**	↓***
HL (n=2,473)	13.12	5.68	13.46	5.61	13.46	5.54	↑*	=	↑*
ASC (n=2,499)	9.48	1.94	9.27	2.02	9.15	2.00	↓***	↓**	↓***

The decreasing trend of life satisfaction had been reported by Shek and Liu (2014)
"↓" means decreasing trend, "=" means no change, "↑" means increasing trend
LS life satisfaction, *HL* hopelessness, *ASC* academic and school competence
*p<.05, **p<.01, ***p<.001

Table 4 Correlations of all variables at the three time points

	T1LS	T1HL	T1ASC	T2LS	T2HL	T2ASC	T3LS	T3HL	T3ASC	T3PNSC
T1LS	1									
T1HL	–.281***	1								
T1ASC	.331***	–.285***	1							
T2LS	.547***	–.280***	.282***	1						
T2HL	–.296***	.446***	–.233***	–.311***	1					
T2ASC	.277***	–.230***	.545***	.354***	–.260***	1				
T3LS	.489***	–.233***	.243***	.581***	–.284***	.291***	1			
T3HL	–.260***	.411***	–.222***	–.317***	.533***	–.274***	–.278***	1		
T3ASC	.232***	–.186***	.462***	.268***	–.230***	.577***	.338***	–.298***	1	
T3PNSC	.169***	–.158***	.190***	.228***	–.205***	.265***	.313***	–.310***	.352***	1

LS life satisfaction, *HL* hopelessness, *ASC* academic and school competence, *PNSC* perceptions of the new school curriculum, *T1* Time 1, *T2* Time 2, *T3* Time 3

*** $p<.001$

Table 5 Gender comparisons on all variables at the three time points

		Male		Female		
		Mean	SD	Mean	SD	*t*
Time 1	LS	19.780	5.650	19.725	5.421	.279
	HL	13.781	6.143	12.933	5.560	4.067***
	ASC	9.220	2.099	9.503	1.901	−4.001***
Time 2	LS	19.115	5.571	18.919	5.459	1.054
	HL	14.058	6.041	13.594	5.601	2.357*
	ASC	9.108	2.154	9.173	2.001	−.912
Time 3	LS	18.602	5.448	18.800	5.246	−1.169
	HL	14.148	5.968	13.283	5.336	4.839***
	ASC	9.027	2.156	9.050	1.915	−.358
	PNSC	10.230	2.055	9.936	1.855	4.762***

LS life satisfaction, *HL* hopelessness, *ASC* academic and school competence, *PNSC* perceptions of the new school curriculum
$^{*}p<.05$, $^{***}p<.001$

At each time point, no significant difference in life satisfaction was found between boys and girls. However, boys displayed a significantly lower sense of hope than did girls. Much worse, boys' hopelessness continuously increased with time.

Regarding gender differences in the relationship between life satisfaction and hopelessness, the interaction effects of gender and life satisfaction on hopelessness at all three time points were significant (Time 1: $b=-.226$, $t=-6.162$, $p<.001$; Time 2: $b=-.196$, $t=-5.769$, $p<.001$; Time 3: $b=-.161$, $t=-4.946$, $p<.001$). It implied that the negative effects of life satisfaction on hopelessness were stronger for adolescent girls (Time 1: $b=-.423$, $t=-15.714$, $p<.001$; Time 2: $b=-.434$, $t=-17.602$, $p<.001$; Time 3: $b=-.386$, $t=-15.966$, $p<.001$) than for adolescent boys (Time 1: $b=-.197$, $t=-7.944$, $p<.001$; Time 2: $b=-.238$, $t=-10.172$, $p<.001$; Time 3: $b=-.225$, $t=-10.321$, $p<.001$) in the junior secondary school years. In short, the findings gave support to Hypothesis 3.

Results showed that the academic and school competence of girls was higher than boys' at all three time points. However, such differences in school competence between girls and boys gradually became smaller and nonsignificant over time (differences reduced from 0.283 to 0.023), which probably explained why boys held more positive views on the new school curriculum than did girls at Time 3 ($t=4.762$, $p<.001$).

Table 4 showed that academic and school competence was positively related to life satisfaction but negatively related to hopelessness at all three time points. After controlling for life satisfaction at Time 1 and Time 2, academic and school competence at Time 1 significantly and positively predicted life satisfaction at Time 3 ($\beta=.037$, $t=2.153$, $p<.05$), suggesting that academic and school competence predicts life satisfaction over time, although the effect size was not big. Besides, gender did not moderate the relationship between academic and school competence and life satisfaction at all three waves ($ps>.05$).

After controlling for hopelessness at Time 1 and Time 2, academic and school competence at Time 1 significantly and negatively predicted hopelessness at Time 3

($\beta=-.066$, $t=-3.751$, $p<.001$). The findings gave support to Hypothesis 4. Moreover, gender has moderating effects on the relationship from academic and school competence to hopelessness at both Time 1 ($b=-.723$, $t=-10.766$, $p<.001$ for males and $b=-.966$, $t=-12.615$, $p<.001$ for females, respectively) and Time 2 ($b=-.596$, $t=-9.660$, $p<.001$ for males and $b=-.905$, $t=-13.114$, $p<.001$ for females, respectively) except Time 3 ($p>.05$). The findings showed that compared to males, females with lower academic and school competence had a higher sense of hopelessness.

Regarding the relationship between subjective well-being and the perceptions of the new school curriculum, it was found that a higher level of life satisfaction and a lower level of hopelessness were positively related to the positive views on the new school curriculum. Across the three time points, the correlation between personal well-being and the perceptions of the new school curriculum was strengthened gradually (βs from .169 to .313 for life satisfaction; βs from −.158 to −.310 for hopelessness), and the correlation between school competence and the perceptions of the new school curriculum was also strengthened gradually (βs from .190 to .352). These findings clearly suggested that subjective well-being and school competence influenced students' attitudes to the new school curriculum. However, academic and school competence had the strongest effects on students' perceptions of the new school curriculum at all three time points. In short, Hypothesis 5 was supported.

Results showed that 38.4 % of the students ($n=1{,}819$) participated in at least one kind of tutoring at Time 3. There were 246 students (5.2 %) participating in in-school tutorial classes, 1,031 students (21.8 %) participated in outside-of-school tutorial classes, and 830 students (17.5 %) participated in private tutoring. The majority of students ($n=1{,}527$) only participated in one kind of tutoring. However, 5.4 % of students ($n=257$) participated in two kinds of tutoring, and 0.5 % of students ($n=25$) even participated in all three kinds of tutoring. Correspondingly, many students spent more or less time and money in tutoring. Most students spent either 2 h ($n=418$) or 3 h ($n=319$) in tutoring per week. Surprisingly, ten students spent 39 h per week in tutoring, which implied that he or she spent as much time in tutoring as school study. Additionally, most students spent HK$1,000 in tutoring per month, and the average expense was HK$1,377 with a high standard deviation (SD=HK$1,983 per month), suggesting that huge range existed in students' tutorial expenses.

Results revealed that students participating in tutoring had higher life satisfaction than did those who did not ($t=-3.667$, $p<.001$), while nonsignificant difference in hopelessness was found ($t=1.171$, $p>.05$). Interestingly, among students who participated in tutoring, a significant relationship was observed between time expenditure in tutoring and hopelessness ($r=.067$, $p<.01$), but was not observed between time expenditure and life satisfaction ($r=.018$, $p>.05$). Hypothesis 6 was partially supported.

Discussion

An understanding of adolescents' subjective well-being would enable researchers to appreciate the role of the quality of life in adolescent psychological health and school adjustment (Lyons, Huebner, Hills, & Van Horn, 2013). Previous studies (e.g., Proctor et al., 2009) reported that life satisfaction and hopelessness could be regarded as two components of psychological well-being. The present study further provides support for this view which lends credence to the validity of the two-factor structure of subjective well-being including life satisfaction and hopelessness (i.e., Hypothesis 1).

In alignment with earlier research (e.g., Shek, 1998), this study provides support for the negative association between life satisfaction and hopelessness (i.e., Hypothesis 2). Besides, adolescent life satisfaction showed a clear declining trend, which has been reported in the work of Shek and Liu (2014), suggesting that perceived life satisfaction becomes lower as adolescents mature. Similarly, adolescent hopelessness significantly increased across the three time points, suggesting adolescents' sense of hope becomes lower and lower. One possible explanation is that life becomes complicated in the eyes of adolescents as they have deeper understanding on people and environment as a result of their cognitive maturity (Shek & Liu, 2014). Another possible explanation is that emotional distress increases in the transition of adolescence (Yeo et al., 2007).

Although nonsignificant difference was detected in life satisfaction between boys and girls, boys were found to be more hopeless than girls. This may be due to the fact that Chinese people have higher expectations for boys, who are expected to bear more stress and reach higher achievements (Shek & Liu, 2014), which in turn makes boys easily feel incapable and hopeless. Besides, the present finding showed that gender difference was found in the prediction from life satisfaction to hopelessness, and this negative prediction was stronger for adolescent girls than for adolescent boys (i.e., Hypothesis 3). It implied that when girls felt dissatisfied with life, they were more likely to become hopeless than boys. A possible explanation is that girls have a lower level of psychosocial resilience (Tusaie, Puskar, & Sereika, 2007) and they are more vulnerable to emotional distress (Yeo et al., 2007).

In contrast to the findings that academic performance was not related to life satisfaction in the United States (Bradley & Corwyn, 2004), a positive relationship between school competence and life satisfaction and a negative relationship between school competence and hopelessness were observed in this study (i.e., Hypothesis 4). The significant findings may be due to the fact that academic achievement is valued above other forms of success in Chinese society and Chinese children are under tremendous pressure to achieve academic excellence (Li, Chan, Chung, & Chui, 2010). Thus, academic success fosters the desirable and satisfactory outcomes for adolescents (Vecchio et al., 2007), and life satisfaction of most Chinese students is governed by academic achievement to great extent. Since disadvantaged people usually perceive themselves unable to change their situations and improve their well-being (Kolarcik et al., 2012), students without good school competence are likely to feel hopeless. Unfortunately, school competence of both boys and girls significantly declined from Secondary 1 to 3, which was consistent with prior studies (e.g., Leung et al., 2004; Vecchio et al., 2007). An obvious reason is that the depth of knowledge is advanced and the school tasks are more challenging with the school years (Schunk & Pajares, 2002); thus, increasing demand on students' school competence is placed, and it is more difficult for students to reach a high level of academic performance.

It should be noted that the negative correlation between school competence and hopelessness was stronger for adolescent girls than for adolescent boys. Perhaps girls are more sensitive than boys to the adverse effect of failure (Rudolph & Flynn, 2007), and they are more likely to feel disappointed and hopeless if they cannot reach satisfying academic achievement.

Given that tremendous emphasis on academic achievement has been given to students in senior secondary schools and curriculum reform is a new initiative in Hong Kong, it is no doubt that adolescents face numerous stressors and challenges when they enter into senior secondary schools (Chow, 2008). Against this background, we especially examine adolescents' perceptions of the new high school curriculum. As expected, many factors such as life satisfaction, hopelessness, and school competence influence students' perceptions of the new school curriculum, but school competence was the most influential one (i.e., Hypothesis 5). Obviously, adolescents with higher life satisfaction tend to hold optimistic views, while adolescents with a lower sense of hope tend to hold pessimistic views on uncertain future study. Compared to subjective well-being, students' school competence has greater influences on their perceptions of the new school curriculum. It is normal that students with good school competence not only have stronger competence to adapt the changes and challenges brought from the new school curriculum, but they are also more confident to proceed to a higher level of study. Thus, good school competence is the essential of the adaptation of reformed curriculum. Here we have observed that girls' perceptions of the new school curriculum were more negative than the perceptions of boys. Three explanations may illustrate this phenomenon. First, girls have greater worries about self than did boys (Yeo et al., 2007). Second, although the school competence of girls was always higher than that of boys from Secondary 1 to 3, the fact that girls' advantage in academics over boys became smaller and nonsignificant with time was found in this study. Third, girls' academic competence decreased faster than did boys', which may lead girls to face the challenges of future study without solid confidence and then form more negative views on the new school curriculum.

The tutoring industry is expanding, and tutoring schools are widespread in Hong Kong, resulting in over one third of students being involved in the different kinds of tutoring. Such a finding was congruent with the conclusion of a comparative study (Newman et al., 2007) that Chinese students spent more time in academics compared to their Western counterparts. Interestingly, students involved in tutoring were found to have higher life satisfaction than those who did not participate in any kind of tutoring. However, this finding is not consistent with the previous finding in Canada (Chow, 2008); tutoring may increase the confidence of the students in Hong Kong, hence leading to the observed effect. Under the highly competitive school environment, many students desire to consolidate their school competence by participating in tutoring; thus, students may feel worried if they do not participate in tutoring. However, too much time spent in tutoring increased the hopelessness of students who participated in tutoring (i.e., Hypothesis 6). On the one hand, longtime tutoring makes students tired through reducing their available time in leisure activities (e.g., sports, gathering with friends). On the other hand, a long time spent in tutoring may damage students' self-confidence in academic competence. In short, students who spent more time in tutoring would feel more hopeless because they suffered from more stress and fatigue (Cantor, Norem, Niedenthal, Langston, & Brower, 1987).

Although this study is a pioneering one in the Chinese context, several limitations should be noted. Firstly, although many students were involved in the study, other stakeholders (e.g., students' parents, teachers) could be invited to understand the related phenomena from different perspectives. Secondly, as only life satisfaction and hopelessness were employed to measure adolescents' subjective well-being, other indicators (e.g., family support, peer interaction) influencing subjective well-being should be taken into account to get a more comprehensive understanding on students' personal well-being. Thirdly, although the sample size of this study was large, caution should be exercised to generalize the findings to other regions, like Mainland China and other Asian countries. Despite these limitations, the present findings substantially enrich the literature on the relationship between subjective well-being and school adjustment among junior secondary school students in Hong Kong.

Acknowledgment The preparation for this work and the Project P.A.T.H.S. were financially supported by the Hong Kong Jockey Club Charities Trust.

References

Abramson, L. Y., Metalsky, G. I., & Alloy, L. B. (1989). Hopelessness depression: A theory-based subtype of depression. *Psychological Review, 96*(2), 358–372.

Beck, A. T., Weissman, A., Lester, D., & Trexler, L. (1974). The measurement of pessimism: The hopelessness scale. *Journal of Consulting and Clinical Psychology, 42*(6), 861–865.

Bolland, J. M. (2003). Hopelessness and risk behaviour among adolescents living in high-poverty inner-city neighbourhoods. *Journal of Adolescence, 26*(2), 145–158.

Bradley, R. H., & Corwyn, R. F. (2004). Life satisfaction among European American, African American, Chinese American, Mexican American, and Dominican American adolescents. *International Journal of Behavioral Development, 28*(5), 385–400.

Cantor, N., Norem, J. K., Niedenthal, P. M., Langston, C. A., & Brower, A. M. (1987). Life tasks, self-concept ideals, and cognitive strategies in a life transition. *Journal of Personality and Social Psychology, 53*(6), 1178–1191.

Chan, B. (2006). *No brain drain, please*. Hong Kong: South China Morning Post Publishers.

Chen, J. J. (2005). Relation of academic support from parents, teachers, and peers to Hong Kong adolescents' academic achievement: The mediating role of academic engagement. *Genetic, Social & General Psychology Monographs, 131*(2), 77–127.

Chow, H. P. (2008). The determinants of life satisfaction: High school students in Regina. *The Alberta Journal of Educational Research, 54*(4), 477–481.

de Castro, B. V., & de Guzman, A. B. (2014). From scratch to notch understanding private tutoring metamorphosis in the Philippines from the perspectives of cram school and formal school administrators. *Education and Urban Society, 46*(3), 287–311.

Diener, E. (2009). Assessing subjective well-being: Progress and opportunities. In E. Diener (Ed.), *Assessing well-being* (pp. 25–65). Dordrecht, The Netherlands: Springer.

Diener, E., Emmons, R. A., Larsen, R. J., & Griffin, S. (1985). The satisfaction with life scale. *Journal of Personality Assessment, 49*(1), 71–75.

Diener, E., Oishi, S., & Lucas, R. E. (2003). Personality, culture, and subjective well-being: Emotional and cognitive evaluations of life. *Annual Review of Psychology, 54*(1), 403–425.

Eccles, J. S. (1999). The development of children ages 6 to 14. *The Future of Children, 9*(2), 30–44.

Gilman, R., & Huebner, E. S. (2006). Characteristics of adolescents who report very high life satisfaction. *Journal of Youth and Adolescence, 35*(3), 293–301.

Han, X. Y., & Shek, D. T. L. (2012). Socio-demographic and family correlates of hopelessness among adolescents in Shanghai, China. *International Journal on Disability and Human Development, 11*(2), 113–119.

Hankin, B. L., Mermelstein, R., & Roesch, L. (2007). Sex differences in adolescent depression: Stress exposure and reactivity models. *Child Development, 78*(1), 279–295.

Heisel, M. J., & Flett, G. L. (2004). Purpose in life, satisfaction with life, and suicide ideation in a clinical sample. *Journal of Psychopathology and Behavioral Assessment, 26*(2), 127–135.

Huebner, E. S. (2004). Research on assessment of life satisfaction of children and adolescents. *Social Indicators Research, 66*(1–2), 3–33.

Huebner, E. S., Antaramian, S. P., Hills, K. J., Lewis, A. D., & Saha, R. (2011). Stability and predictive validity of the Brief Multidimensional Students' Life Satisfaction Scale. *Child Indicators Research, 4*(1), 161–168.

Kolarcik, P., Geckova, A. M., Reijneveld, S. A., & van Dijk, J. P. (2012). Social support, hopelessness and life satisfaction among Roma and non-Roma adolescents in Slovakia. *International Journal of Public Health, 57*(6), 905–913.

Kwan, Y. K. (2010). Life satisfaction and self-assessed health among adolescents in Hong Kong. *Journal of Happiness Studies, 11*(3), 383–393.

Leung, J., & Leung, K. (1992). Life satisfaction, self-concept, and relationship with parents in adolescence. *Journal of Youth and Adolescence, 21*(6), 653–665.

Leung, C. Y. W., McBride-Chang, C., & Lai, B. P. Y. (2004). Relations among maternal parenting style, academic competence, and life satisfaction in Chinese early adolescents. *The Journal of Early Adolescence, 24*(2), 113–143.

Lewis, A. D., Huebner, E., Malone, P. S., & Valois, R. F. (2011). Life satisfaction and student engagement in adolescents. *Journal of Youth and Adolescence, 40*(3), 249–262.

Li, H. C. W., Chan, S. L. P., Chung, O. K. J., & Chui, M. L. M. (2010). Relationships among mental health, self-esteem and physical health in Chinese adolescents: An exploratory study. *Journal of Health Psychology, 15*(1), 96–106.

Long, R. F., Huebner, E. S., Wedell, D. H., & Hills, K. J. (2012). Measuring school-related subjective well-being in adolescents. *American Journal of Orthopsychiatry, 82*(1), 50–60.

Lucas, R. E., Diener, E., & Suh, E. (1996). Discriminant validity of well-being measures. *Journal of Personality and Social Psychology, 71*(3), 616–628.

Lyons, M. D., Huebner, E. S., Hills, K. J., & Van Horn, M. L. (2013). Mechanisms of change in adolescent life satisfaction: A longitudinal analysis. *Journal of School Psychology, 51*(5), 587–598.

Ma, C. Q., & Huebner, E. S. (2008). Attachment relationships and adolescents' life satisfaction: Some relationships matter more to girls than boys. *Psychology in the Schools, 45*(2), 177–190.

McKnight, C. G., Huebner, E. S., & Suldo, S. (2002). Relationships among stressful life events, temperament, problem behavior, and global life satisfaction in adolescents. *Psychology in the Schools, 39*(6), 677–687.

Newman, J., Bidjerano, T., Özdoğru, A. A., Kao, C. C., Özköse-Biyik, Ç., & Johnson, J. J. (2007). What do they usually do after school? A comparative analysis of fourth-grade children in Bulgaria, Taiwan, and the United States. *The Journal of Early Adolescence, 27*(4), 431–456.

Noddings, N. (2003). *Happiness and education*. Cambridge, UK: Cambridge University Press.

Park, S., Morash, M., & Stevens, T. (2010). Gender differences in predictors of assaultive behavior in late adolescence. *Youth Violence and Juvenile Justice, 8*(4), 314–331.

Pavot, W., Diener, E., Colvin, C. R., & Sandvik, E. (1991). Further validation of the satisfaction with life scale: Evidence for the cross-method convergence of well-being measures. *Journal of Personality Assessment, 57*(1), 149–161.

Proctor, C., Linley, P., & Maltby, J. (2009). Youth life satisfaction: A review of the literature. *Journal of Happiness Studies, 10*(5), 583–630.

Pun, S. S. (2013). The politics of hope and cynicism in the realization of the vision of the 334 education reform in Hong Kong. *Asia Pacific Education Review, 14*, 55–65.

Roeser, R. W., Eccles, J. S., & Freedman-Doan, C. (1999). Academic functioning and mental health in adolescence patterns, progressions, and routes from childhood. *Journal of Adolescent Research, 14*(2), 135–174.

Rudolph, K. D., & Flynn, M. (2007). Childhood adversity and youth depression: Influence of gender and pubertal status. *Development and Psychopathology, 19*(2), 497–521.

Schunk, D. H., & Pajares, F. (2002). The development of academic self-efficacy. In A. Wigfield & J. Eccles (Eds.), *Development of achievement motivation* (pp. 16–31). San Diego, CA: Academic.

Shek, D. T. L. (1992). "Actual-ideal" discrepancies in the representation of self and significant-others and psychological well-being in Chinese adolescents. *International Journal of Psychology, 27*(3), 229.

Shek, D. T. L. (1993). Measurement of pessimism in Chinese adolescents: The Chinese Hopelessness Scale. *Social Behavior and Personality, 21*(2), 107–119.

Shek, D. T. L. (1997). The relation of parent-adolescent conflict to adolescent psychological well-being, school adjustment, and problem behavior. *Social Behavior and Personality, 25*(3), 277–290.

Shek, D. T. L. (1998). A longitudinal study of the relations between parent-adolescent conflict and adolescent psychological well-being. *The Journal of Genetic Psychology, 159*(1), 53–67.

Shek, D. T. L. (2005). Perceived parental control processes, parent-child relational qualities, and psychological well-being in Chinese adolescents with and without economic disadvantage. *The Journal of Genetic Psychology, 166*(2), 171–188.

Shek, D. T. L. (2007). A longitudinal study of perceived parental psychological control and psychological well-being in Chinese adolescents in Hong Kong. *Journal of Clinical Psychology, 63*(1), 1–22.

Shek, D. T. L. (2008). Economic disadvantage, perceived family life quality, and emotional well-being in Chinese adolescents: A longitudinal study. *Social Indicators Research, 85*(2), 169–189.

Shek, D. T. L., & Lee, T. Y. (2007). Family life quality and emotional quality of life in Chinese adolescents with and without economic disadvantage. *Social Indicators Research, 80*(2), 393–410.

Shek, D. T. L., & Liu, T. T. (2014). Life satisfaction in junior secondary school students in Hong Kong: A 3-year longitudinal study. *Social Indicators Research, 117*(3), 777–794.

Shek, D. T. L., & Yu, L. (2012). Longitudinal impact of the project PATHS on adolescent risk behavior: What happened after five years? *The Scientific World Journal, 2012*, 1–13.

Suh, E., Diener, E., Oishi, S., & Triandis, H. C. (1998). The shifting basis of life satisfaction judgments across cultures: Emotions versus norms. *Journal of Personality and Social Psychology, 74*(2), 482–493.

Suldo, S. M., & Huebner, S. E. (2006). Is extremely high life satisfaction during adolescence advantageous? *Social Indicators Research, 78*(2), 179–203.

Sun, R. C., & Shek, D. T. L. (2012). Positive youth development, life satisfaction and problem behaviour among Chinese adolescents in Hong Kong: A replication. *Social Indicators Research, 105*(3), 541–559.

Tam, V. C., & Chan, R. M. (2010). Hong Kong parents' perceptions and experiences of involvement in homework: A family capital and resource management perspective. *Journal of Family and Economic Issues, 31*(3), 361–370.

Taris, T. W. (2000). *A primer in longitudinal data analysis*. London: Sage.

Telzer, E. H., & Fuligni, A. J. (2013). Positive daily family interactions eliminate gender differences in internalizing symptoms among adolescents. *Journal of Youth and Adolescence, 42*(10), 1498–1511.

Tusaie, K., Puskar, K., & Sereika, S. M. (2007). A predictive and moderating model of psychosocial resilience in adolescents. *Journal of Nursing Scholarship, 39*(1), 54–60.

Valois, R. F., Zullig, K. J., Huebner, E. S., & Drane, J. W. (2004). Life satisfaction and suicide among high school adolescents. *Social Indicators Research, 66*(1–2), 81–105.

Vecchio, G. M., Gerbino, M., Pastorelli, C., Del Bove, G., & Caprara, G. V. (2007). Multi-faceted self-efficacy beliefs as predictors of life satisfaction in late adolescence. *Personality and Individual Differences, 43*(7), 1807–1818.

Xu, F., Ware, R. S., Lap, A. T., Wang, Z., Hong, X., Song, A., et al. (2012). A school-based comprehensive lifestyle intervention among Chinese kids against obesity (CLICK-Obesity): Rationale, design and methodology of a randomized controlled trial in Nanjing city, China. *BMC Public Health, 12*(1), 316–323.

Yeo, L. S., Ang, R. P., Chong, W. H., & Huan, V. S. (2007). Gender differences in adolescent concerns and emotional well-being: Perceptions of Singaporean adolescent students. *Journal of Genetic Psychology, 168*(1), 63–80.

Development of Delinquent Behavior in Early Adolescents in Hong Kong

Daniel T.L. Shek and Li Lin

Abstract The delinquent behavior of early adolescents in Hong Kong was examined. A sample of adolescents ($N = 3,328$ students at Wave 1) responded to a validated measure of delinquency on three occasions in their junior secondary school years. Prevalence findings showed that delinquent behavior was not prevalent, except in the areas of cheating, speaking foul language, damaging others' properties, and engaging in assault. Regarding demographic correlates of delinquent behavior, it increased across time and adolescent boys showed more delinquent behavior than did adolescent girls. While economic disadvantage did not predict delinquent behavior, family intactness was associated with delinquent behavior across three waves concurrently. Generally speaking, higher levels of positive youth development and family functioning predicted lower delinquency in the junior secondary school years.

Keywords Delinquency • Positive youth development • Family functioning • Chinese adolescents • Chinese

Introduction

Increasing rates of norm-breaking and antisocial behavior (e.g., stealing, fighting, and cheating) are often observed in adolescence (Arnett, 1999; Boyer, 2006). In Hong Kong, youth problem behavior like shoplifting, steeling, smoking, and underage sex has aroused wide attention of researchers and practitioners (Shek, 2006a). Much effort was thus made in identifying protective factors that can lower the proneness of youth delinquent behavior and risk factors that would enhance its likelihood. Family characteristics including family economic status, family structure, family dyadic relationship, and systematic functioning play a significant role in misconduct of youth (Deković, Janssens, & As, 2003; Hoeve et al., 2009; Hoeve et al., 2012). In addition, higher levels of positive youth development attributes such

D.T.L. Shek, Ph.D., B.B.S., S.B.S., J.P. (✉) • L. Lin, Ph.D.
Department of Applied Social Sciences, The Hong Kong Polytechnic University, Hunghom, Hong Kong
e-mail: daniel.shek@polyu.edu.hk

D.T.L. Shek et al. (eds.), *Chinese Adolescents in Hong Kong*,
Quality of Life in Asia 5, DOI 10.1007/978-981-287-143-5_7

as psychosocial competencies, confidence, positive social connection, character strength, and care (Lerner, Fisher, & Weinberg, 2000; Roth & Brooks-Gunn, 2003) were associated with less misconduct of youth (Lewin-Bizan, Bowers, & Lerner, 2010; Sun & Shek, 2010, 2013).

Unfortunately, while much work has been done to examine risk and protective factors of delinquency in Western contexts, relatively less research has been conducted in different Chinese contexts (Shek, Ma, & Sun, 2011). To fill up this gap, the current study examined the descriptive profile and psychosocial correlates of delinquent behavior with a large sample of Hong Kong junior secondary school students across three waves of assessments.

Ascending Trend of Delinquent Behavior

Previous research in Western youth has yielded rich evidence suggesting a rising tendency of delinquent behavior during adolescence (e.g., Overbeek, Vollebergh, Meeus, Engels, & Luijpers, 2001). Cognitive immaturity, emotional impulsivity, parenting practices (e.g., monitoring), peer relationship, and some psychobiological transformations during adolescence may impinge upon this trend (Boyer, 2006). The salient increase of delinquent behavior starts from early adolescence and usually reaches its peak at mid-adolescence (e.g., Farrell, Sullivan, Esposito, Meyer, & Valois, 2005). Unfortunately, research on the course of delinquent behavior in Chinese youth is almost nonexistent, although it was noted that Chinese youth reported a lower rate of delinquent behavior than Western youth (Jessor et al., 2003). For an exception, using individual growth curve models, Shek and Yu (2012) found an upward trend in delinquency in junior secondary school students of Hong Kong. Shek and Lin (2014) similarly reported significant time effect using repeated measure analysis. Based on these findings, it was hypothesized that delinquent behavior would increase during early adolescence of Hong Kong youth.

Family Influence

Given the increasing severity of delinquent behavior during adolescence, a large body of research has examined family protective and risk factors involved (e.g., Deković et al., 2003). Family characteristics including parenting practices, parent-child relationship, family systematic functioning, family structure, and economic status are well documented to be relevant to misconduct of youth (Deković et al., 2003; Hoeve et al., 2009, 2012).

To begin with, background family characteristics such as family economic status and family structure are associated with youth delinquency. Family poverty was found to be associated with a higher rate of delinquent behavior. According to the

Family Stress Model (e.g., Conger, Ge, Elder, Lorenz, & Simons, 1994; Mistry, Vandewater, Houston, & McLoyd, 2002), poverty-related stress would disrupt family dynamics (e.g., parent-child relationship, marriage relationship) or parents' adaptive functioning (e.g., parents' mental health), which further enhances the rate of externalizing problem of children. However, mixed findings were observed with regard to Hong Kong youth. While Shek's (2003) study on poor Hong Kong adolescents demonstrated the positive association between parents' and adolescents' perceived economic stress and adolescents' engagement in risk behavior, Shek and Lin's (2014) research on Hong Kong youth did not find any difference in delinquent behavior between poor youth and nonpoor youth.

In addition, family intactness also predicts youth delinquency. In the social control theory (Hirschi, 1969), it is asserted that family restructuring (e.g., divorce or remarriage) tends to weaken the bonding between parent and child, diminish parental monitoring, which eventually increases the risk behavior of adolescent children. The detrimental effect of broken family on proneness of youth delinquency was observed in many studies. Based on a sample of 720 UK adolescents, Jolliffe (2013) found that adolescents residing in non-intact families (not living with biological parents) reported higher rates of delinquent behavior than did those living in intact families. Shek and Leung's (2013) research on Hong Kong youth also echoed this finding.

On top of the background family factors, more proximal factors like parental support, monitoring, and attachment to parents were identified as protective factors of youth problem behavior (Hoeve et al., 2009, 2012). However, relatively fewer studies have examined family as a context where multiple family members were involved. The notion of family functioning pertains to how well the family functions as a system or as a whole (e.g., communication of family members and mutual support among family members) rather than simple dyadic relationship (e.g., parental support and parenting practices; Gorman-Smith, Tolan, Zelli, & Huesmann, 1996; Shek, 2002; Shek & Lin, 2014). Prior research has shown that adaptive family functioning was reversely associated with youth delinquency (e.g., Gorman-Smith et al., 1996; Schwartz, Pantin, Prado, Sullivan, & Szapocznik, 2005). Family context where there is no warmth, support, communication, or appropriate control but conflicts is likely to render deviant behavior engagement of youth directly or render deviant peer involvement which further increases the rate of youth individual delinquency (e.g., Henry, Tolan, & Gorman-Smith, 2001).

Research on the Hong Kong youth sample echoed these findings by revealing the negative association between family functioning and youth delinquency as well as problem behavior intention (Shek, Ma, & Tang, 2012). Nevertheless, whether family functioning can exert longitudinal effect over delinquency of Hong Kong youth is still unclear, which requires further research adopting a longitudinal approach. Lastly, the aforementioned family characteristics might interweave with each other, which gives rise to a possibility that some aspects of family characteristics may be only spuriously related to youth delinquent behavior (Deković et al., 2003). As such, it is necessary to test their relative contribution in a single statistical model.

Positive Youth Development

Healthy development of adolescents was usually conceived in terms of absence of psychosocial symptoms and problem behavior. Nevertheless, the traditional conceptualization of adolescent development has been challenged by the positive youth perspective (Lerner et al., 2000; Roth & Brooks-Gunn, 2003; Shek, 2006a; Shek, Siu, & Lee, 2007). By focusing on the potentials and abilities rather than problems of youth, researchers claimed that nurturing adolescent developmental assets, abilities, and potentials would help them "navigate adolescence in a healthy way" (Roth & Brooks-Gunn, 2003, p. 94). Catalano, Berglund, Ryan, Lonczak, and Hawkins (2004) identified 15 positive youth development constructs from the effective positive youth development programs which include bonding, resilience, cognitive competence, emotional competence, social competence, behavioral competence, moral competence, self-determination, self-efficacy, clear and positive identity, belief in the future, spirituality, development of prosocial norms, opportunities for prosocial involvement, and recognition for positive behavior. Empirical research has shown that youth problem behavior can be reduced by promoting their positive youth development attributes, including psychosocial competencies (Haegerich & Tolan, 2008), character (Parker, Nelson, & Burns, 2010), or overall positive youth development attributes (Lewin-Bizan et al., 2010). In the Chinese context, a series of studies showed that positive youth development attributes were negatively associated with problem behavior intention, substance abuse, and delinquent behavior (e.g., Shek & Ma, 2011; Shek & Yu, 2011; Sun & Shek, 2010, 2013).

The Current Study

Against the above background, a longitudinal study was conducted to examine delinquent behavior among junior secondary school students in Hong Kong. Several research questions were asked in this study:

1. What is the prevalence of delinquent behavior in junior secondary school students in Hong Kong?
2. Does delinquent behavior change with time in Hong Kong Chinese youth? Based on the previous studies (Overbeek et al., 2001; Shek & Yu, 2012), it was hypothesized that adolescent delinquent behavior would increase in the early adolescent years (Hypothesis 1).
3. Are background family characteristics related to youth delinquent behavior? Based on the existing literature, it was hypothesized that:
   (a) Adolescent boys would have more delinquent behavior than did adolescent girls (Jessor et al., 2003; Hypothesis 2a).
   (b) Adolescents experiencing economic disadvantage would have more delinquent behavior than did adolescents without economic disadvantage (Conger et al., 1994; Hypothesis 2b).

(c) Adolescents from non-intact families would have more delinquent behavior than did adolescents from intact families (Jolliffe, 2013; Shek & Leung, 2013; Hypothesis 2c).

4. Is family functioning related to delinquent behavior? Based on the existing findings (Schwartz et al., 2005; Shek et al., 2012), the general expectation was that family functioning would be negatively related to delinquency (Hypothesis 3).
5. Is positive youth development related to delinquent behavior? Based on the existing evidence (Lewin-Bizan et al., 2010; Sun & Shek, 2010, 2013), it was expected that positive youth development would be negatively related to delinquency.

Methods

The data were derived from three consecutive waves of a 6-year longitudinal study assessing adolescents' psychosocial development and their families in Hong Kong. A total of 3,328 Secondary One students (age = 12.59 ± 0.74 years) from 28 randomly selected secondary schools participated in the Wave 1 assessment. Among them, 52.3 % were male and 78.1 % were born in Hong Kong. In addition, 84.4 % of them were from intact families while others were from non-intact families with parents separated, divorced, remarried, or with other reasons. Finally, 5.8 % of them reported receiving financial aid from the Hong Kong government (Comprehensive Social Security Assistance: CSSA) during the assessment, which indicates they were experiencing family poverty. The second assessment was administrated 1 year later with a total of 3,638 Secondary Two students (age = 13.64 ± 0.75 years) recruited. The third assessment was conducted 2 years later with a total of 4,106 Secondary Three students (14.65 years ± 0.80 year) involved. Across the assessment period, a total of 2,667 students completed three waves of assessment, which indicated an acceptable attrition rate of 19.9 %. Other demographic information about the participants is shown in Table 1.

Parental and student consent had been obtained prior to data collection. During the data collection, the purpose of the study and confidentiality of the data were repeatedly emphasized to all participants. Students finished the questionnaire in a self-report manner with sufficient time. A trained research assistant was present throughout the administration process.

Instruments

Delinquent Behavior

Participants' delinquent behavior was measured by 12-item delinquent behavior scale. Respondents filled in the scale by indicating how frequent they engaged in 12 delinquent behaviors in the past year, ranging from 0 (never) to 6 (more than 10

Table 1 Demographic profile of the participants

	Wave 1		Wave 2		Wave 3	
	N	%	*N*	%	*N*	%
Gender						
Male	1,718	52.3	1,864	52.1	2,185	53.7
Female	1,570	47.7	1,716	47.9	1,885	46.3
Place of birth						
Hong Kong	2,589	78.1	2,806	77.9	3,195	79.4
Others	724	15.3	795	22.1	904	22.1
Family economic status						
Not receiving CSSA	2,932	81.2	2,605	79.1	3,308	81.4
Receiving CSSA	208	5.8	225	6.8	212	5.2
Others (don't know)	472	13.1	463	9.8	545	13.4
Parents' marital status						
Intact marriage	2,779	84.4	2,985	82.7	3,372	82.5
Non-intact family	514	15.6	624	17.3	715	17.5

Note. The cases with missing data were not included

[a]Intact family refers to family of first marriage; non-intact family refers to family with parents separated, divorced, remarried, or with other reasons

times). The delinquent behaviors included stealing, cheating, truancy, running away from home, vandalism, assault, engaging in sexual relationship with others, gang fighting, speaking foul language, staying away from home without parental consent, strong-arming others, and breaking into residences. The reliabilities of the scale across three waves were satisfactory, αs > .70 (see Table 2).

The Chinese Positive Youth Development Scale (CPYDS)

Participants' positive youth development was assessed by the short form of the Chinese Positive Youth Development Scale (CPYDS; Shek et al., 2007). The CPYDS consists of 15 subscales which assess adolescents' functioning in bonding (BO), resilience (RE), social competence (SC), recognition for positive behavior (PB), emotional competence (EC), cognitive competence (CC), behavioral competence (BC), moral competence (MC), self-determination (SD), self-efficacy (SE), clear and positive identity (CPI), beliefs in the future (BF), prosocial involvement (PI), prosocial norms (PN), and spirituality (SP). Each subscale was measured by a 6-point scale except SP that was measured by a 7-point scale. Participants were required to indicate the extent they agree with the statements in the questionnaire. Shek and Ma's (2010) multigroup confirmatory factor analyses (MCFA) revealed that four higher-order factors can be derived from the 15 subscales, which are cognitive-behavioral competencies (CBC), prosocial attributes (PA), positive identity (PIT), and general positive youth development qualities (GPYDQ). In the current study, we used a composite score by averaging all the items across 15 subscales,

Table 2 Descriptive statistics of key variables and internal consistency coefficients of scales (Wave 1–3)

	Mean (SD)			Cronbach's α		
	W1	W2	W3	W1	W2	W3
Family functioning						
Mutuality	3.89 (.89)	3.80 (.90)	3.82 (.87)	.87	.88	.89
Harmony	3.81 (.92)	3.73 (.93)	3.70 (.92)	.76	.78	.79
Communication	3.51 (1.01)	3.41 (.96)	3.43 (.93)	.81	.81	.81
CFAIALL	3.73 (.81)	3.65 (.81)	3.65 (.79)	.90	.90	.90
Positive youth development						
CBC	4.45 (.75)	4.42 (.74)	4.43 (.70)	.87	.89	.89
PA	4.50 (.89)	4.38 (.86)	4.39 (.82)	.83	.84	.83
GPYDQ	4.58 (.71)	4.51 (.71)	4.52 (.67)	.93	.93	.93
PIT	4.24 (.96)	4.16 (.96)	4.14 (.93)	.87	.89	.89
PYD	4.51 (.70)	4.43 (.69)	4.44 (.65)	.96	.96	.96
Delinquent behavior						
Overall	.39 (.47)	.47 (.58)	.46 (.55)	.70	.76	.72
Male	.43 (.51)	.52 (.60)	.52 (.60)	–	–	–
Female	.35 (.42)	.43 (.55)	.39 (.46)	–	–	–
Families without economic disadvantage	.39 (.46)	.47 (.56)	.46 (.51)	–	–	–
Families with economic disadvantage	.41 (.42)	.53 (.63)	.50 (.63)	–	–	–
Intact families	.37 (.46)	.45 (.57)	.43 (.48)	–	–	–
Non-intact families	.48 (.52)	.56 (.60)	.60 (.78)	–	–	–

Note. W1 Wave 1, *W2* Wave 2, *W3* Wave 3, *CFAIALL* total score of family functioning, *CBC* cognitive-behavioral competencies, *PA* prosocial attributes, *GPYDQ* general positive youth development, *PIT* positive identity, *PYD* total score of positive youth development. Intact family refers to family of first marriage; non-intact family includes family with parents separated, divorced, remarried, or with other reasons

with higher scores indicating better positive youth development. The reliabilities of the whole scale across three waves were satisfactory, $\alpha s > .96$ (see Table 2).

The Chinese Family Assessment Instrument (CFAI)

Participants' family functioning was evaluated by the simplified version of the Chinese Family Assessment Instrument with nine items (Shek, 2002). This scale assesses perceived family functioning in three dimensions: mutuality (mutual support, love, and concern among family members), communication (frequency and nature of interaction among family members), as well as conflicts (presence of conflicts in the family). Mean scores were calculated after scores of items assessing conflicts were reversed. Higher scores indicate better family functioning. The reliabilities of the whole scale across three waves were satisfactory, $\alpha s > .90$ (see Table 2).

Basic Family Characteristics

Participants' family economic status was indicated by whether they received financial aids (CSSA) from the Hong Kong government or not. Those who reported receiving CSSA were regarded as experiencing family poverty. In addition, the current marital status of participants' parents was recorded (1 = divorced, 2 = separated, 3 = first marriage, 4 = second marriage, 5 = others). In this study, participants whose parents were in first marriage were grouped into the category of intact family while others were grouped into the category of non-intact family.

Data Analytic Plan

The first objective of the current study was to provide descriptive profile of different types of delinquent behaviors among junior secondary school students in Hong Kong. Therefore, the numbers and proportions of youths who have never attempted misconduct, attempted less than 6 times, and attempted more than 6 times were presented. The second objective was to investigate the trend of delinquent behavior during junior secondary school years. Therefore, a mixed ANOVA analysis was conducted with delinquent behavior as repeated measure while gender as a between-subject variable. The last objective was to examine whether positive youth development, family functioning, and other family demographic factors (i.e., family economic status and family intactness) were predictive of adolescent delinquent behavior in a longitudinal approach. We first examined which factors would contribute to the severity of delinquent behavior. As such, multiple regression analyses were conducted, in which participants' characteristics at Wave 1 predicted their delinquent behavior at Wave 2 and Wave 3, respectively, while gender was controlled. As the distribution of delinquent behavior was not normal, with most of the respondents reporting nonoccurrence on many types of delinquent behaviors, we also examined which factors would account for their involvement in delinquent behavior. As such, the mean scores of delinquent behavior were re-coded as dichotomous variable with "0" indicating "never conducted any delinquent behavior in the past year" and "1" indicating "have conducted at least one type of delinquent behavior in the past year." Then, the occurrence of delinquent behavior at Wave 2 and Wave 3 was regressed on positive youth development and family factors, controlling gender, and initial occurrence of delinquent behavior, respectively.

Results

Descriptive Profiles

The prevalence of delinquent behavior among Hong Kong youth is presented in Table 3. The proportions of students who have conducted delinquent behavior were generally low across junior secondary school years. For example, more than 90 %

Table 3 Delinquent behaviors in the past year

	Never			Attempted (1–6 times)			Attempted (6 times or above)		
	N (%)			*N* (%)			*N* (%)		
	Wave 1	Wave 2	Wave 3	Wave 1	Wave 2	Wave 3	Wave 1	Wave 2	Wave 3
1. Stealing	2,980 (89.6)	3,273 (90.0)	3,662 (89.2)	318 (9.6)	318 (8.7)	284 (6.9)	16 (0.5)	41 (1.1)	27 (0.7)
2. Cheating	1,298 (39.0)	1,378 (37.9)	1,644 (40.0)	1,602 (48.2)	1,678 (46.1)	1,625 (39.6)	410 (12.3)	565 (15.5)	690 (16.8)
3. Truancy	3,205 (96.4)	3,438 (94.5)	3,731 (90.9)	96 (2.9)	164 (4.5)	210 (5.1)	13 (0.4)	30 (0.8)	28 (0.7)
4. Running away from home	3,182 (95.7)	3,455 (95.0)	3,784 (92.2)	127 (3.8)	161 (4.4)	174 (4.2)	5 (0.2)	11 (0.3)	13 (0.3)
5. Damaging others' properties	2,861 (86.0)	3,164 (87.0)	3,593 (87.5)	417 (12.5)	419 (11.5)	337 (8.2)	27 (0.8)	46 (1.3)	38 (0.9)
6. Assault	2,922 (87.9)	3,226 (88.7)	3,633 (88.5)	342 (10.3)	341 (9.4)	276 (6.7)	46 (1.4)	60 (1.6)	58 (1.4)
7. Having sexual intercourse with others	3,290 (98.9)	3,572 (98.2)	3,903 (95.1)	20 (0.6)	37 (1.0)	40 (1.0)	2 (0.1)	17 (0.5)	29 (0.7)
8. Group fighting	3,182 (95.7)	3,477 (95.6)	3,841 (93.5)	96 (2.9)	103 (2.8)	88 (2.1)	14 (0.4)	30 (0.8)	26 (0.6)
9. Speaking foul language	1,000 (30.1)	1,041 (28.6)	1,259 (30.7)	1,458 (43.8)	1,335 (36.7)	1,234 (30.1)	802 (24.1)	1,244 (34.2)	1,459 (35.5)
10. Staying outside overnight without parents' consent	3,177 (95.5)	3,462 (95.2)	3,772 (91.9)	80 (2.4)	124 (3.4)	142 (3.5)	19 (0.6)	34 (0.9)	42 (1.0)
11. Strong arming others	2,762 (83.1)	3,082 (84.7)	3,545 (86.3)	436 (13.1)	435 (12.0)	319 (7.8)	77 (2.3)	111 (3.1)	102 (2.5)
12. Trespasses	3,139 (94.4)	3,501 (96.2)	3,853 (93.8)	112 (3.4)	102 (2.8)	87 (2.1)	11 (0.3)	19 (0.5)	29 (0.7)

Table 4 Results of mixed effect ANOVAs on life satisfaction

Source of variation	df	F	p	η_p^2
Time	(2, 2270)	44.68	.000	.038
Gender[a]	(1, 2271)	22.78	.000	.010
Time × gender	(2, 2270)	5.11	.006	.004

[a]Male = 1; female = 0

of the respondents had never engaged in truancy, running away from home, sexual intercourse with others, group fighting, staying out overnight without parents' consent, and trespasses. Yet, cheating (>50 %) and speaking foul language (>60 %) were more prevalent among respondents. Moreover, quite a proportion of adolescents ever damaged others' properties and engaged in assault (>10 %).

Variation of Delinquent Behavior with Time

In order to examine the changes of delinquent behavior during junior secondary school years by gender, we performed one mixed ANOVA analysis with time as repeated measure and gender as a between-subject variable. As shown in Table 4, the main effects of time ($F(2, 2270) = 44.68$, $p < .001$, $\eta_p^2 = .038$) and gender were observed ($F(1, 2271) = 22.78$, $p < .001$, $\eta_p^2 = .010$), and the interaction effect between time and gender ($F(2, 2270) = 5.11$, $p < .01$, $\eta_p^2 = .004$) was also significant.

Bonferroni post hoc comparisons further revealed that delinquent behavior significantly increased from Wave 1 assessment to Wave 2 assessment while remained stable from Wave 2 assessment to Wave 3 assessment (Wave 1 vs. Wave 2: $p < .001$; Wave 1 vs. Wave 3: $p < .001$; Wave 2 vs. Wave 3: ns.). Though the interaction effect was significant, further tests did not uncover notably divergent patterns between boys and girls. For boys, their delinquent behavior significantly increased from Wave 1 assessment to Wave 2 assessment while remained stable from Wave 2 assessment to Wave 3 assessment (Wave 1 vs. Wave 2: $p < .001$; Wave 1 vs. Wave 3: $p < .001$; Wave 2 vs. Wave 3: ns.). For girls, their delinquent behavior significantly increased from Wave 1 assessment to Wave 2 assessment yet showed an insignificantly declining trend from Wave 2 assessment to Wave 3 assessment (Wave 1 vs. Wave 2: $p < .001$; Wave 1 vs. Wave 3: $p < .01$; Wave 2 vs. Wave 3: ns.). Boys consistently reported higher levels of delinquent behavior than girls (Wave 1: $p < .01$; Wave 2: $p < .001$; Wave 3: $p < .001$).

Psychosocial Correlates of Delinquent Behavior

The zero-order correlations of delinquent behavior with positive youth development and family factors are presented in Tables 5, 6, and 7. Family economic status was not related to delinquent behavior across three waves, while family

Table 5 Correlations of delinquent behavior at three waves with positive youth development and family factors at Wave 1

	1	2	3	4	5	6	7	8	9	10	11	12	13	14	15
1. DE	1.00														
2. SDE	.57	1.00													
3. TDE	.47	.57	1.00												
4. CFAIM	–.29	–.23	–.18	1.00											
5. CFAIH	–.25	–.24	–.19	.61	1.00										
6. CFAICOM	–.31	–.25	–.19	.77	.49	1.00									
7. CFAIALL	–.33	–.28	–.21	.92	.80	.88	1.00								
8. CBC	–.21	–.17	–.14	.39	.20	.38	.37	1.00							
9. PA	–.35	–.25	–.19	.42	.26	.42	.42	.60	1.00						
10. GPYDQ	–.34	–.26	–.22	.54	.36	.53	.55	.80	.74	1.00					
11. PIT	–.23	–.15	–.13	.43	.26	.41	.42	.71	.63	.75	1.00				
12. PYD	–.33	–.26	–.21	.52	.34	.52	.53	.88	.82	.97	.84	1.00			
13. Gender	.08	.08	.11	.05	–.05	.08	.04	.02[n]	–.14	–.07	.01[n]	–.05	1.00		
14. SFES	.01[n]	.07	.04	–.07	.08	–.08	–.10	–.03[n]	–.03[n]	–.03[n]	–.07	–.05	–.03[n]	1.00	
15. SFI	–.08	–.07	–.07	.19	.17	.15	.19	.07	.09	.10	.08	.10	.01[n]	–.35	1.00

Note. DE delinquent behavior at Wave 1, *SDE* delinquent behavior at Wave 2, *TDE* delinquent behavior at Wave 3, *CFAIM* family mutuality, *CFAIH* family harmony, *CFAICOM* family communication, *CFAIALL* total score of family functioning, *CBC* cognitive behavior competencies, *PA* prosocial attribute, *GPYDQ* general positive youth development, *PIT* positive identity, *PYD* total score of positive youth development, *SFES* family economic status (*0* not receiving CSSA, *1* receiving CSSA), *SFI* family intactness (*0* non-intact family, *1* intact family)

[n]The correlations were not significant at $p < .05$ level

Table 6 Correlations of delinquent behavior with positive youth development and family functioning at Wave 2

	1	2	3	4	5	6	7	8	9	10	11	12	13
1. SDE	1.00												
2. SCFAIM	–.27	1.00											
3. SCFAIH	–.21	.61	1.00										
4. SCFAICOM	–.25	.78	.49	1.00									
5. SCFAIALL	–.28	.92	.81	.88	1.00								
6. SCBC	–.22	.38	.18	.36	.35	1.00							
7. SPA	–.29	.41	.26	.40	.41	.60	1.00						
8. SGPYDQ	–.31	.52	.33	.51	.52	.80	.75	1.00					
9. SPIT	–.17	.40	.22	.40	.39	.71	.63	.75	1.00				
10. SPYD	–.29	.50	.30	.49	.50	.88	.81	.97	.84	1.00			
11. SGender	.08	.05	–.01[n]	.09	.05	.04	–.14	–.06	.03	–.03[n]	1.00		
12. SFES	.03[n]	–.08	–.08	–.07	–.09	–.01[n]	–.03[n]	–.04	–.05	–.05	–.02[n]	1.00	
13. SFI	–.07	.18	.13	.15	.18	.05	.07	.08	.05	.08	.02[n]	–.28	1.00

Note. SDE delinquent behavior, *SCFAIM* family mutuality, *SCFAIH* family harmony, *SCFAICOM* family communication, *SCFAIALL* total score of family functioning, *SCBC* cognitive behavior competencies, *SPA* prosocial attribute, *SGPYDQ* general positive youth development, *SPIT* positive identity, *SPYD* total score of positive youth development, *SFES* family economic status (*0* not receiving CSSA, *1* receiving CSSA), *SFI* family intactness (*0* non-intact family, *1* intact family)

[n]The correlations were not significant at $p < .05$ level

Table 7 Correlations of delinquent behavior with positive youth development and family functioning at Wave 3

	1	2	3	4	5	6	7	8	9	10	11	12	13
1. TDE	1.00												
2. TCFAIM	−.23	1.00											
3. TCFAIH	−.19	.63	1.00										
4. TCFAICOM	−.22	.77	.49	1.00									
5. TCFAIALL	−.25	.92	.81	.87	1.00								
6. TCBC	−.13	.34	.18	.35	.33	1.00							
7. TPA	−.23	.37	.23	.37	.38	.57	1.00						
8. TGPYDQ	−.22	.49	.31	.49	.50	.79	.72	1.00					
9. TPIT	−.13	.35	.21	.38	.36	.70	.61	.74	1.00				
10. TPYD	−.22	.47	.29	.48	.48	.87	.79	.97	.84	1.00			
11. TGender	.11	.01[n]	−.04[n]	.06	.01[n]	.05	−.13	−.04	.07	−.02[n]	1.00		
12. SFES	.02[n]	−.08	−.05	−.06	−.07	−.01[n]	−.01[n]	−.04	−.04	−.03	−.02	1.00	
13. SFI	−.12	.17	.13	.13	.17	.03[n]	.05	.05	.03[n]	.04	.03[n]	−.28	1.00

Note. TDE delinquent behavior, *TCFAIM* family mutuality, *TCFAIH* family harmony, *TCFAICOM* family communication, *TCFAIALL* total score of family functioning, *TCBC* cognitive behavior competencies, *TPA* prosocial attribute, *TGPYDQ* general positive youth development, *TPIT* positive identity, *TPYD* total score of positive youth development, *SFES* family economic status (*0* not receiving CSSA, *1* receiving CSSA), *SFI* family intactness (*0* non-intact family; *1* intact family)

[n]The correlations were not significant at $p<.05$ level

Table 8 Multiple regression analyses on delinquent behavior at Wave 2

	Model 1 (controlling DE)				Model 2 (not controlling DE)			
Predictors at Wave 1	Beta	*p*	R^2 change	*p*	Beta	*p*	R^2 change	*p*
Step 1			.329	.000	–	–	–	–
DE	.532	.000			–	–	–	–
Step 2			.002	.021			.006	.001
Gender[a]	.051	.008			.080	.000		
Step 3			.003	.011			.007	.002
Family economic disadvantage[b]	.045	.028			.036	.126		
Family intactness[c]	.000	.996			−.003	.892		
Step 4			.009	.000			.098	.000
CFAIALL	−.089	.000			−.204	.000		
PYD	−.021	.363			−.158	.000		

Note. DE delinquent behavior at Wave 1, *CFAIALL* total score of family functioning, *PYD* total score of positive youth development
[a]Male = 1, Female = 0
[b]Receiving CSSA = 1, Not receiving CSSA = 0
[c]Intact = 1, Non-intact = 0

intactness was negatively associated with delinquent behavior across three waves to a minor degree. The concurrent associations also indicated that better family functioning and positive youth development were associated with a lower level of delinquent behavior. As the correlations of different factors of positive youth development with delinquent behavior were consistent, we used a composite score of positive youth development (PYD) across all 15 subscales for further analyses. Similarly, a composite score of family functioning across three dimensions was employed for the following analyses.

To further examine the overtime effect of positive youth development, family functioning, and other family factors, four sets of multiple regression analyses were conducted after controlling gender, with the first two sets analyzing the 1-year overtime effects while another two sets analyzing the 2-year overtime effects. As shown in Table 8, when respondents' characteristics at Wave 1 predicted delinquent behavior at Wave 2, the prediction of family functioning ($\beta = -.204$, $p < .001$) and positive youth development ($\beta = -.158$, $p < .001$) was significant, respectively. Adolescents who experienced better positive youth development and family functioning reported low levels of delinquent behavior 1 year later. However, initial family economic status and family intactness did not predict delinquent behavior 1 year later. When initial level of delinquent behavior was controlled, only family functioning significantly predicted delinquent behavior 1 year later ($\beta = -.089$, $p < .001$). Similarly, as shown in Table 9, initial state of family functioning ($\beta = -.147$, $p < .001$) and positive youth development ($\beta = -.145$, $p < .001$) significantly predicted youths' delinquent behavior 2 years later. However, only family functioning ($\beta = -.050$, $p < .05$) was significantly predictive of youths' delinquent behavior to a small degree 2 years later with initial state of delinquent behavior controlled.

Table 9 Multiple regression analyses on delinquent behavior at Wave 3

	Model 1 (controlling DE)				Model 2 (not controlling DE)			
Predictors at Wave 1	Beta	*p*	R^2 change	*p*	Beta	*p*	R^2 change	*p*
Step 1			.229	.000	–	–	–	–
DE	.441	.000			–	–	–	–
Step 2			.012	.000			.020	.000
Gender[a]	.115	.000			.145	.000		
Step 3			.001	.188			.005	.008
Family economic disadvantage[b]	.017	.443			.017	.486		
Family intactness[c]	−.017	.464			−.025	.313		
Step 4			.005	.005			.064	.000
CFAIALL	−.050	.048			−.147	.000		
PYD	−.036	.145			−.145	.000		

Note. DE delinquent behavior at Wave 1, *CFAIALL* total score of family functioning, *PYD* total score of positive youth development
[a]Male = 1, Female = 0
[b]Receiving CSSA = 1, Not receiving CSSA = 0
[c]Intact = 1, Non-intact = 0

Regarding the question about the predictors of occurrence of delinquent behavior, we performed two sets of logistic regression analyses, controlling gender and initial occurrence of delinquent behavior (see Tables 10 and 11). The results showed that adolescents who demonstrated delinquent behavior at Wave 1 were 6.680 times more likely to conduct delinquent behavior at Wave 2, while 5.447 times at Wave 3. Next, when controlling the influence of initial occurrence of delinquent behavior, respondents' Family Functioning significantly predicted the likelihood of misconduct at Wave 3, but not at Wave 2. Specifically, the occurrence of delinquent behavior at Wave 3 (having delinquent behavior) was associated with worse family functioning (OR = .814, $p < .05$) and weaker positive youth development (OR = .755, $p < .05$) at Wave 1, to a small degree.

Discussion

The overarching objectives of the current study were to investigate the youth delinquent behavior across three consecutive years and its psychosocial correlates. Based on a large sample of Hong Kong junior secondary school students, we found that, generally, the prevalence rates of youth delinquency were low. It is in line with previous studies conducted in mainland China revealing that Chinese youth reported a lower rate of delinquency than Western youth (e.g., Greenberger, Chen, Beam, Whang, & Dong, 2000; Jessor et al., 2003). Compared with another study on Hong Kong early adolescent sample (Lau & Kan, 2010), more adolescents in our study

Table 10 Logistic regression analyses on delinquent behavior[a] at Wave 2

Predictors at Wave 1	*B*	Wald X^2	*p*	Odds ratio (OR)	95 % C.I. Lower	95 % C.I. Upper
Step 1						
DE	1.899	179.754	.000	6.680	5.060	8.817
Step 2						
Gender[b]	.018	.018	.895	1.018	.785	1.319
Step 3						
Family economic disadvantage[c]	.423	1.905	.168	1.526	.837	2.783
Family intactness[d]	.184	.802	.370	1.202	.804	1.797
Step 4						
CFAIALL	−.110	1.139	.286	.895	.731	1.097
PYD	−.129	1.145	.285	.879	.695	1.113

Note. DE delinquent behavior at Wave 1, *CFAIALL* total score of family functioning, *PYD* total score of positive youth development

[a]Having at least one type of delinquent behavior = 1, Not having any delinquent behavior =0

[b]Male = 1, Female = 0

[c]Receiving CSSA = 1, Not receiving CSSA = 0

[d]Intact = 1, Non-intact = 0

Table 11 Logistic regression analyses on delinquent behavior[a] at Wave 3

Predictors at Wave 1	*B*	Wald X^2	*p*	Odds ratio (OR)	95 % C.I. Lower	95 % C.I. Upper
Step 1						
DE	1.695	145.959	.000	5.447	4.137	7.171
Step 2						
Gender[b]	−.118	.846	.358	.889	.692	1.142
Step 3						
Family economic disadvantage[c]	.151	.243	.622	1.163	.638	2.118
Family intactness[d]	.083	.159	.690	1.086	.724	1.629
Step 4						
CFAIALL	−.206	4.233	.040	.814	.668	.990
PYD	−.281	5.667	.017	.755	.599	.952

Note. DE delinquent behavior at Wave 1, *CFAIALL* total score of family functioning, *PYD* total score of positive youth development

[a]Having at least one type of delinquent behavior = 1, Not having any delinquent behavior = 0

[b]Male = 1, Female = 0

[c]Receiving CSSA = 1, Not receiving CSSA = 0

[d]Intact = 1, Non-intact = 0

reported nonengagement in delinquent behavior (i.e., sex intercourse: 98.9 % vs. 92.1 %; running away: 95.7 % vs. 88.2 %; property damaging: 86.0 % vs. 73.4 %). However, it is worth noting that cheating and speaking foul language appear popular among Hong Kong youth. As academic achievement is highly emphasized in Hong

Kong society, it is not uncommon for students to take risk to cheat on the examination for a desirable grade. Additionally, the peer culture is tolerant of this kind of academic dishonesty (see Nora & Zhang, 2010). Yet, it is argued that cheating may dampen students' motivation for learning (Cizek, 2003). Therefore, more efforts are required to examine the detriment of cheating. The prevalence of using foul language is similar to the finding of the Youth Opinion Survey (72.2 %; Hong Kong Federation of Youth Groups, 2009). Speaking foul language might have become a subculture of youth, which is acceptable among the peers.

An increasing trend of delinquent behavior was witnessed in our study, which is consistent with prior studies in Western (Overbeek et al., 2001) and Hong Kong youth (Shek & Yu, 2012). A significant escalation was observed during the transition from Secondary One to Secondary Two, which indicates a critical period when intervention can be provided for risky adolescents. In line with much extant literature (e.g., Jessor et al., 2003), boys reported higher rates of delinquent behavior than girls. However, boys did not notably differ from girls in the pattern of delinquency growth notwithstanding the significant interaction effect of gender and time. Such findings are in congruent with Farrell et al.'s (2005) study in which gender made difference in the initial level of delinquency yet not in the trajectory of change. A possible explanation for gender difference may lie in parenting monitoring and deviant peer involvement that exert primary influence on youth delinquency (O'Donnell, Richards, Pearce, & Romero, 2012), as boys tend to have looser parental monitoring yet more alliance with delinquent peers than girls (Kerr & Stattin, 2000; Liu & Kaplan, 1999).

As far as family characteristics were concerned, poor adolescents unexpectedly did not report higher levels of delinquent behavior than their nonpoor counterparts. As we used the receipt of CSSA as the index of family poverty, it is possible that those receiving social welfare were still not the poorest ones. Also, some poor families could not get the governmental financial aid due to various reasons (Census and Statistics Department, 2013). Since the Hong Kong government published the first official poverty line recently (Ip, 2013), it may be better to refer to the poverty line when categorizing family economic status in the future.

Looking at the concurrent associations, adolescents from intact families reported lower rates of delinquency than those from non-intact families. The non-intact structure of family implies more problems, such as problems in parenting practices and parent-child relationship (Shek, 2007), which possibly enhances the deviant involvement of youth. However, family structure was not predictive of both severity and presence of delinquent behavior longitudinally when other family characteristics were concerned. Back to the questions regarding the relative effects of different family characteristics (Deković et al., 2003), the current findings suggest that the effect of family intactness may be weaker than family functioning or other proximal family factors in predicting youth deviant involvement. It is also possible that the effect of family structure is mediated by family functioning, which requires further evidence.

The findings with respect to family functioning generally supported the hypothesis notwithstanding some insignificant effects. The findings together with the previous study in Hong Kong (Shek et al., 2012) suggest that healthy family functioning is relevant to minimizing the severity and presence of Hong Kong youth delinquency. Moreover, the longitudinal findings can be construed as a positive response to the call for longitudinal research in Chinese family process (Shek, 2006b). However, as initial status of family functioning predicted delinquent behavior in Wave 3 but not that in Wave 2, the effect of family function may be time dependent.

Akin to prior research, the concurrent associations of the current study showed that positive youth development was related with less delinquent involvement. Also, the longitudinal result revealed that Hong Kong early adolescents with better positive youth development were less likely to engage in delinquent behavior 2 years later. Suggested by Sun and Shek (2013), positive youth development attributes can be construed as developmental assets to protect youth from vulnerability to risks. On the other hand, positive youth development did not predict the severity of youth delinquency when initial level of positive youth development was controlled. As multiple predictors were included in the regression model, it is possible that the effect was reduced when shared variance was excluded. It is noted that positive youth development was moderately associated with family functioning across the three waves (rs = .48 to .51). It is also possible that positive youth development exerts indirect effect over time. As the findings are not definitive, further endeavor is still needed, for example, to explore if there is any mediator that could transfer the influence of positive youth development to youth delinquency (e.g., life satisfaction; Sun & Shek, 2013).

To summarize, the current study has made several contributions to the existing documents about youth delinquency. First, it clarifies the prevalence of youth delinquency in Hong Kong across 3 years. Meanwhile, it arouses our concerns toward popular youth phenomena of cheating and foul language. Moreover, the heightened delinquent behavior among male adolescents and those from non-intact families is still worthy of attention. Lastly, it basically supports theoretical prediction on the role of family functioning and positive youth development, which provides evidence to carry out intervention project enhancing family functioning and positive youth development of Hong Kong adolescents (e.g., the Project P.A.T.H.S.; Shek, 2006a). Taken together, the current findings help to build up theoretical model of youth delinquency in the Chinese context.

Limitations

Despite the contributions, the findings of the current study should be interpreted cautiously because of several notable limitations. Firstly, self-report was employed in this study. Although it is a common practice to employ self-administered data in studying youth delinquency, it cannot exclude the possibility that social desirability hinders respondents from reporting the true frequency of delinquent behavior. We encourage obtaining different perspectives like peer reports, teacher reports, and parent reports in future studies, not only for gathering delinquent information but also for assessing family characteristics and positive youth development. Secondly, the sample is restricted in Hong Kong society, which has socioeconomic and even cultural differences from other Chinese societies (e.g., mainland China, Taiwan). It should be cautious to generalize the current findings to other Chinese societies. Lastly, the current study is based on quantitative data, leaving several questions unresolved. For instance, why do Hong Kong adolescents receiving CSSA not demonstrate more delinquent behavior? In-depth qualitative research, like interview, can be exploited to explore economic status, family process, and youth development underlying the superficial phenomenon (Leung & Shek, 2011).

Acknowledgment The preparation for this work and the Project P.A.T.H.S. were financially supported by the Hong Kong Jockey Club Charities Trust.

References

Arnett, J. J. (1999). Adolescent storm and stress, reconsidered. *American Psychologist, 54*(5), 317–326.

Boyer, T. W. (2006). The development of risk-taking: A multi-perspective review. *Developmental Review, 26*(3), 291–345.

Catalano, R. F., Berglund, M. L., Ryan, J. A. M., Lonczak, H. S., & Hawkins, J. D. (2004). Positive youth development in the United States: Research findings on evaluations of positive youth development programs. *The Annals of the American Academy of Political Social Science, 591*, 98–124.

Census and Statistics Department. (2013). *Hong Kong poverty situation report 2012*. Hong Kong: Government of the Hong Kong SAR.

Cizek, G. J. (2003). *Detecting and preventing classroom cheating: Promoting integrity in assessment*. Thousand Oaks, CA: Sage.

Conger, R. D., Ge, X., Elder, G. H., Lorenz, F. O., & Simons, R. L. (1994). Economic stress, coercive family process, and developmental problems of adolescents. *Child Development, 65*(2), 541–561.

Deković, M., Janssens, J. M., & As, N. (2003). Family predictors of antisocial behavior in adolescence. *Family Process, 42*(2), 223–235.

Farrell, A. D., Sullivan, T. N., Esposito, L. E., Meyer, A. L., & Valois, R. F. (2005). A latent growth curve analysis of the structure of aggression, drug use, and delinquent behaviors and their interrelations over time in urban and rural adolescents. *Journal of Research on Adolescence, 15*(2), 179–204.

Gorman-Smith, D., Tolan, P. H., Zelli, A., & Huesmann, L. R. (1996). The relation of family functioning to violence among inner-city minority youths. *Journal of Family Psychology, 10*(2), 115.

Greenberger, E., Chen, C., Beam, M., Whang, S., & Dong, Q. (2000). The perceived social contexts of adolescents' misconduct: A comparative study of youths in three cultures. *Journal of Research on Adolescence, 10*, 365–388.

Haegerich, T. M., & Tolan, P. H. (2008). Core competencies and the prevention of adolescent substance use. *New Directions for Child and Adolescent Development, 2008*(122), 47–60.

Henry, D. B., Tolan, P. H., & Gorman-Smith, D. (2001). Longitudinal family and peer group effects on violence and nonviolent delinquency. *Journal of Clinical Child Psychology, 30*(2), 172–186.

Hirschi, T. (1969). *Causes of delinquency*. Berkeley, CA: University of California Press.

Hoeve, M., Dubas, J. S., Eichelsheim, V. I., van der Laan, P. H., Smeenk, W., & Gerris, J. R. (2009). The relationship between parenting and delinquency: A meta-analysis. *Journal of Abnormal Child Psychology, 37*(6), 749–775.

Hoeve, M., Stams, G. J. J., Van Der Put, C. E., Dubas, J. S., van der Laan, P. H., & Gerris, J. R. (2012). A meta-analysis of attachment to parents and delinquency. *Journal of Abnormal Child Psychology, 40*(5), 771–785.

Hong Kong Federation of Youth Groups. (2009). *The deviant behaviour of youth in Hong Kong*. Hong Kong. Retrieved from http://www.hkfyg.org.hk/yrc/chinese/yr-p184c.html

Ip, K. (2013, September 30). Poverty strategy in the works, says Lam. *The Standard*, p. P02.

Jessor, R., Turbin, M. S., Costa, F. M., Dong, Q., Zhang, H., & Wang, C. (2003). Adolescent problem behavior in China and the United States: A cross-national study of psychosocial protective factors. *Journal of Research on Adolescence, 13*(3), 329–360.

Jolliffe, D. (2013). Exploring the relationship between the Five-Factor Model of personality, social factors and self-reported delinquency. *Personality and Individual Differences, 55*, 47–52.

Kerr, M., & Stattin, H. (2000). What parents know, how they know it, and several forms of adolescent adjustment: Further support for a reinterpretation of monitoring. *Developmental Psychology, 36*(3), 366.

Lau, M., & Kan, M. Y. (2010). Prevalence and correlates of problem behaviors among adolescents in Hong Kong. *Asia-Pacific Journal of Public Health, 22*(3), 354–364.

Lerner, R. M., Fisher, C. B., & Weinberg, R. A. (2000). Applying developmental science in the 21st century: International scholarship for our times. *International Journal of Behavioral Development, 24*(1), 24–29.

Leung, J. T. Y., & Shek, D. T. L. (2011). Quantitative and qualitative approaches in the study of poverty and adolescent development: Separation or integration? *International Journal of Adolescent Medicine and Health, 23*(2), 115–121.

Lewin-Bizan, S., Bowers, E. P., & Lerner, R. M. (2010). One good thing leads to another: Cascades of positive youth development among American adolescents. *Development and Psychopathology, 22*(4), 759–770.

Liu, X., & Kaplan, H. B. (1999). Explaining the gender difference in adolescent delinquent behavior: A longitudinal test of mediating mechanisms. *Criminology, 37*(1), 195–216.

Mistry, R. S., Vandewater, E. A., Houston, A. C., & McLoyd, V. C. (2002). Economic well-being and children's social adjustment: The role of family process in an ethnically diverse low income sample. *Child Development, 73*(3), 935–951.

Nora, W. L. Y., & Zhang, K. C. (2010). Motives of cheating among secondary students: The role of self-efficacy and peer influence. *Asia Pacific Education Review, 11*(4), 573–584.

O'Donnell, P., Richards, M., Pearce, S., & Romero, E. (2012). Gender differences in monitoring and deviant peers as predictors of delinquent behavior among low-income urban African American youth. *The Journal of Early Adolescence, 32*(3), 431–459.

Overbeek, G., Vollebergh, W., Meeus, W., Engels, R., & Luijpers, E. (2001). Course, co-occurrence, and longitudinal associations of emotional disturbance and delinquency from adolescence to young adulthood: A six-year three-wave study. *Journal of Youth and Adolescence, 30*(4), 401–426.

Parker, D. C., Nelson, J. S., & Burns, M. K. (2010). Comparison of correlates of classroom behavior problems in schools with and without a school-wide character education program. *Psychology in the Schools, 47*(8), 817–827.

Roth, J. L., & Brooks-Gunn, J. (2003). What exactly is a youth development program? Answers from research and practice. *Applied Developmental Science, 7*(2), 94–111.

Schwartz, S. J., Pantin, H., Prado, G., Sullivan, S., & Szapocznik, J. (2005). Family functioning, identity, and problem behavior in Hispanic immigrant early adolescents. *The Journal of Early Adolescence, 25*(4), 392–420.

Shek, D. T. L. (2002). Assessment of family functioning in Chinese adolescents: The Chinese family assessment instrument. *International Perspectives on Child and Adolescent Mental Health, 2*, 297–316.

Shek, D. T. L. (2003). Economic stress, psychological well-being and problem behavior in Chinese adolescents with economic disadvantage. *Journal of Youth and Adolescence, 32*(4), 259–266.

Shek, D. T. L. (2006a). Adolescent developmental issues in Hong Kong: Relevance to positive youth development programs in Hong Kong. *International Journal of Adolescent Medicine and Health, 18*(3), 341–354.

Shek, D. T. L. (2006b). Chinese family research puzzles, progress, paradigms, and policy implications. *Journal of Family Issues, 27*(3), 275–284.

Shek, D. T. L. (2007). Intact and non-intact families in Hong Kong: Differences in perceived parental control processes, parent-child relational qualities, and adolescent psychological well-being. *Journal of Divorce & Remarriage, 47*(1–2), 157–172.

Shek, D. T. L., & Leung, H. (2013). Positive youth development, life satisfaction and problem behaviors of adolescents in intact and non-intact families in Hong Kong. *Frontiers in Pediatrics, 1*, 1–7.

Shek, D. T. L., & Lin, L. (2014). Personal well-being and family quality of life of early adolescents in Hong Kong: Do economic disadvantage and time matter? *Social Indicators Research, 117*, 795–809. doi:10.1007/s11205-013-0399-3.

Shek, D. T. L., & Ma, C. M. S. (2010). Dimensionality of the Chinese positive youth development scale: Confirmatory factor analyses. *Social Indicators Research, 98*(1), 41–59.

Shek, D. T. L., & Ma, C. M. S. (2011). Substance abuse in junior secondary school students in Hong Kong: Prevalence and psychosocial correlates. *International Journal of Child Health and Human Development, 4*(4), 433–442.

Shek, D. T. L., Ma, H. K., & Sun, R. C. F. (2011). A brief overview of adolescent developmental problems in Hong Kong. *The Scientific World Journal, 11*, 2243–2256.

Shek, D. T. L., Ma, C. M. S., & Tang, C. Y. P. (2012). Delinquency and problem behavior intention among early adolescents in Hong Kong: Profiles and psychosocial correlates. *International Journal on Disability and Human Development, 11*(2), 151–158.

Shek, D. T. L., Siu, A. M. H., & Lee, T. Y. (2007). The Chinese positive youth development scale: A validation study. *Research on Social Work Practice, 17*(3), 380–391.

Shek, D. T. L., & Yu, L. (2011). Descriptive profiles and correlates of substance use in Hong Kong adolescents: A longitudinal study. *International Journal of Child Health and Human Development, 4*(4), 443–460.

Shek, D. T. L., & Yu, L. (2012). Longitudinal impact of the Project PATHS on adolescent risk behavior: What happened after five years? *The Scientific World Journal, 2012*. doi:10.1100/2012/316029.

Sun, R. C. F., & Shek, D. T. L. (2010). Life satisfaction, positive youth development, and problem behaviour among Chinese adolescents in Hong Kong. *Social Indicators Research, 95*(3), 455–474.

Sun, R. C. F., & Shek, D. T. L. (2013). Longitudinal influences of positive youth development and life satisfaction on problem behaviour among adolescents in Hong Kong. *Social Indicators Research, 114*, 1171–1197. doi:10.1007/s11205-012-0196-4.

Substance Abuse in Junior Secondary School Students in Hong Kong

Daniel T.L. Shek and Janet T.Y. Leung

Abstract Based on three waves of longitudinal data collected from 2,667 secondary school students over the junior secondary school years, the prevalence of substance abuse behaviors among Hong Kong adolescents and the sociodemographic, familial, and psychosocial correlates of adolescent substance abuse were examined in the study. Results showed that drug use in the areas of smoking, drinking, and organ solvent deserves our attention. Results also showed that socioeconomic status as well as family conflicts and communication predicted adolescent substance abuse. At the same time, positive youth development attributes were negatively associated with adolescent substance abuse. The contributions of family functioning and positive youth development to the reduction of adolescent substance abuse are discussed.

Keywords Adolescent substance abuse • Economic disadvantage • Family functioning • Longitudinal study • Positive youth development

Introduction

Substance abuse is a growing social issue in Hong Kong and the global context. From the World Drug Report 2012 issued by the United Nations Office on Drugs and Crimes (2012), it was found that 5 % of the world's adult population was estimated to have used an illicit drug at least once in 2010. This implies that among 20 persons aged between 15 and 64, one has had the experience of drug abuse (i.e., ever use). Problem drug users were estimated to occupy about 0.6 % of the world's adult population. The illicit drugs have killed 0.245 million people each year and have brought misery to thousands of the families. They also contributed to crime, instability, health problems such as hepatitis B and C, and spread of HIV and

D.T.L. Shek, Ph.D., B.B.S., S.B.S., J.P. (✉)
Department of Applied Social Sciences, The Hong Kong Polytechnic University, Hunghom, Hong Kong
e-mail: daniel.shek@polyu.edu.hk

J.T.Y. Leung, Ph.D.
Department of Applied Social Sciences, City University of Hong Kong, Hong Kong, Hong Kong

D.T.L. Shek et al. (eds.), *Chinese Adolescents in Hong Kong*, Quality of Life in Asia 5, DOI 10.1007/978-981-287-143-5_8

further hindered social and economic development (United Nations Office on Drugs and Crimes, 2012). Global estimates of the prevalence of tobacco and alcohol are also alarming. It was estimated that 25 % and 42 % of the world's population aged 15 and above have had tobacco and alcohol use in the past month (United Nations Office on Drugs and Crimes, 2012).

Regarding adolescent use of drugs, it has also become a social problem in recent years (United Nations Office on Drugs and Crimes, 2012). From the 2012 Monitoring the Future (MTF) National Survey Report measuring the drug, alcohol, and tobacco use among the 8th, 10th, and 12th graders in the USA, the lifetime prevalence of alcohol, cigarettes, and illicit drug use among the adolescents (combined figures of 8th, 10th, and 12th graders) were 50.0 %, 27.0 %, and 34.1 %, respectively. It seems a good news that there has been a significant decline of alcohol and cigarette use since the peak at 1991 (80.1 % and 53.5 % of alcohol and cigarette use) and the trends were dropping steadily. However, the use of illicit drugs among adolescents has been rising since 2008 (32.6 %). Among the illicit drugs, marijuana was the most popular drug that adolescents use (37.9 %). Moreover, the trends in 30-day prevalence of the use of alcohol, cigarettes, and illicit drug use among adolescents were 25.9 %, 10.6 %, and 16.8 %, respectively, which remained high in figures (Johnston, O'Malley, Bachman, & Schulenberg, 2013). In Europe, adolescent use of illicit drugs was also a major social concern. The school surveys conducted by the European School Survey Project on Alcohol and Other Drugs in 35 European countries in 2007 identified that among 15- and 16-year-old students, 23 % of male and 17 % of female students had used drugs at least once (i.e., lifetime prevalence, Hibell et al., 2009).

Based on the reports of the Central Registry of Drug Abuse (CRDA) monitored by the Narcotics Division of the Hong Kong Special Administrative Region, there were two peaks of the substance abuse in the past 10 years. The first peak was in the early 2000s which was contributed by the rave party culture. The second peak happened in 2008–2009 when ketamine abuse was rapidly spread in secondary schools. It was found that young people under the age of 21 who had abused drugs rose by 49.0 % from 2005 to 2009, though there was a prominent decrease of 19.1 % and 28.6 % in 2010 and 2011, respectively. The percentage of adolescent drug abusers among all reported drug abusers increased from 14.0 % in 2003 to 24.4 % in 2008, with a decrease of 22.4 % and 8.5 % in 2010 and 2011, respectively (Narcotics Division, 2012).

Shek and Leung (2013) highlighted four significant observations based on the analyses of the statistics and trends of drug abuse in Hong Kong. First, the prevalence of psychotropic substance abuse was alarming. According to the "2008/09 Survey of Drug Use among Students" conducted by Narcotics Division (2010), the lifetime prevalence rates among different student groups were 1.6 % for upper primary school students, 4.3 % for secondary school students, 2.9 % for undergraduate students, and 5.4 % for other postsecondary school students. Second, there was a decrease in age of first drug taking. It was found that 14 % of the drug-taking students took drug when they were 10 years old or even younger (Narcotics Division, 2010). Third, there were difficulties in the identification of drug abusers. Based on the statistics of the Central Registry of Drug Abuse in 2011 (Narcotics Division, 2012), 41.8 % of drug abusers aged under 21 reported to have drugs taken mostly at home and/or at friend's home in 2011. Last but not least, there was a growing belief among teenagers that psychotropic substance abuse was a choice of life rather than as an addictive behavior (Shek, Ma, & Sun, 2011).

The emergence of adolescent substance abuse raises the question of what factors contribute to the occurrence of the related problems. According to the ecological perspective (Bronfenbrenner, 1979, 1986), while there are risk factors that increase one's likelihood of using drugs, there are also protective factors that decrease one's risk for substance abuse. Shek (2007) identified five groups of ecological factors that contribute to adolescent substance abuse in Hong Kong, including factors in the personal (e.g., curiosity, lack of psychosocial competencies and coping skills, hopelessness, emptiness), interpersonal (e.g., undesirable peer influence), school (e.g., underachievement, undesirable after-school activities), family (e.g., marital disruption and parental absence, loose parental supervision, acute decline in family solidarity), and societal (growing addiction culture, availability of drug, growing up in poverty) domains. The identification of the risk and protective factors is critical in guiding the early identification and preventive mechanisms to prevent the adolescents from taking drugs, as well as developing intervention strategies that may help those adolescents with substance abuse (Shek, 2007).

Among the possible risk and protective factors that are related to adolescent substance abuse, there are three aspects that are worth noting. First, economic disadvantage has been identified as one of the risk factors that contribute to adolescent substance abuse (Shek, 2005; Unger, Sun, & Johnson, 2007). There are several explanations of how poverty influenced adolescent drug abuse. First, poverty has a negative impact on the identity formation process of poor adolescents. Phillips and Pittman (2003) pointed out that "stress, social stigma or marginalization, and the nature of the opportunity structures faced by many poor adolescents conspire to create a context that is not conducive to exploring identity issues" (p. 123). Poor adolescents who experience self-derogation may lead to exploring deviant behaviors (including drug abuse) and identifying deviant groups in order to escape from self-devaluing experiences (Kaplan, Martin, & Robbins, 1982). Furthermore, poverty has indirect influence on adolescent drug abuse via ecological factors of family processes, neighborhood, and peer influence. According to the family stress model, economic disadvantage negatively influences adolescent psychosocial adjustment via poor parents' mental health, marital relationship, and disruptive parenting (Conger & Conger, 2008). Last but not least, Jencks and Mayer (1990) suggested that neighborhood poverty influences adolescent problem behaviors via peer influences (the "epidemic" theories) and the neighborhood role models (collective socialization).

Second, while some family processes such as family conflicts are regarded as risk factors of adolescent substance abuse (Shek, 2007), some positive family processes such as mutual care are regarded as protective factors. Jessor and Jessor (1977) commented that externalizing problems (including smoking, drinking, substance abuse) were the results from the interaction between the risk factors and protective factors in the family system. There was evidence that both family structure and practices influenced adolescent substance abuse (Griffin, Botvin, Scheier, Diaz, & Miller, 2000; Ledoux, Miller, Choquet, & Plant, 2002; Mak et al., 2010). Lee and Goddard (1989) identified five family risk factors that may lead to adolescent substance abuse, including lack of emotional closeness, lack of parent involvement in children's activities, inconsistent or inadequate discipline, poor communication, and parental modeling. Moreover, there was evidence that family systems influenced adolescent substance abuse via the mediation of maladjustment (Frojd, Kaltiala-Heino, & Rimpla, 2007; Roustit, Chaix, & Chauvin, 2007). On the other hand, family processes such as smooth communication and mutual care can help to prevent adolescents from engaging in substance abuse.

Third, positive youth development has been regarded as an important protective factor that protects adolescents from substance abuse (Shek & Yu, 2011a). Positive youth development represents not only a positive appraisal of self-worth and self-mastery, which are important indicators of adolescent positive identity, it also helps to build up the human capital (such as improving their problem-solving capabilities) and social capital (i.e., the connections with other people and the community) which is fundamental in times of threats and adversity (Masten, Monn, & Supkoff, 2011). Unfortunately, the studies that examined the relationships between positive youth development and adolescent substance abuse in the Chinese context were lacking (Shek & Ma, 2011).

Against this background, the study aimed at identifying the sociodemographic (such as socioeconomic status, family intactness) and familial factors (such as family conflicts) that may increase the risks of adolescents to take drugs. At the same time, the familial and psychosocial protective factors that reduce adolescents from the use of drugs are also examined.

Several research questions are addressed in this chapter as follows:

1. What is the prevalence of substance abuse with reference to different types of drugs?
2. Does adolescent drug abuse change across time? Based on the previous empirical studies (e.g., Shek & Yu, 2011a) and the statistics of drug abusers from the Central Registry of Drug Abuse (Narcotics Division, 2012), it was expected that adolescent substance abuse increased across time (Hypothesis 1).
3. Do adolescents experiencing economic disadvantage differ from adolescents not experiencing economic disadvantage in terms of substance abuse? Based on the self-derogation thesis of poor adolescents (Kaplan et al., 1982), family stress model (Conger & Conger, 2008), and the influence of neighborhood poverty (Jencks & Mayer, 1990), it was expected that adolescents experiencing economic disadvantage would take more drugs than do adolescents not experiencing economic disadvantage (Hypothesis 2).
4. Do adolescents growing up in an intact family differ from adolescents growing up in a non-intact family in terms of substance abuse? Based on the previous literature (Frojd et al., 2007; Mak et al., 2010; Roustit et al., 2007), it was expected that adolescents growing up in a non-intact family would take more drugs than do adolescents growing up in an intact family (Hypothesis 3).
5. Is family functioning related to adolescent substance abuse? Based on the familial risk factors identified by Lee and Goddard (1989), and the previous empirical studies (Griffin et al., 2000; Ledoux et al., 2002), it was generally expected that

family functioning would be negatively associated with adolescent substance abuse (Hypothesis 4).

6. Are positive youth development attributes related to adolescent substance abuse? Based on the resilience literature (Masten et al., 2011) and previous empirical studies (Shek & Yu, 2011a), it was generally expected that positive youth development attributes would be negatively associated with adolescent substance abuse (Hypothesis 5).

Methods

Procedures and Participants

The data were derived from Wave 1, Wave 2, and Wave 3 of a 6-year longitudinal study assessing adolescent psychosocial development in Hong Kong. A total of 28 secondary schools in Hong Kong were randomly selected to participate in the study. At Wave 1, 3,325 secondary 1 students were invited to respond to the questionnaires containing the psychosocial and family attribute measures. The students were invited to respond to the same questionnaire in Wave 2 and Wave 3 in two consecutive years, having 2,904 and 2,885 students responded in the study, respectively. There were totally 2,667 students responding to all three waves of assessment, and the data were used in the study.

During data collection, the purpose of the study was introduced and confidentiality was repeatedly ensured to all participants. Parental and student consent was obtained. All participants responded to the questionnaires containing the related measures in a self-administration format. Adequate time was provided for the participants to fill up the questionnaire. A trained research assistant was present throughout the data collection process.

Based on the data of Wave 3, there were 2,185 (53.7 %) male and 1,885 (46.3 %) female respondents. The mean age of the students was 14.65 years (SD = .80 year). Majority of the respondents were born locally in Hong Kong (79.4 %), while the others were born in Mainland China (18.9 %) and other places (1.7 %). There were 212 respondents (5.2 %) who were recipients of Comprehensive Social Security Assistance (CSSA). There were 629 respondents (15.3 %) coming from the non-intact families. The demographic information of the respondents is listed in Table 1.

Instruments

Substance Abuse Scale

Eight items were used to assess the participants' frequency of using different types of substance (i.e., alcohol, tobacco, ketamine, cannabis, cough mixture, organic solvent, heroin, and pills such as ecstasy and methaqualone) during the last year.

Table 1 Sociodemographic profiles of respondents at Wave 3

	N	%
Gender		
Male	2,185	53.7
Female	1,885	46.3
Place of birth		
Hong Kong	3,195	79.4
Mainland	762	18.9
Others	68	1.7
Family economic status		
Not receiving CSSA	3,308	81.4
Receiving CSSA	212	5.2
Others (don't know)	525	13.4
Parents' marital status		
First marriage	3,372	82.5
Divorced	345	8.4
Separated	95	2.3
Remarried	189	4.6
Others (don't know)	86	2.1

Participants rated the occurrence of the behaviors on a 6-point Likert scale (0="never," 1="1–2 times," 2="3–5 times," 3="more than 5 times," 4="several times a month," 5="several times a week," 6="everyday"). A composite score was calculated averaging all eight item scores to obtain the mean of overall substance abuse. Moreover, separate analyses were carried out by combining "smoking" and drinking" into one indicator ("smoking and drinking") and aggregation of other drugs into another indicator ("other substance abuse"). The justification is that alcohol and cigarettes are commercially available drugs where other drugs are basically illegal drugs.

The Chinese Positive Youth Development Scale (CPYDS)

The Chinese Positive Youth Development Scale (CPYDS) was used to assess the positive youth development of adolescents in the study. The CPYDS has 15 subscales, including bonding (BO), resilience (RE), social competence (SC), recognition for positive behavior (PB), emotional competence (EC), cognitive competence (CC), behavioral competence (BC), moral competence (MC), self-determination (SD), self-efficacy (SE), clear and positive identity (SI), prosocial norms (PN), and spirituality (SP) (Shek, Siu, & Lee, 2007). The respondents are requested to rate their score in a 6-point Likert scale (1="strongly agree" to 6="strongly disagree"). The CPYDS showed good reliability and validity in previous validation studies (Shek & Ma, 2010a; Shek et al., 2007). A composite score was calculated by averaging all item scores to obtain the mean of overall positive youth development.

The Chinese Family Assessment Instrument (CFAI)

The Chinese Family Assessment Instrument (CFAI) was used to assess family functioning. In the present study, three subscales, family mutuality (mutual care, support, and concern among family members), family communication (quality of interaction among family members), and family conflicts (presence of conflicts among family members), were examined. The respondents responded to a 5-point Likert scale (1 = "very dissimilar," 2 = "somewhat dissimilar," 3 = "neither similar nor dissimilar," 4 = "somewhat similar," 5 = "very similar"). The reliability and validity of the CFAI were supported in previous validation studies (Shek, 2002; Shek & Ma, 2010b). A higher score on the subscales indicates higher levels of family mutuality, communication, and conflicts, respectively.

Sociodemographic Information

Two items were designed to investigate the family background of the respondents. The first item is to understand whether the students' families were currently receiving Comprehensive Social Security Assistance (CSSA), which served as an effective indicator of economic status of the families. The second item asked the students to indicate the marital status of their parents (1 = "divorced," 2 = "separated," 3 = "first marriage," 4 = "second marriage," 5 = "others"). Family intactness was indexed by parental marital status, with students whose parents were in their first marriage were regarded as living in intact families, while the other marital statuses (e.g., divorced, separated, remarried) were considered as non-intact families (Shek & Liu, 2013).

Results

Regarding Research Question 1, the prevalence of substance abuse among Hong Kong adolescents is shown in Table 2. It is not surprising that most adolescents reported that they had never use illicit drugs over the years. However, it is still alarming that 5.1 % and 34.2 % of adolescents reported that they smoked and drank during the past year in Wave 3, respectively. Among them, 1.7 % and 4.7 % were frequent users of tobacco and alcohol, respectively. Moreover, there were growing trends of adolescent tobacco and alcohol users from Wave 1 to Wave 3, with increasing rates of 0.5 % and 7.1 % in smoking and drinking, respectively. Among substance abuse, it was found that the frequencies of substance abuse were quite stable in Waves 1 and 2, with a slight increase in Wave 3. Among the different psychotropic substance types, it was found that organic solvent and cough mixture were the two most common psychotropic substances abused by the adolescents. Generally speaking the findings supported Hypothesis 1.

Table 2 Numbers and percentages of past year substance abuse among adolescents across waves

	0	1	2	3	4	5	6
	(Never)	(1–2 times)	(3–5 times)	(More than 5 times)	(Several times a month)	(Several times a week)	(Everyday)
Smoking							
W1 (*n*=2,661)	2,537 (95.1 %)	80 (3.0 %)	21 (0.8 %)	16 (0.6 %)	3 (0.1 %)	1 (0 %)	3 (0.1 %)
W2 (*n*=2,667)	2,511 (94.2 %)	80 (3.0 %)	20 (0.7 %)	22 (0.8 %)	7 (0.3 %)	11 (0.4 %)	10 (0.4 %)
W3 (*n*=2,667)	2,439 (91.5 %)	60 (2.2 %)	13 (0.5 %)	18 (0.7 %)	12 (0.4 %)	15 (0.6 %)	20 (0.7 %)
Drinking							
W1 (*n*=2, 667)	1,924 (72.1 %)	394 (14.8 %)	129 (4.8 %)	150 (5.6 %)	43 (1.6 %)	9 (0.3 %)	0 (0.0 %)
W2 (*n*=2, 667)	1,744 (65.4 %)	451 (16.9 %)	178 (6.7 %)	190 (7.1 %)	74 (2.8 %)	12 (0.4 %)	2 (0.1 %)
W3 (*n*=2, 667)	1,654 (62 %)	409 (15.3 %)	182 (6.8 %)	197 (7.4 %)	91 (3.4 %)	29 (1.1 %)	6 (0.2 %)
Ketamine							
W1 (*n*=2,649)	2,652 (99.4 %)	2 (0.1 %)	1 (0.0 %)	0 (0.0 %)	0 (0.0 %)	0 (0.0 %)	0 (0.0 %)
W2 (*n*=2, 667)	2,652 (99.4 %)	2 (0.1 %)	1 (0.0 %)	1 (0.0 %)	1 (0.0 %)	0 (0.0 %)	1 (0.0 %)
W3 (*n*=2, 667)	2,568 (96.3 %)	4 (0.1 %)	0 (0.0 %)	2 (0.1 %)	2 (0.1 %)	1 (0.0 %)	1 (0.0 %)
Cannabis							
W1 (*n*=2,667)	2,657 (99.6 %)	0 (0.0 %)	0 (0.0 %)	0 (0.0 %)	0 (0.0 %)	0 (0.0 %)	0 (0.0 %)
W2 (*n*=2, 667)	2,661 (99.8 %)	0 (0.0 %)	0 (0.0 %)	0 (0.0 %)	0 (0.0 %)	0 (0.0 %)	1 (0.0 %)
W3 (*n*=2, 667)	2,573 (96.5 %)	1 (0.0 %)	2 (0.1 %)	2 (0.1 %)	0 (0.0 %)	0 (0.0 %)	1 (0.0 %)
Cough mixture							
W1 (*n*=2,667)	2,640 (99.0 %)	8 (0.3 %)	2 (0.1 %)	4 (0.1 %)	0 (0.0 %)	0 (0.0 %)	0 (0.0 %)
W2 (*n*=2,667)	2,652 (99.4 %)	7 (0.3 %)	0 (0.0 %)	1 (0.0 %)	0 (0.0 %)	0 (0.0 %)	1 (0.0 %)

W3 (n=2,667)	2,568 (96.3 %)	7 (0.3 %)	2 (0.1 %)	1 (0.0 %)	0 (0.0 %)	0 (0.0 %)	1 (0.0 %)
Organic solvents							
W1 (n=2,667)	2,607 (97.8 %)	32 (1.2 %)	4 (0.1 %)	9 (0.3 %)	1 (0.1 %)	2 (0.1 %)	0 (0.0 %)
W2 (n=2,667)	2,629 (98.6 %)	25 (0.9 %)	2 (0.1 %)	4 (0.1 %)	1 (0.0 %)	0 (0.0 %)	1 (0.0 %)
W3 (n=2,667)	2,545 (95.4 %)	18 (0.7 %)	8 (0.3 %)	2 (0.1 %)	2 (0.1 %)	0 (0.0 %)	1 (0.0 %)
Pills (e.g., ecstasy and methaqualone)							
W1 (n=2,667)	2,655 (99.6 %)	0 (0.0 %)	0 (0.0 %)	0 (0.0 %)	0 (0.0 %)	0 (0.0 %)	0 (0.0 %)
W2 (n=2,667)	2,661 (99.8 %)	1 (0.0 %)	0 (0.0 %)	0 (0.0 %)	0 (0.0 %)	0 (0.0 %)	1 (0.0 %)
W3 (n=2,667)	2,570 (96.4 %)	1 (0.0 %)	1 (0.0 %)	1 (0.0 %)	0 (0.0 %)	1 (0.0 %)	1 (0.0 %)
Heroin							
W1 (n=2,667)	2,657 (99.6 %)	0 (0.0 %)	0 (0.0 %)	0 (0.0 %)	0 (0.0 %)	0 (0.0 %)	0 (0.0 %)
W2 (n=2,667)	2,653 (99.5 %)	1 (0.0 %)	0 (0.0 %)	0 (0.0 %)	0 (0.0 %)	0 (0.0 %)	1 (0.0 %)
W3 (n=2,667)	2,568 (96.3 %)	2 (0.1 %)	0 (0.0 %)	0 (0.0 %)	0 (0.0 %)	0 (0.0 %)	3 (0.1 %)

W1 Wave 1, *W2* Wave 2, *W3* Wave 3

Table 3 Results of mixed effect ANOVAs on adolescent substance abuse

Source of variation	df (hypothesis df, error df)	*F*	$\eta^2 p$
Economic disadvantage	1, 2,003	.87 ns	.000
Time	2, 2,002	28.92***	.028
Time × economic disadvantage	2, 2,002	5.23**	.005
Family intactness	1, 2,483	20.88***	.008
Time	2, 2,482	48.85***	.038
Time × family intactness	2, 2,482	11.83***	.009

Note: *F* values for time in the two ANOVAs are not the same because the missing values in the two analyses are not the same
$^{**}p<.01$; $^{***}p<.000$

A two-way mixed ANOVA was performed to examine the effects of time (Wave 1, Wave 2, and Wave 3) and economic disadvantage (families receiving CSSA and families not receiving CSSA) on adolescent substance abuse across time. Results showed that there was no difference between the poor group (those received CSSA) and the nonpoor group (those who did not receive CSSA) on the occurrence of adolescent substance abuse. However, there were main effects of time emerged on adolescent substance abuse, with $F(2,2002)=28.92$, $p<.001$, and partial $\eta^2=0.028$. Furthermore, there was significant interaction effect of group X time on adolescent substance abuse, with $F(2,2002)=5.23$, $p<.01$, and partial $\eta^2=0.005$. The results of post hoc pairwise comparisons suggested that there was significant difference between poor and nonpoor groups in adolescent substance abuse in Wave 3, but not in Waves 1 and 2. Besides, there was significant difference of adolescent substance abuse across time period of Waves 1, 2, and 3 within the poor group, but there was no significant difference of substance abuse among Waves 2 and 3 within nonpoor group. Table 3 showed the mixed two-way ANOVA between poor and nonpoor groups on adolescent substance abuse. The findings supported Hypothesis 2. Figure 1 showed the mean distributions of substance abuse between the two groups (poor and nonpoor) in Waves 1, 2, and 3.

Regarding the effects of family intactness and time on adolescent substance abuse, a mixed two-way ANOVA was conducted to test the hypothesis with group (intact and non-intact families) as the between-subject factor and time (Wave 1, Wave 2, Wave 3) as the within-subject factor. There was significant difference between adolescents from intact families and non-intact families on the occurrence of adolescent substance abuse, with $F(1,2483)=20.88$, $p<.001$, and partial $\eta^2=0.008$. There were main effects of time emerged on adolescent substance abuse, with $F(2,2482)=48.85$, $p<.001$, and partial $\eta^2=0.038$. There was also significant interaction effect of group X time on adolescent substance abuse, with $F(2,2482)=5.23$, $p<.01$, and partial $\eta^2=0.009$. The results of post hoc pairwise comparisons suggested that there was significant difference between intact and non-intact family groups in adolescent substance abuse in Waves 2 and 3, but not in Wave 1. Besides, there were significant differences of adolescent substance abuse

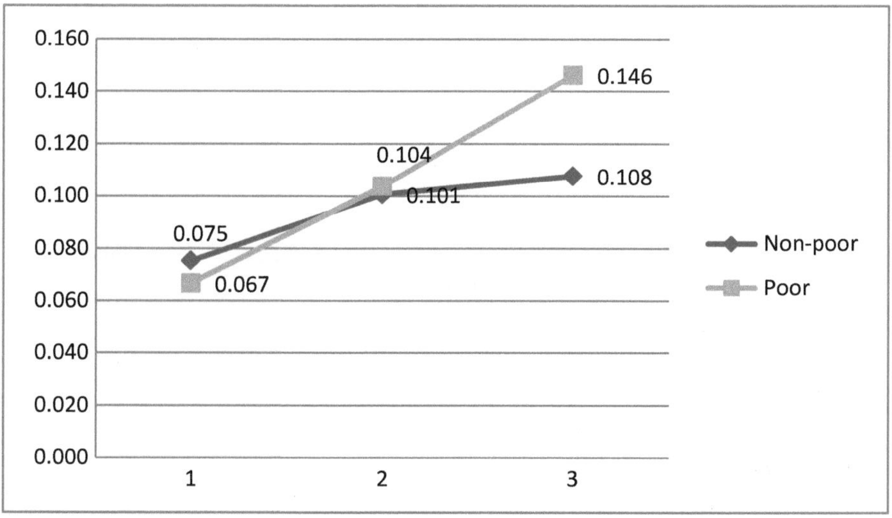

Post hoc comparison:	Mean difference (P–N)			Mean difference (across time)		
	W1	W2	W3	W1 - W2	W2 - W3	W1 - W3
Poor (P) vs. Non-poor (N)	-.009ns	.003ns	.038*			
Poor Group				-.007*	-.042*	-.079***
Non-poor group				-.025***	-.007ns	-.032***

*p<.05, **p<.01,***p<.000

W1= Wave 1; W2=Wave 2; W3=Wave 3

Fig. 1 Adolescent drug use between poor and nonpoor groups across time

across time period of Waves 1, 2, and 3 within the non-intact family group, but there was no significant difference of substance abuse across time period of Waves 2 and 3 within intact family group. The findings provided support for Hypothesis 3. Table 3 showed the mixed two-way ANOVA of intact and non-intact family groups on adolescent substance abuse. Figure 2 showed the mean distributions of substance abuse between the two groups (intact and non-intact families) in Waves 1, 2, and 3.

To examine the relationships between sociodemographic characteristics, family functioning, positive youth development, and adolescent substance abuse, correlational analyses of demographic characteristics, family intactness, family functioning, positive youth development at Wave 1, and adolescent substance abuse at Wave 3 were performed. It was found that age, gender, economic disadvantage, and migrant status at Wave 1 were correlated with overall substance abuse at Wave 3, with elder students, boys, more economic disadvantage, and migrant adolescents were more

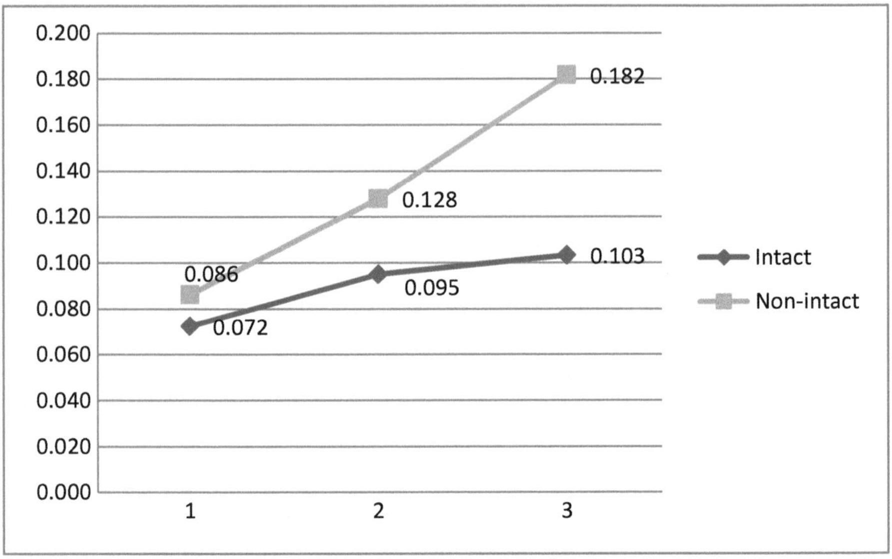

Post hoc comparison:	Mean difference (I–N)			Mean difference (across time)		
	W1	W2	W3	W1 - W2	W2 - W3	W1 - W3
Intact (I) vs. Non-intact (N)	-.014ns	.033**	.078***			
Intact family group				-.042***	-.054***	-.095***
Non-intact family group				-.023***	-.008ns	-.031***

*p<.05, **p<.01,***p<.000

W1= Wave 1; W2=Wave 2; W3=Wave 3

Fig. 2 Adolescent drug use between intact and non-intact families across time

likely to have substance abuse. Regarding family characteristics, it was found that family intactness, family mutuality, and family communication were negatively related to overall substance abuse, whereas family conflicts were positively related to overall substance abuse. Finally, it was found that positive youth development was negatively associated with overall substance abuse. Table 4 shows the correlational analyses of the variables.

To examine the relative contribution of different predictors to adolescent substance abuse across time, hierarchical multiple regression analyses of predictor variables at Wave 1 to adolescent substance abuse at Wave 3 were performed. Sociodemographic factors (adolescents' age, gender, economic disadvantage, migrant status, and family intactness), family functioning factors (mutuality, family conflicts, family communication), and positive youth development were entered into separated hierarchical blocks. Among the sociodemographic factors, it was found

Table 4 Correlations among demographic, family functioning, and positive youth development correlates at Wave 1 on overall substance abuse, smoking and drinking, and other substance abuse at Wave 3

	Age	Gender	Economic disadvantage	Migrant status	Family intactness	Family mutuality	Family conflicts	Family communication	Positive youth development	Overall substance abuse	Drinking and smoking	Other substance[a]
Age	–											
Gender	–.02											
Economic disadvantage	.09***	.02										
Migrant status	.35***	.04	.16***									
Family intactness	–.06**	.00	–.36***	–.07**								
Family mutuality	–.05**	–.07**	–.08***	–.08***	.18***							
Family conflicts	–.09***	–.04	.11***	.08***	–.15***	–.66***						
Family communication	–.04*	–.01***	–.09***	–.1***	.14***	.76***	–.53***					
Positive youth development	.02	.05*	–.02*	–.00	.08***	.52***	–.35***	.51***				
Overall substance abuse	.12***	–.04*	.02*	.06**	–.05**	–.15***	.15***	–.17***	–.13***			
Drinking and smoking	.11***	–.02**	.05*	.04*	–.07**	–.17***	.17***	–.17***	–.15***	.90***		
Other substance	.06**	–.01	.03	.06**	.01	–.04*	.04*	–.02	.01	.59***	.18***	–

W1 Wave 1, *W2* Wave 2, *W3* Wave 3

*$p<.05$; **$p<.001$; ***$p<.000$

[a]Ketamine, cannabis, cough mixture, organic solvent, pills, and heroin

that economic disadvantage predicted adolescent substance abuse, with $\beta=0.06$ ($p<0.05$). Among family and psychosocial factors (family mutuality, family conflicts, family communication, positive youth development), it was found that family conflicts at Wave 1 positively predicted adolescent substance abuse, with $\beta=0.07$ ($p<0.05$), whereas family communication and positive youth development negatively influenced adolescent substance abuse, with $\beta=-0.12$ and -0.08 ($p<0.001$), respectively. The familial and psychosocial factors explained 4 % of the total variance of adolescent substance abuse. The findings generally supported Hypothesis 4 and Hypothesis 5. Table 5 shows the hierarchical multiple regression analyses of the sociodemographic, familial, and psychosocial correlates at Wave 1 on its influence of adolescent substance abuse at Wave 3. As a summary, it was found that age of adolescents, economic disadvantage, and family conflicts at Wave 1 positively predicted adolescent substance abuse at Wave 3, whereas family communication and positive youth development attributes at Wave 1 negatively predicted adolescent substance abuse at Wave 3.

Discussion

There were several unique features in the study. First, a large sample size was used which could generate findings with high generalizability. Second, different substances were examined in the study, including both legal substances (e.g., tobacco and alcohol) and illicit drugs (e.g., psychotropic drugs and heroin). Third, as a longitudinal research design was used, the impact of demographic and psychosocial factors on adolescent substance abuse across time could be described. Last but not the least, an array of sociodemographic (e.g., economic disadvantage, family intactness), familial (e.g., family functioning), and personal factors (i.e., positive youth development) were studied which can provide a more comprehensive picture for social scientists, researchers, and policy makers to tackle the problem of adolescent substance abuse.

In the present study, the rates of substance abuse among Hong Kong adolescents seemed to be lower when compared with the global trends (United Nations Office on Drugs and Crimes, 2012), those of the USA (Johnston et al., 2013), and the European countries (Hibell et al., 2009). However, the growing numbers of students who smoked and drank should deserve the attention of researchers, social workers, and policy makers. Smoking among adolescents has been regarded as a powerful predictor for the use of illicit drugs (Fleming, Leventhal, Glynn, & Ershler, 1989; Kandel, Yamaguchi, & Chen, 1992). Torabi, Bailey, and Majd-Jabbari (1993) termed cigarette smoking as a "gateway drug" that inferred the likelihood of children and adolescents to alcohol and illicit drug use. Lau and Kan (2010) found that smoking and drinking among adolescents were associated with other problem behaviors such as truancy, gambling, gang involvement, sexual activities, etc. Clearly, drug abuse has indelible harmful effects on adolescents by damaging their physical and mental health, and the prevention and early identification of adolescent drug abuse in Hong Kong is necessary.

Table 5 Regression analyses based on demographic, sociodemographic, family functioning, and positive youth development correlates at Wave 1 on substance abuse at Wave 3

	Overall substance abuse			Smoking and drinking			Other substance abuse[a]		
	Step 1	Step 2	Step 3	Step 1	Step 2	Step 3	Step 1	Step 2	Step 3
	β	β	β	β	β	β	β	β	β
Demographic factors									
Age	.04 ns	.05 ns	.05*	.05 ns	.05*	.05*	.00 ns	–.01 ns	–.01 ns
Gender	–.01 ns	–.01 ns	–.02 ns	–.01 ns	–.01 ns	–.02 ns	.01 ns	.01 ns	.00 ns
Sociodemographic factors									
Economic disadvantage		.07*	.06*		.06*	.05 ns		.05 ns	.05 ns
Migrant status		–.03 ns	–.04 ns		–.04 ns	–.05 ns		.03 ns	.03 ns
Family intactness		–.01 ns	.02 ns		–.01 ns	.01 ns		.02 ns	.03 ns
Familial and psychosocial factors									
Family mutuality			.01 ns			.02 ns.			–.04 ns
Family conflicts			.07*			.09*			.02 ns
Family communication			–.12**			–.13**			–.01 ns
Positive youth development			–.08**			–.08**			–.04 ns
F	1.64 ns	2.26*	9.45***	1.76 ns	2.21 ns	9.99***	.03 ns	1.03 ns	1.34 ns
R	.05	.08	.23	.05	.08	.23	.01	.06	.09
R^2	.00	.01	.05	.00	.01	.05	.00	.00	.01
ΔR^2		.01	.04		.01	.05		.00	.00

*$p<.05$; **$p<.001$; ***$p<.000$

[a]Ketamine, cannabis, cough mixture, organic solvent, pills, and heroin

Echoing the poverty studies (Shek, 2005; Unger et al., 2007) that economic disadvantage was one of the predictors of adolescent substance abuse, the present study also showed that economic disadvantage was a risk factor for adolescent substance abuse. However, research findings indicated that there was an interaction effect of economic disadvantage and time in adolescent substance abuse. It was found that poor adolescents were more likely to commit smoking, drinking, and substance abuse across time, when compared with the nonpoor adolescents when they were in the higher grades. This observation is in line with the explanation of identity formation of adolescents experiencing economic disadvantage (Phillips & Pittman, 2003). As suggested by Rosenberg (1979), individual's psychological well-being is shaped by the messages one receives from one's status in society through reflected appraisals and social comparison. It is posited that the "social meanings" of being socioeconomically disadvantaged are more salient in adolescents than children, resulting in poor psychosocial adjustment (McLoyd et al., 2009). Adolescents in lower socioeconomic strata will have a negative appraisal of self-worth, with a sense of resentment, powerlessness, and loss of control. This is magnified by the stigmatizing conditions and circumstances precipitated by socioeconomic disadvantage (Lindheim & Syme, 1983). Thus, poor adolescents are more prone to substance abuse with increase in age, when they experience more social inequalities in the social stratification systems and result in lower self-esteem (Rosenberg & Pearlin, 1978).

The research findings support the previous studies (Barrett & Turner, 2006; Ledoux et al., 2002; Mak et al., 2010) that adolescents from non-intact families were more prone to smoke, drink alcohol, and use drugs, when compared with the non-intact families. Adolescents may experience the lack of parental supervision and monitoring due to parental absence (Shek & Yu, 2011a). Also, the weakening of emotional bonds and modeling from parents may contribute to the risk factors of substance abuse (Lee & Goddard, 1989).

Regarding the influence of family functioning, the present study suggested that family conflicts positively predicted adolescent drug abuse, while family communication negatively predicted drug abuse of adolescents. The results are in line with the previous research. McCubbin, Needle, and Wilson (1985) further explained adolescent health risk behaviors (cigarette smoking, liquor drinking, and marijuana smoking) in relation to family patterns of dealing with stress. When adolescents' needs exceed the family's capability to meet their demands, adolescents may experience stress and distress. Some adolescents who fail to obtain the support from their families appeared to "turn to the use of these substances as a way to numb the sensations they feel and hence, cope" (McCubbin et al., 1985, p. 60). Thus, harmonious family relationship and good parent-child communication are protective factors of adolescents against drug abuse.

Last but not the least, research findings indicated that positive youth development attributes negatively predicted adolescent substance abuse over time. The results were consistent with the previous findings that positive youth development was a protective factor against adolescent problem behaviors (Catalano, Berglund, Ryan, Lonczak, & Hawkins, 2004; Sun & Shek, 2012). The findings are also consistent with the previous studies that when compared with the control group, students who had joined the Project P.A.T.H.S. took drugs slower in their growth trajectories. This provides invaluable insight for researchers, social workers, and policy makers to identify the preventive measures in protecting the adolescents from attempting cigarettes, alcohol, and drugs.

The present study has theoretical and practical implications. Theoretically, the research identified some risk factors (e.g., economic disadvantage) and protective factors (e.g., positive youth development) of adolescent substance abuse in the Chinese context. Besides, different ecological factors were used to identify the sociodemographic (e.g., economic disadvantage), familial (e.g., family intactness, conflicts, and communication), and psychosocial (e.g., positive youth development) factors that may contribute to adolescent substance abuse. The results were in line with the Western literature in understanding adolescent developmental needs and problems. Obviously, research in the Western and Chinese contexts suggests that family functioning and positive youth development attributes are important determinants of adolescent substance abuse over time.

Practically, in view of the hazardous effects of drugs to adolescents, identifying effective strategies to prevent adolescents from drug abuse is of paramount importance. As commented by Shek (2007), tackling the issue of adolescent substance abuse should call for a multipronged approach. Employing the ecological perspective, the present study suggests three important strategies in preventing the adolescents from drug abuse. First, as positive youth development is a powerful protective factor against adolescent substance abuse, positive youth development programs such as Project P.A.T.H.S. should be widely developed and implemented in primary and secondary schools. There was evidence on the effectiveness of Project P.A.T.H.S. not only to foster the psychosocial competencies of the participants (Shek, 2010; Shek & Sun, 2010) but also prevent adolescents from problem behaviors such as substance abuse and delinquent behaviors (Shek & Yu, 2011b, 2012). In North America, Catalano et al. (2004) assessed the 25 well-evaluated positive youth development programs and found that 96 % of those programs decreased the occurrence of problem behaviors of adolescents. Other studies also showed that positive development programs helped to reduce adolescent problem behaviors (Scales & Leffert, 1999; Wilson & Lipsey, 2006). As such, the importance of using positive youth development strategies to prevent adolescents from risk behaviors is indisputable.

Second, family plays an important role in protecting adolescents against the risk of drug abuse. Family life education and parenting enhancement programs should be developed to build up family competence to support adolescents. However, the substantial drop in family solidarity of the Social Development Index (The Hong Kong Council of Social Service, 2013) and the increase of divorce rate in recent years in Hong Kong have put an alarm on adolescent substance abuse, as family non-intactness and conflicts are regarded as risk factors contributing to the problems. In view of family breakdown and dysfunctions having detrimental effects to adolescent development, marital counseling and postdivorced parenting education programs are also necessary.

Third, economic disadvantage has been one of the predictors of adolescent drug abuse. Supportive service for the poor adolescents and their families would be important to enhance the competencies of adolescents, as well as to build a nurturing ecological environment for the adolescents to develop healthily. In fact, it is not just a question of providing more financial resource for them. Instead, it is important to promote the holistic development of adolescents at the same time.

Though the present study has theoretical and practical implications, there are also several limitations. First, as the findings presented in the study were based on adolescents in Hong Kong, there is a need to assess the generalizability of the findings in different Chinese communities (e.g., mainland China) and Chinese adolescents living in non-Chinese contexts (e.g., Chinese–Americans). Second, as the research findings are based solely on quantitative methods and the number of students who reported taking illicit drugs was relatively small, it would be methodologically superior to use multiple methods in future study. Qualitative methodologies such as focus groups and in-depth interviews should be employed to gain a more comprehensive view of the issue. Third, as the assessment of drug abuse, family functioning, and positive youth development was based on self-reported measures of adolescents, the inclusion of different information sources from parents and teachers may create a fuller picture of the phenomenon.

Despite these limitations, the present study enriches our understanding of the phenomenon of adolescent substance abuse in Hong Kong, which provides important insights for researchers, social workers, educators, and policy makers in tackling the problems of adolescent substance abuse. As suggested by the United Nations Office of Drugs and Crime (2012) that "prevention, treatment, rehabilitation, reintegration and health all have to be recognized as key elements in the global strategy to reduce drug demand" (p. iv), the present study is an active response to the quest.

Acknowledgment The preparation for this paper was financially supported by the Hong Kong Jockey Club Charities Trust. The authorship is equally shared between the first author and second author.

References

Barrett, A. E., & Turner, R. J. (2006). Family structure and substance use problems in adolescence and early adulthood: Examining explanations for the relationship. *Addiction, 101*(1), 109–120.

Bronfenbrenner, U. (1979). *The ecology of human development: Experiments by nature and design*. Cambridge, MA: Harvard University Press.

Bronfenbrenner, U. (1986). Ecology of the family as a context for human development: Research perspectives. *Developmental Psychology, 22*(6), 723–742.

Catalano, R. F., Berglund, M. L., Ryan, J. A. M., Lonczak, H. S., & Hawkins, J. D. (2004). Positive youth development in the United States: Research findings on evaluation of positive youth development programs. *Annals of the American Academy of Political and Social Science, 591*, 98–124.

Conger, R. D., & Conger, K. J. (2008). Understanding the processes through which economic hardship influences families and children. In D. R. Crane & T. B. Heaton (Eds.), *Handbook of families and poverty* (pp. 64–81). Los Angeles: Sage.

Fleming, R., Leventhal, H., Glynn, K., & Ershler, J. (1989). The role of cigarettes in the initiation and progression of early substance use. *Addictive Behaviors, 14*, 261–272.

Frojd, S., Kaltiala-Heino, R., & Rimpela, M. (2007). The association of parental monitoring and family structure with diverse maladjustment outcomes in middle adolescent boys and girls. *Nordic Journal of Psychiatry, 61*(4), 296–303.

Griffin, K. W., Botvin, G. J., Scheier, L. M., Diaz, T., & Miller, N. L. (2000). Parenting practices as predictors of substance use, delinquency, and aggression among urban minority youth: Moderating effects of family structure and gender. *Psychology of Addictive Behaviors, 14*(2), 174–184.

Hibell, B., Guttormsson, U., Ahlström, S., Balakireva, O., Bjarnason, T., Kokkevi, A., et al. (2009). *The 2007 ESPAD report: Substance Use among students in 35 European Countries*. Stockholm: Swedish Council for Information on Alcohol and Other Drugs.

Jencks, C., & Mayer, S. (1990). The social consequences of growing up in a poor neighbourhood. In L. Lynn & M. McGeary (Eds.), *Inner city poverty in the United States* (pp. 111–186). Washington, DC: National Academy Press.

Jessor, R., & Jessor, S. L. (1977). *Problem behavior and psychosocial development: A longitudinal study of youth*. San Diego, CA: Academic.

Johnston, L. D., O'Malley, P. M., Bachman, J. G., & Schulenberg, J. E. (2013). *Monitoring the Future: National results on drug use 2012 overview – Key findings on adolescent drug use*. Ann Arbor, MI: Institute for Social Research, The University of Michigan. Retrieved December 16, from http://monitoringthefuture.org//pubs/monographs/mtf-overview2012.pdf

Kandel, D. B., Yamaguchi, K., & Chen, K. (1992). Stages of progression in drug involvement from adolescence to adulthood: Further evidence for the gateway theory. *Journal of Studies of Alcohol and Drugs, 53*, 447–457.

Kaplan, H. B., Martin, S. S., & Robbins, C. (1982). Application of a general theory of deviant behavior: Self-derogation and adolescent drug use. *Journal of Health and Social Behavior, 23*, 274–294.

Lau, M., & Kan, M. Y. (2010). Prevalence and correlates of problem behaviors among adolescents in Hong Kong. *Asia-Pacific Journal of Public Health, 22*(3), 354–364.

Ledoux, S., Miller, P., Choquet, M., & Plant, M. (2002). Family structure, parent-child relationships, and alcohol and other drug use among teenagers in France and the United Kingdom. *Alcohol and Alcoholism, 37*(1), 52–60.

Lee, T. R., & Goddard, H. W. (1989). Developing family relationship skills to prevent substance abuse among high-risk youth. *Family Relations, 38*(3), 301–305.

Lindheim, R., & Syme, S. L. (1983). Environments, people and health. *Annual Reviews of Public Health, 4*, 335–359.

Mak, K. K., Ho, S. Y., Thomas, G. N., Schooling, C. M., McGhee, S. M., & Lam, T. H. (2010). Family structure, parent-child conversation time and substance use among Chinese adolescents. *Public Health, 10*, 503–511.

Masten, A. S., Monn, A. R., & Supkoff, L. M. (2011). Resilience in children and adolescents. In S. M. Southwick, B. T. Litz, D. Charney, & M. J. Friedman (Eds.), *Resilience and mental health: Challenges across the lifespan* (pp. 103–119). New York: Cambridge University Press.

McCubbin, H. I., Needle, R. H., & Wilson, M. (1985). Adolescent health risk behaviors: Family stress and adolescent coping as critical factors. *Family Relations, 34*(1), 51–62.

McLoyd, V. C., Kaplan, R., Purtell, K. M., Bagley, E., Hardaway, C. R., & Smalls, C. (2009). Poverty and socioeconomic disadvantage in adolescence. In R. M. Lerner & L. Steingberg (Eds.), *Handbook of adolescent psychology* (Contextual influences on adolescent development, Vol. 2, pp. 444–491). Hoboken, NJ: Wiley.

Narcotics Division. (2010). *The 2008/09 survey of drug use among students*. Hong Kong: Narcotics Division, Security Bureau, Government of Hong Kong Special Administrative Region.

Narcotics Division. (2012). *Central registry of drug abuse sixty-first report: 2002–2011*. Hong Kong: Narcotics Division, Security Bureau, Government of Hong Kong Special Administrative Region.

Phillips, T. M., & Pittman, J. F. (2003). Identity processes in poor adolescents: Exploring the linkages between economic disadvantage and the primary task of adolescence. *Identity: An International Journal of Theory and Research, 3*(2), 115–129.

Rosenberg, M. (1979). *Conceiving the self*. New York: Basic Books.

Rosenberg, M., & Pearlin, L. (1978). Social class and self-esteem among children and adults. *American Journal of Sociology, 84*, 53–77.

Roustit, C., Chaix, B., & Chauvin, P. (2007). Family breakup and adolescents' psychosocial maladjustment: Public health implications of family disruptions. *Pediatrics, 120*(4), e984–991.

Scales, P. C., & Leffert, N. (1999). *Developmental assets: A synthesis of the scientific research on adolescent development*. Minneapolis, MN: Search Institute.

Shek, D. T. L. (2002). Assessment of family functioning Chinese adolescents: The Chinese family assessment instrument. In N. N. Singh, T. Ollen-dick, & A. N. Singh (Eds.), *International perspectives on child and adolescent mental health* (pp. 297–316). Amsterdam: Elsevier.

Shek, D. T. L. (2005). A longitudinal study of perceived family functioning and adolescent adjustment in Chinese adolescents with economic disadvantage. *Journal of Family Issues, 26*(4), 518–543.

Shek, D. T. L. (2007). Tackling adolescent substance abuse in Hong Kong: Where we should and should not go. *TheScientificWorldJOURNAL: TSW Child Health & Human Development, 19*(7), 2021–2030.

Shek, D. T. L. (2010). Objective outcome evaluation of the Project P.A.T.H.S. in Hong Kong: Findings based on individual growth curve models. *TheScientificWorldJOURNAL: TSW Child Health & Human Development, 10*, 182–191.

Shek, D. T. L., & Leung, J. T. Y. (2013). Adolescent developmental issues in Hong Kong: Phenomena and implications for youth service. In D. T. L. Shek & R. C. F. Sun (Eds.), *Development and evaluation of Positive Adolescent Training through Holistic Social Programs (P.A.T.H.S.)* (pp. 1–14). Singapore: Springer.

Shek, D. T. L., & Liu, T. T. (2013). Life satisfaction in junior secondary school students in Hong Kong: A 3-year longitudinal study. *Social Indicators Research*. doi: 10.1007/s11205-013-0398-4.

Shek, D. T. L., & Ma, C. M. S. (2010a). Dimensionality of the Chinese Positive Youth Development Scale: Confirmatory factor analyses. *Social Indicators Research, 98*, 41–59.

Shek, D. T. L., & Ma, C. M. S. (2010b). The Chinese Family Assessment Instrument (C-FAI): Hierarchical confirmatory factor analyses and factorial invariance. *Research on Social Work Practice, 20*(1), 112–123.

Shek, D. T. L., & Ma, C. M. S. (2011). Substance abuse in junior secondary school students in Hong Kong: Prevalence and psychosocial correlates. A longitudinal study. *International Journal of Child Health and Human Development, 4*(4), 433–442.

Shek, D. T. L., Ma, H. K., & Sun, R. C. F. (2011). A brief overview of adolescent developmental problems in Hong Kong. *TheScientificWorldJOURNAL, 11*, 2243–2256.

Shek, D. T. L., Siu, A. M. H., & Lee, T. Y. (2007). The Chinese Positive Youth Development Scale: A validation study. *Research on Social Work Practice, 17*, 380–391.

Shek, D. T. L., & Sun, R. C. F. (2010). Effectiveness of the Tier 1 Program of Project P.A.T.H.S.: Findings based on three years of program implementation. *TheScientificWorldJOURNAL: TSW Child Health & Human Development, 10*, 1509–1519.

Shek, D. T. L., & Yu, L. (2011a). Descriptive profiles and correlates of substance use in Hong Kong adolescents: A longitudinal study. *International Journal of Child Health and Human Development, 4*(4), 443–460.

Shek, D. T. L., & Yu, L. (2011b). Prevention of adolescent problem behavior: Longitudinal impact of the Project P.A.T.H.S. in Hong Kong. *TheScientificWorldJOURNAL: TSW Child Health & Human Development, 11*, 546–567.

Shek, D. T. L., & Yu, L. (2012). Longitudinal impact of the Project P.A.T.H.S. on adolescent risk behavior: What happened after five years. *TheScientificWorldJOURNAL, 2012*, Article ID 316029, 13 pp. doi: 10.1100/2012/316029.

Sun, R. C. F., & Shek, D. T. L. (2012). Positive youth development, life satisfaction and problem behavior among Chinese adolescents in Hong Kong: A replication. *Social Indicators Research, 105*(3), 541–559.

The Hong Kong Council of Social Service. (2013). *Social development index report 2012* [in Chinese]. Hong Kong: The Hong Kong Council of Social Service. Retrieved December 16 at http://www.socialindicators.org.hk/sites/default/files/shares/files/general/SDI_Report_2012.pdf

Torabi, M. R., Bailey, W. J., & Majd-Jabbari, M. (1993). Cigarette smoking as a predictor of alcohol and other drug use by children and adolescents: Evidence of the "gateway drug effect". *The Journal of School Health, 63*, 302–306.

Unger, J. B., Sun, P., & Johnson, C. A. (2007). Socioeconomic correlates of smoking among an ethnically diverse sample of 8th grade adolescents in Southern California. *Preventive Medicine, 44*, 323–327.

United Nations Office on Drugs and Crimes. (2012). *World drug report 2012*. New York: United Nations (online). Retrieved December 16, 2013, from http://www.unodc.org/unodc/en/data-and-analysis/WDR-2012.html

Wilson, S. J., & Lipsey, M. (2006). *The effects of school-based social information processing interventions on aggressive behavior, Part I: Universal programs*. Nashville, TN: Center for Evaluation Research and Methodology, Vanderbilt Institute for Public Policy Studies, Vanderbilt University.

A Longitudinal Study on Deliberate Self-Harm and Suicidal Behaviors Among Chinese Adolescents

Ben M.F. Law and Daniel T.L. Shek

Abstract This longitudinal study examined deliberate self-harm and suicidal behaviors among adolescents in junior secondary schools in Hong Kong. With specific reference to adolescents in Grade 9, the prevalence of deliberate self-harm behavior was 21.9 %, with preventing wounds from healing, self-scratching, and wrist cutting being the most prevalent self-harm behaviors; the prevalence of self-harm behavior was higher in girls than in boys. The prevalence of suicide attempts was 3.4 %, with girls manifesting more suicidal behaviors than boys. A path model with family functioning (mutuality, communication, and conflicts) at Time 1, positive youth development qualities at Time 2, and self-harm and suicidal behaviors at Time 3 was tested. The following results were obtained: (a) mutuality and communication at Time 1 predicted self-harm and suicidal behaviors at Time 3 via positive youth development at Time 2; (b) mutuality at Time 1 directly predicted self-harm behavior at Time 3; (c) family conflicts at Time 1 directly predicted suicidal behavior at Time 3. The proposed overall model was not entirely gender invariant. Although the paths were gender invariant, family conflicts at Time 1 predicted suicidal behavior at Time 3 for girls but not boys. The theoretical and applied implications of the findings are discussed in this work.

Keywords Deliberate self-harm • Suicidal behavior • Positive youth development • Family functioning • Path model

B.M.F. Law, Ph.D. (✉)
Department of Social Work and Social Administration, The University of Hong Kong, Pokfulam Road, Hong Kong
e-mail: blaw@hku.hk

D.T.L. Shek, Ph.D., B.B.S., S.B.S., J.P.
Department of Applied Social Sciences, The Hong Kong Polytechnic University, Hunghom, Hong Kong

D.T.L. Shek et al. (eds.), *Chinese Adolescents in Hong Kong*,
Quality of Life in Asia 5, DOI 10.1007/978-981-287-143-5_9

Introduction

Using the data derived from a 3-year longitudinal study, this work examines the prevalence of deliberate self-harm and suicidal behaviors among Grade 9 Chinese adolescents as well as the related predictors. A causal model with family functioning at Wave 1 and positive youth development (PYD) qualities at Wave 2 as predictors as well as self-harm and suicidal behaviors at Wave 3 was tested. As gender differences are commonly found for deliberate self-harm and suicidal behaviors, the gender invariance of the proposed model is also tested.

Deliberate self-harm is an intentional act by an individual to harm himself or herself physically (Isacsson & Rich, 2001). Self-harm is more prevalent among adolescents than among adults (Fox & Hawton, 2004). Methods of self-harm include drug overdose, self-hitting, pinching, scratching, biting, self-cutting, burning, jumping from a high place, or self-poisoning (Yip, Ngan, & Lam, 2003). A study involving a large sample of adolescents in China (Wan, Hu, Hao, Sun, & Tao, 2011) showed that 17.0 % had harmed themselves in the past 12 months. The most common form of self-harm is self-hitting. In a recent study, Law and Shek (2013) reported that 23.5 % of Grade 8 students in Hong Kong had attempted deliberate self-harm in the past 12 months.

Self-harm behaviors are closely related to suicide. The percentage of people who have attempted suicide was 0.7 % of those who have exhibited self-harm behaviors during the past year; this value was 66 times higher than the suicide rate in the general population during the same period (Hawton, 2005). According to the World Health Organization (2008), almost one million people die from suicide yearly, with a mortality rate of 16 per 100,000. The suicide rates among young people have been increasing in the last 45 years. Youth suicide is currently at the highest risk of mortality in a third of all countries worldwide. Suicide is the second leading cause of death for those aged between 10 and 24 years. In Hong Kong, the suicide rates among adolescents are comparatively low. The suicide rate for young people under the age of 15 decreased from 1.0 to 0.3 % per 100,000 from 2000 to 2009, whereas the rate for those aged 15–24 years increased from 7.7 to 8.5 % per 100,000 (World Health Organization, 2008). The values of the 12-month prevalence of suicidal ideation and attempt across the three Asian cities of Taipei, Shanghai, and Hanoi were 8.4 % (Blum, Sudhinaraset, & Emerson, 2012). In a recent study, Law and Shek (2013) reported that almost 13 % of Grade 8 adolescents in Hong Kong had manifested suicidal thoughts, 5 % had made suicidal plans, and 4 % had attempted suicide. The figure in Hong Kong is relatively higher than the international figures.

Self-harm and suicidal behaviors have personal and social correlates. On the individual level, alcohol or substance use (Tuisku et al., 2014), difficulties in regulating personal emotions (Pisani et al., 2013), coping problems or impulsivity (Zhang, Li, Tu, Xiao, & Jia, 2011), depression or hopelessness (Mustanski & Liu, 2013), and history of abuse (Mota et al., 2012) are factors related to self-harm and suicidal behaviors. On the interpersonal level, peer support (Czyz, Liu, & King, 2012; Samuel & Sher, 2013; Tuisku et al., 2014), trusted adults (Pisani et al., 2013), and family support (Chan et al., 2009; Maimon, Browning, & Brooks-Gunn, 2010) could prevent self-harm and suicidal behaviors. One study concluded that family, school, and peer relationships are significant protective factors. Another study found that social isolation predicts suicide attempts (Hall-Lande, Eisenberg, Christenson, & Neumark-Sztainer, 2007).

To reduce self-harm and suicidal behaviors, individual protective factors with psychosocial intervention implications have been explored in many studies. Among all protective factors, self-esteem is most widely studied in the area of adolescent suicide (Sharaf, Thompson, & Walsh, 2010). Strategies that promote good general coping skills and prevention efforts are highly needed (Lubell & Vetter, 2006). Psychosocial adjustment skills and adolescent resilience are likewise necessary in preventing self-harm and suicidal behaviors (Rew, Thomas, Horner, Resnick, & Beuhring, 2001; Zweig, Phillips, & Lindberg, 2002).

Several observations regarding studies on adolescent self-harm and suicidal behaviors have been noted. First, although several methods have been employed to study self-harm and suicidal behaviors, which consist of suicidal ideations, plans, or attempts, descriptive profiles of such behaviors among adolescents have not been systematically examined. Second, studies on self-harm among Chinese adolescents are rarely reported. In fact, most of the literature in the last 10 years has focused on suicidal behaviors, with the awareness of self-harm behavior emerging only in the last few years. Third, few longitudinal studies exploring the changes in or stability of self-harm and suicidal behaviors among adolescents have been conducted (e.g., Tuisku et al., 2014). Without longitudinal studies, we cannot examine the causal relationships among variables. Fourth, although self-harm and suicidal behaviors are closely related, no study has differentiated the possible different predictors or correlates involved. One possible reason for this knowledge gap is that most studies explore either self-harm or suicidal behaviors, while a few studies examine both behaviors (e.g., Tuisku et al., 2014). Fifth, many researchers (e.g., Chan et al., 2009) highlighted the importance of family functioning in preventing self-harm and suicidal behaviors. However, no studies to date have explored the critical domains within family functioning that can cause self-harm or suicidal behaviors. Sixth, although studies have highlighted the necessity of individual protective factors, such as self-esteem, optimism, and resilience, such studies are fragmented and have thus increased the need to propose an encompassing factor that can include all critical individual protective factors with psychosocial intervention implications. One possibility is the construct of PYD, which encompasses different PYD qualities. Seventh, although family functioning and PYD are equally important in affecting the prevalence of self-harm or suicidal behaviors, no study has explored these domains together.

In view of the above observations, the present study attempted to explore the descriptive profiles of self-harm and suicidal behaviors among junior secondary school students in Hong Kong. A longitudinal approach was adopted to examine how family functioning and PYD contribute to self-harm and suicidal behaviors over time.

One crucial issue addressed in this study is how family functioning predicts self-harm and suicidal behaviors. Family functioning is important in influencing the destructive thinking and behavior of adolescents. Siu and Shek (2005) suggested that mutuality among family members, communication and cohesiveness, conflict and harmony, parental concern, and parental control are significant dimensions in understanding family atmosphere in Chinese communities. Destructive family dynamics can upset adolescent development, which may in turn result in self-harm and suicidal behaviors among adolescents. Conceptually speaking, good family functioning can be regarded as a protective factor that reduces the occurrence of deliberate self-harm and suicide in adolescents.

Another issue addressed in this study was how PYD relates to adolescent development. Along the line of positive psychology, the whole doctrine of PYD argues that "problem-free" is not adequate for youth development (Sun & Hui, 2007) and that youth workers must focus on the youth as resources. Benson (1997) proposed 40 developmental internal and external assets. The internal assets include commitment to learning, positive values, social competence, and positive identity. The external assets include positive family communication and support, parental involvement, other adult relationships, caring neighborhood and school climate, empowerment (e.g., from the community), youth as resources, family and school boundaries, and peer influence. In a large youth promotion program in Hong Kong, Shek, Sun, and Merrick (2013) highlighted the importance of 15 PYD qualities, namely, promotion of bonding, resilience, social competence, emotional competence, cognitive competence, behavioral competence, moral competence, self-determination, spirituality, self-efficacy, positive identity, belief in the future, recognition of positive behavior, prosocial involvement, and prosocial norms. In the present study, PYD qualities were hypothesized as capable of reducing self-harm and suicidal behaviors. Taken as a whole, a conceptual framework was tested in this study. Under this framework, family functioning was proposed to influence the development of PYD qualities, which would further affect deliberate self-harm and suicidal behaviors. Specifically, family functioning at Time 1 was proposed to affect PYD at Time 2, which would in turn influenced adolescent self-harm and suicidal behaviors at Time 3.

Another issue related to the understanding of adolescent self-harm and suicidal behaviors is gender issue. As the number of girls exhibiting self-harm and suicidal behaviors is greater than that of boys (Evans, Smith, Hill, Albers, & Neufeld, 1996; Lee, 2011), we must ask whether the proposed model is equally applicable to males and females. Thus, we enhance our understanding of the proposed model by examining its gender invariance.

Method

Participants and Procedures

The data reported in this paper were derived from the first three waves of a 6-year longitudinal study on adolescents' development and their families in Hong Kong. Schools were randomly sampled based on the list of secondary schools in Hong Kong as issued by the Hong Kong Education Bureau. At Wave 1, 3,325 Secondary 1 students (Grade 7) from 28 schools participated in the study. The mean age of

Table 1 Description of demographic variables ($n=2{,}489$)

	Overall %/ mean (SD)	Male ($n=1{,}231$) %/mean (SD)	Female ($n=1{,}258$) %/mean(SD)	Statistical test	Cohen's *d*
Gender		–	–	–	–
Male	49.5 %				
Female	50.5 %				
Age (in years)	12.56 (.70)	12.58 (.72)	12.54 (.68)	$t(2{,}464)=1.45$	.06
Age range	10–17	10–17	11–16		
Household income (in HK$)					–
≤$10,000	19.5 %	18.3 %	20.9 %	$\chi^2(6)=16.07$*	
$10,001–$20,000	30.1 %	25.2 %	35.7 %		
$20,001–$30,000	15.2 %	14.3 %	16.3 %		
$30,001–$40,000	8.9 %	10.6 %	6.8 %		
$40,001–$50,000	6.7 %	7.3 %	6.1 %		
$50,001–$60,000	5.3 %	6.6 %	3.8 %		
≥ $60,001	14.3 %	17.7 %	10.4 %		

Note: Valid cases ranged from 2,239 to 2,489. Valid percentages are reported because of missing data
*$p<.05$

the participants was 12.6 years old (SD=.70). The demographic information of the respondents at Wave 3 is shown in Table 1. A total of 2,667 participants completed the questionnaires in all three waves. Only those who had completed all three waves were included in the analysis ($n=2{,}667$). However, cases with missing gender information ($n=28$) as well as those that lack all dependent variables ($n=8$) and any predictor variable ($n=142$) were excluded. Therefore, the final sample size was 2,489.

During data collection, the purpose of the study was mentioned, and the confidentiality of the collected data was assured. School, parental, and student consents had been obtained prior to data collection. All participants responded to all scales in the self-administered questionnaire within the adequate time provided.

Instruments

The Chinese Positive Youth Development Scale (CPYDS): The CPYDS was developed to assess PYD attributes (Shek, Siu, & Lee, 2007). The CPYDS has 15 subscales, namely, bonding, resilience, social competence, recognition of positive behavior, emotional competence, cognitive competence, behavioral competence, moral competence, self-determination, self-efficacy, clear and positive identity, beliefs in the future, prosocial involvement, prosocial norms, and spirituality. A 6-point Likert scale (from 1 = strongly disagree to 6 = strongly agree) was used to assess the responses of the participants. Existing research findings showed that the CPYDS is a valid and reliable instrument. A composite score was calculated to obtain the mean scores of the 15 PYD constructs. The internal consistency of this scale was .96 for all three waves.

The Chinese Family Assessment Instrument (CFAI): The CFAI (Shek & Ma, 2010) was used to assess family functioning. Three subscales, namely, mutuality (mutual support, love, and concern among family members), communication (frequency and nature of interaction among family members), and conflicts and harmony (presence of conflicts and harmonious behavior in the family) were used to index family functioning. The five response options were "very similar," "somewhat similar," "neither similar nor dissimilar," "somewhat dissimilar," and "very dissimilar." A high total score on the subscales indicated a high level of positive family functioning. The reliability and validity of the CFAI have been verified in previous studies. Three composite scores were computed to obtain the average scores of the three subscales of family functioning. All Cronbach alphas were at least .76 (i.e., mutuality .87, conflict .76, and communication .81 at Time 1; mutuality .86, conflict .78, and communication .81 at Time 2; mutuality .88, conflict .79, and communication .81 at Time 3).

Deliberate Self-Harm Behavior Checklist: A checklist of self-harm behavior was used. The list included wrist cutting, burning with cigarette or fire, carving words or marks on the body, self-scratching, self-biting, rubbing sandpaper against the body, acid dripping, bleach scrubbing, putting sharp objects into the body, rubbing glass against the body, breaking bones, head banging, self-punching, and preventing wounds from healing. The response options were "yes (within the past 12 months)" or "no (within the past 12 months)." The Cronbach alphas at Time 1, Time 2, and Time 3 were .83, .84, and .82, respectively.

Suicidal Behavior Checklist: Suicidal behaviors were assessed in terms of suicidal thoughts, plans, and attempts. The response options were "yes (within the past 12 months)" or "no (within the past 12 months)." The Cronbach alphas at Time 1, Time 2, and Time 3 were .68, .70, and .68, respectively.

Data Analysis

Descriptive statistics of self-harm and suicidal behaviors are reported in this paper with consideration of gender invariance. The path analyses were conducted using Mplus 7 (Muthén & Muthén, 1998–2012). Full information maximum likelihood estimation was employed to deal with missing data. The path analyses were conducted to examine the relationships among the four study variables. Specifically, we hypothesized a fully mediated model with family functioning variables at Wave 1 as the predictors, PYD qualities at Wave 2 as the mediator, and self-harm and suicidal behavior at Wave 3 as the outcome variables (see Fig. 1). The model would be revised based on modification indices and initial findings. As we anticipated that

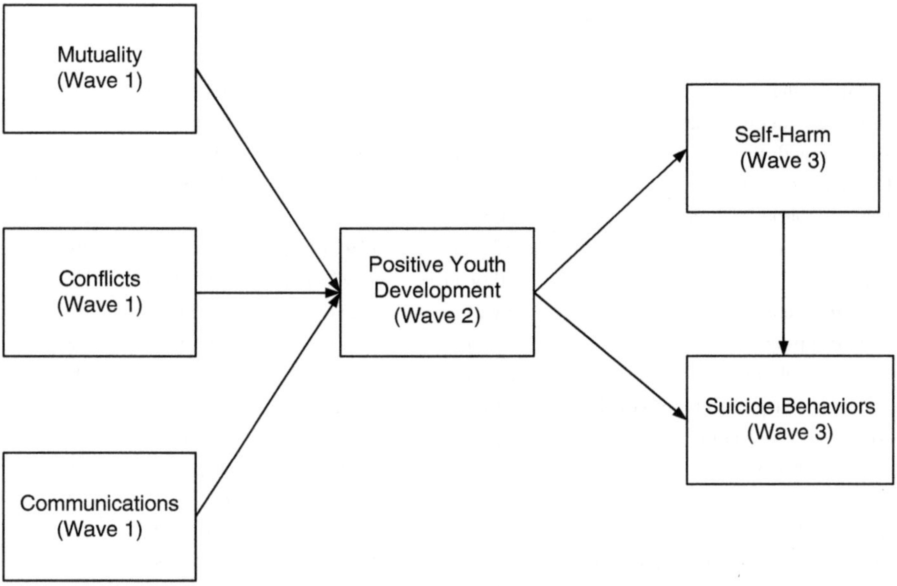

Fig. 1 Conceptual relationships among family functioning, positive youth development qualities, self-harm, and suicidal behaviors

gender might moderate the relationships among the study variables, we performed a multiple group path analysis to test the model across genders. Then, we conducted a series of invariance tests to determine whether each path was successively held invariant across genders.

Results

Among the 2,489 participants, approximately 49.5 % were male, and approximately 49.6 % reported that their household income was below HK$20,000. The average age was 12.56 years (SD = .70), with ages ranging from 10 years to 17 years. Table 1 shows the demographic characteristics.

Profile of Self-Harm and Suicidal Behaviors

Table 2 presents the self-harm behavior of the participants. The prevalence for deliberate self-harm behavior at Grade 9 was 21.9 %, with the top three forms being *preventing wounds from healing* (9.5 %), *self-scratching* (9.1 %), and *wrist cutting* (6.9 %). The participants seldom performed acid dropping (0.2 %), bleach

Table 2 Self-harm behavior in the past 12 months by gender ($N=2,489$)

	Male (%)	Female (%)	Total (%)	χ^2
Wrist-cutting	40 (3.2)	134 (10.7)	174 (6.9)	53.09***
Burning with cigarette	7 (.5)	10 (.8)	17 (.7)	49 ns
Burning with fire	13 (1.1)	7 (.6)	20 (.8)	1.89 ns
Carving word on body	26 (2.1)	67 (5.3)	93 (3.7)	18.26***
Carving marks on body	30 (2.4)	63 (5.0)	93(3.7)	11.68***
Self-scratching	67 (5.4)	159 (12.6)	226 (9.1)	39.61***
Biting	50 (4.1)	97 (7.7)	147 (5.9)	15.25***
Rubbing sand paper	3 (.2)	4 (.3)	7 (.3)	.13 ns
Acid dripping	4 (.3)	1 (.1)	5 (.2)	1.85 ns
Bleach scrubbing	2 (.2)	2 (.2)	4 (.2)	.00 ns
Inserting sharp objects into the body	13 (1.1)	24 (1.9)	37 (1.5)	3.15 ns
Rubbing glass against skin	6 (.5)	8 (.6)	14 (.6)	.26 ns
Breaking bones	3 (.2)	1 (.1)	4 (.2)	1.03 ns
Head banging	29 (2.4)	32 (2.5)	61 (2.5)	.11 ns
Self-punching	38 (3.1)	66 (5.2)	104 (4.2)	7.50*
Preventing wounds from healing	96 (7.8)	141 (11.2)	237 (9.5)	8.77*
Other forms of self-harm	32 (2.6)	42 (3.3)	74 (3.0)	1.26 ns
Any form of self-harm	212 (17.2)	334 (26.6)	546 (21.9)	31.56***

*$p<.05$; ***$p<.001$

Table 3 Suicidal behavior in the past 12 months by gender ($N=2,489$)

	Male (%)	Female (%)	Total (%)	χ^2
Suicidal thoughts	94 (7.6)	194 (15.4)	288 (11.6)	37.66***
Suicidal plans	33 (2.7)	69 (5.5)	102 (4.1)	12.71**
Suicidal attempts	25 (2.0)	60 (4.8)	85 (3.4)	14.35***

**$p<.01$; ***$p<.001$

scrubbing (0.2 %), and sandpaper rubbing (0.3 %). The prevalence of self-harm behaviors for girls was higher than that for boys (girls = 26.6 %, boys = 21.97 %, $\chi^2=31.56$, $p<.001$). The girls manifested the following self-harm behaviors more than the boys did: wrist cutting, word or mark carving, self-scratching, biting, self-punching, and preventing wounds from healing ($p<.05$ in all cases). The largest differences were observed in wrist cutting and self-scratching.

The findings on suicidal behaviors are shown in Table 3. Almost 11.6 % of the adolescents manifested suicidal thoughts, 4.1 % made suicidal plans, and 3.4 % attempted suicide. The girls reported significantly more suicidal behaviors, particularly suicidal thoughts, than the boys did (girls = 15.4 %, boys = 7.6 %, $\chi^2=37.66$, $p<.001$).

Path Analysis in Overall Sample

Our hypothesized model (Fig. 1) was tested and found to fit the data adequately given the following indices: $\chi^2(6) = 61.648$, $p < .001$, RMSEA = .061 (90 % CI = .048–.075), CFI = .947, TLI = .893, SRMR = .049. However, modification indices suggested the addition of the path from mutuality at Wave 1 to self-harm at Wave 3 (MI = 35.754). As parents with children who have exhibited self-harm behaviors admitted their lack of skills in parenting adolescents as well as the significant difficulties they face in family communication, in parent–child relationships, and in the area of discipline following self-harm (Byrne et al., 2008), the expression of concern or mutuality might be a key factor that leads to self-harm. This assumption justifies the addition of the path.

The following fit indices improved after the addition of the path: $\chi^2(5) = 21.165$, $p < .001$, RMSEA = .040 (90 % CI = .026–.057), CFI = .981, TLI = .954, SRMR = .024. The modification indices further suggested the addition of the path from conflicts at Wave 1 to suicidal behaviors at Wave 3 (MI = 16.676). As the literature showed that suicide risk increases with high parent–child conflicts (Randell, Wang, Herting, & Eggert, 2006), the addition of the path was again justified. The revised model fitted the data very well after the addition of the path, as could be noted in the following: $\chi^2(4) = 8.237$, $p = .0833$, RMSEA = .021 (90 % CI = .000–.041), CFI = .996, TLI = .988, SRMR = .010. With no other suggestions for improvement from the modification indices, the revised model was finalized (Fig. 2).

The final revised model showed that family functioning at Wave 1 was positively associated with PYD at Wave 2. However, only mutuality ($\beta = .185$, $p < .001$) and communication ($\beta = .226$, $p < .001$) significantly predicted PYD. Mutuality at Wave 1 negatively predicted self-harm at Wave 3 ($\beta = -.132$, $p < .001$). Similarly, conflicts at Wave 1 negatively predicted suicidal behaviors at Wave 3 ($\beta = -.079$, $p < .001$). PYD at Wave 2 was negatively associated with self-harm and suicidal behaviors at Wave 3. The participants who reported an increase in self-harm behaviors tended to exhibit a corresponding increase in suicidal behaviors ($\beta = .415$, $p < .001$).

We also examined the indirect effects among the study variables (see Table 4). We found that mutuality at Wave 1 ($\beta = -.026$, $p < .001$) and communication at Wave 1 ($\beta = -.032$, $p < .001$) were negatively associated with self-harm at Wave 3 via PYD at Wave 2. Mutuality at Wave 1 was negatively associated with suicidal behavior at Wave 3 via (1) PYD at Wave 2 ($\beta = -.011$, $p < .01$), (2) self-harm at Wave 3 ($\beta = -.055$, $p < .01$), and (3) both PYD at Wave 2 and self-harm at Wave 3 ($\beta = -.011$, $p < .001$). Communication at Wave 1 was negatively associated with suicidal behavior via (1) PYD at Wave 2 ($\beta = -.013$, $p < .01$) as well as (2) PYD at Wave 2 and self-harm at Wave 3 ($\beta = -.013$, $p < .001$). In sum, PYD was a mediator of the effects of mutuality and communication on self-harm and suicidal behaviors. No significant indirect effects of the path from conflicts to self-harm and suicidal behaviors via PYD were found.

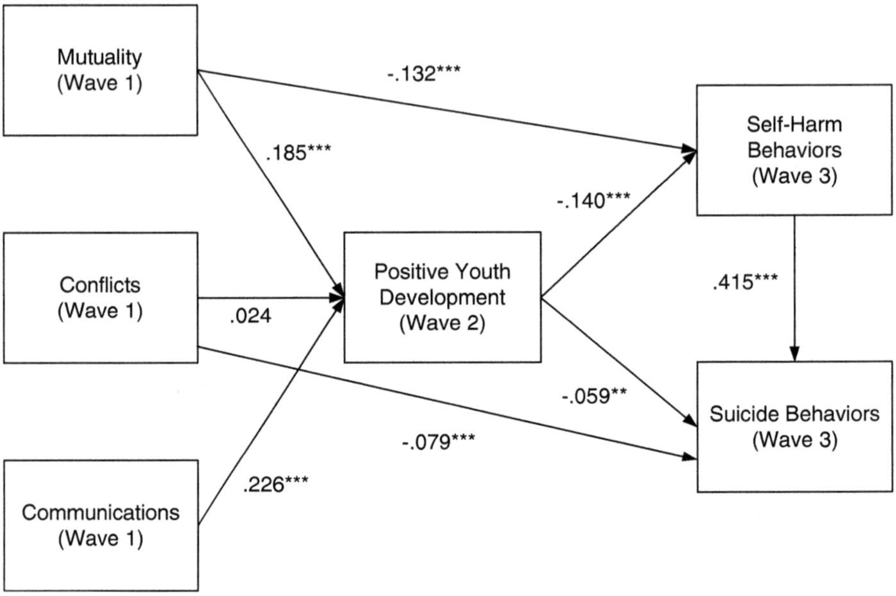

Fig. 2 Standardized coefficients of direct effects among study variables (Note: **$p<.01$; ***$p<.001$)

Table 4 Standardized coefficients of indirect effects

	Standardized coefficients
(1) Time 1 Mutuality → Time 2 PYD → Time 3 Self-Harm Behavior	–.026***
(2) Time 1 Conflicts → Time 2 PYD → Time 3 Self-Harm Behavior	–.003
(3) Time 1 Communication → Time 2 PYD → Time 3 Self-Harm Behavior	–.032***
(4a) Time 1 Mutuality → Time 2 PYD → Time 3 Suicidal Behavior	–.011**
(4b) Time 1 Mutuality → Time 3 Self-Harm Behavior → Time 3 Suicide Behavior	–.055***
(4c) Time 1 Mutuality → Time 2 PYD → Time 3 Self-Harm Behavior → Time 3 Suicidal Behavior	–.011***
(4) Total indirect effects	–.077***
(5a) Time 1 Conflicts → Time 2 PYD → Time 3 Suicidal Behavior	–.001
(5b) Time 1 Conflicts → Time 2 PYD → Time 3 Self-Harm Behavior → Suicide Behavior	–.001
(5) Total indirect effects	–.003
(6a) Time 1 Communication → Time 2 PYD → Time 3 Suicide Behavior	–.013**
(6b) Time 1 Communication → Time 2 PYD → Time 3 Self-Harm Behavior → Time 3 Suicide Behavior	–.013***
(6) Total indirect effects	–.027***

PYD Positive Youth Development
**$p<.01$; ***$p<.001$

Multiple Group Path Analysis Across Genders

We conducted a multiple group path analysis to investigate how gender moderates the relationships among the study variables. The following fit indices indicated that the finalized model (see Fig. 2) fitted the data well across genders: $\chi^2(8) = 19.023$, $p < .05$, RMSEA = .033 (90 % CI = .014–.053), CFI = .989, TLI = .968, SRMR = .013. Figure 3 shows the standardized coefficients of the model. In general, the patterns were similar to that of the model based on the total sample. In terms of gender effects, many parameters were similar across genders. However, two particular paths were quite different between males and females. Specifically, the path from conflicts at Wave 1 to suicidal behaviors at Wave 3 was not significant among males ($\beta = -.024$, $p = ns$) but was significant among females ($\beta = -.126$, $p < .001$). Meanwhile, the path from PYD at Wave 2 to suicidal behaviors at Wave 3 was significant among males ($\beta = -.072$, $p < .05$) but not among females ($\beta = -.057$, $p = ns$) (Table 5).

To determine if the paths estimated across genders were invariant, a fully constrained model (M2 in Table 6) was compared with the freely estimated final revised model presented above (M1). We used the criterion proposed by Cheung and Rensvold (2002) instead of the insignificance of the chi-square difference test between nested models to judge a lack of invariance (i.e., ΔCFI = or < .01) because

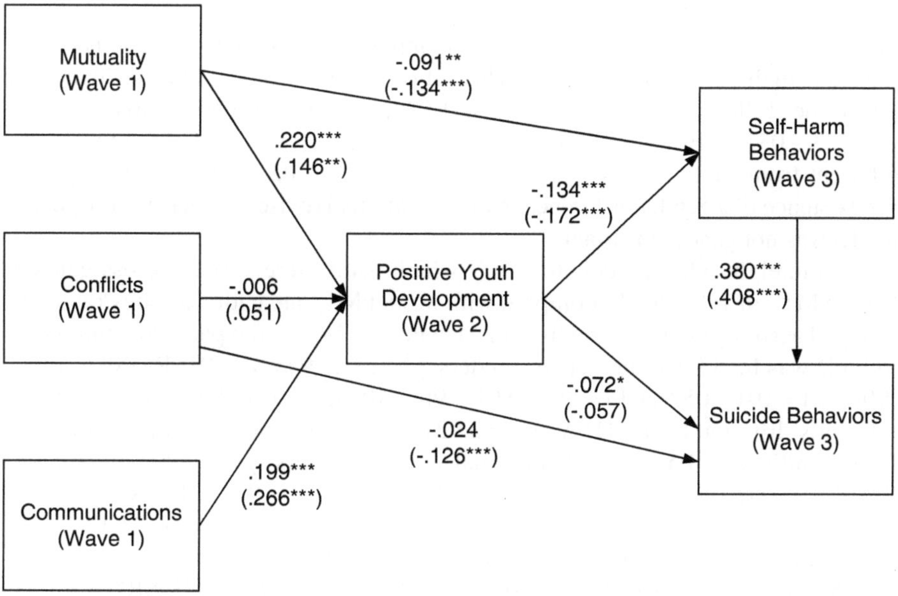

Fig. 3 Standardized coefficients of the final revised model across genders (Coefficients without parentheses represent the results for males. Coefficients with parentheses represent the results for females. $^*p < .05$; $^{**}p < .01$; $^{***}p < .001$)

Table 5 Standardized coefficients of indirect effects across genders

	Male	Female
(1) Time 1 Mutuality → Time 2 PYD → Time 3 Self-Harm Behavior	–.029**	–.025*
(2) Time 1 Conflicts → Time 2 PYD → Time 3 Self-Harm Behavior	.001	–.009
(3) Time 1 Communication → Time 2 PYD → Time 3 Self-Harm Behavior	–.027**	–.046***
(4a) Time 1 Mutuality → Time 2 PYD → Time 3 Suicidal Behavior	–.016*	–.008
(4b) Time 1 Mutuality → Time 3 Self-Harm Behavior → Time 3 Suicidal Behavior	–.035**	–.055***
(4c) Time 1 Mutuality → Time 2 PYD → Time 3 Self-Harm Behavior → Time 3 Suicidal Behavior	–.011**	–.010*
(4) Total indirect effects	–.062***	–.073***
(5a) Time 1 Conflicts → Time 2 PYD → Time 3 Suicidal Behavior	.000	–.003
(5b) Time 1 Conflicts → Time 2 PYD → Time 3 Self-Harm Behavior → Time 3 Suicidal Behavior	.000	–.004
(5) Total indirect effects	.001	–.006
(6a) Time 1 Communication → Time 2 PYD → Time 3 Suicidal Behavior	.014*	–.015
(6b) Time 1 Communication → Time 2 PYD → Time 3 Self-Harm Behavior → Time 3 Suicidal Behavior	–.010**	–.019***
(6) Total indirect effects	–.024**	–.034**

PYD Positive Youth Development
$^{*}p<.05$; $^{**}p<.01$; $^{***}p<.001$

this criterion is unaffected by both model complexity and sample size and is uncorrelated with the overall fit measures. The fully constrained model fitted the data well given the following indices: $\chi^2(16)=51.036$, $p<.001$, RMSEA = .042 (90 % CI = .029–.055), CFI = .966, TLI = .949, SRMR = .061. However, it was significantly different from M1: $\Delta\chi^2(8)=32.013$, $p<.001$, ΔCFI = –.023. This result suggested the existence of a gender difference in the overall final revised model. Therefore, the model was not gender invariant.

We ran eight other models to verify which paths were variant across genders (M3 to M10 in Table 6). To compare with Model M1, one path was constrained to be equal across genders at one time in each model. In M3, the path from mutuality to PYD was held invariant across genders: $\chi^2(9)=21.944$, $p<.01$, RMSEA = .034 (90 % CI = .016–.052), CFI = .987, TLI = .966, SRMR = .014; the path was not significantly different from M1: $\Delta\chi^2(1)=2.921$, $p=ns$, ΔCFI = –.002. In M4, the path from conflicts to PYD was held equal across genders: $\chi^2(9)=20.066$, $p<.05$, RMSEA = .031 (90 % CI = .013–.050), CFI = .989, TLI = .971, SRMR = .014; the path was not significantly different from M1: $\Delta\chi^2(1)=1.043$, $p=ns$, ΔCFI = .000. In M5, the path from communication to PYD was held invariant: $\chi^2(9)=19.200$, $p<.05$, RMSEA = .030 (90 % CI = .011–.049), CFI = .990, TLI = .973, SRMR = .013; the path was not significantly different from M1: $\Delta\chi^2(1)=.177$, $p=ns$, ΔCFI = .001. In M6, the path from mutuality to self-harm was constrained to be equal: $\chi^2(9)=21.442$, $p<.05$, RMSEA = .033 (90 % CI = .015–.052), CFI = .988,

Table 6 Invariance tests across genders

	Parameters constrained	χ^2	df	CFI	$\Delta\chi^2$	Δdf	Δ*p*-value	ΔCFI
M1	None	19.023*	8	.989	–	–	–	–
M2	All	51.036***	16	.966	32.013***	8	<.001	–.023
M3	Mutuality → Positive Youth Development	21.944**	9	.987	2.921	1	.087	–.002
M4	Conflicts → Positive Youth Development	20.066*	9	.989	1.043	1	.307	.000
M5	Communication → Positive Youth Development	19.200*	9	.990	.177	1	.674	.001
M6	Mutuality → Self-Harm Behavior	21.442*	9	.988	2.419	1	.120	–.001
M7	Conflicts → Suicidal Behavior	30.282***	9	.979	11.259***	1	<.001	–.010
M8	Positive Youth Development → Self-Harm Behavior	24.125**	9	.985	5.102*	1	.024	–.004
M9	Positive Youth Development → Suicidal Behavior	19.153*	9	.990	.130	1	.718	.001
M10	Self-Harm Behaviors → Suicidal Behaviors	20.058*	9	.989	1.035	1	.309	.000

Note: M1 is the baseline model in which all parameters were freely estimated. From M2 to M10, the reference model is M1
$^*p<.05$; $^{**}p<.01$; $^{***}p<.001$

TLI = .968, SRMR = .020; the path was not significantly different from M1: $\Delta\chi^2(1) = 2.419$, $p = ns$, ΔCFI = –.001. In M7, the path from conflicts to suicidal behaviors was held invariant: $\chi^2(9) = 30.282$, $p < .001$, RMSEA = .044 (90 % CI = .027–.061), CFI = .979, TLI = .945, SRMR = .021; the path was significantly different from M1: $\Delta\chi^2$ (1) = 11.259, $p < .001$, ΔCFI = –.010. In M8, the path from PYD to self-harm was significantly constrained: $\chi^2(9) = 24.125$, $p < .01$, RMSEA = .037 (90 % CI = .019–.055), CFI = .985, TLI = .961, SRMR = .021; the path was not significantly different from M1: $\Delta\chi^2(1) = 5.102$, $p < .05$, ΔCFI = –.004. In M9, the path from PYD to suicidal behavior was held invariant: $\chi^2(9) = 19.153$, $p < .05$, RMSEA = .030 (90 % CI = .010–.049), CFI = .990, TLI = .974, SRMR = .013; the path was not significantly different from M1: $\Delta\chi^2(1) = .130$, $p = ns$, ΔCFI = .001. In M10, the path from self-harm to suicidal behavior was constrained to be equal: $\chi^2(9) = 20.058$, $p < .05$, RMSEA = .031 (90 % CI = .012–.050), CFI = .989, TLI = .971, SRMR = .017; the path was not significantly different from M1: $\Delta\chi^2(1) = 1.035$, $p = ns$, ΔCFI = .000. In sum, only one parameter (i.e., from conflict to suicidal behavior) was significantly variant across genders.

Table 5 shows the indirect effects across genders. The patterns of indirect effects were similar to those reported above regardless of gender. Only two specific indirect effects were different between males and females. First, the indirect effect of PYD from mutuality to suicidal behavior was significant in males ($\beta = -.016$, $p < .05$) but not in females ($\beta = -.008$, $p = ns$). Second, the indirect effect of PYD from communication to suicidal behavior was also significant in males ($\beta = -.014$, $p < .05$) but not in females ($\beta = -.015$, $p < .05$).

Discussion

The prevalence of self-harm behavior among the Grade 9 adolescents who participated in the study was around 21.9 %, which was lower than the percentage (23.5 %) when these students were in Grade 8 (Law & Shek, 2013). In fact, all kinds of self-harm behaviors among the adolescents decreased as they advanced to Grade 9 from Grade 8. Despite this decrease, the figure remains alarming because it implies that one in four to five adolescents have attempted to self-harm in the past 12 months. This percentage is higher than that in another study in China that reported that almost 17 % of adolescents have manifested self-harm behaviors in the past 12 months (Wan et al., 2011). The most common forms of self-harm among Chinese adolescents in Hong Kong are self-scratching and preventing wounds from healing. This finding varies from that of other studies in mainland China, in which self-hitting was reported as the most prevalent (Wan et al., 2011). The least common form of self-harm involves the use of chemicals. Self-harm does not entail sophisticated methods, and Chinese adolescents are not known to attempt using toxic chemicals.

In the present work, students became much more susceptible to suicidal attempts in Grade 8 than when they were in Grade 7 (Law & Shek, 2013). When they reached Grade 9, the percentage of suicidal behaviors decreased. The suicide rate among Hong Kong adolescents is relatively low and can be explained in terms of the social and economic environment. In general, the strongest predictive factors of population suicide rate are economic prosperity and political stability (World Health Organization, 2008). As Hong Kong has experienced economic prosperity and freedom for decades, not many adolescents have been exposed to economic hardships. Moreover, Hong Kong's educational system promotes moral education and PYD programs.

The lack of studies that explain the tendency of the prevalence of self-harm and suicidal behaviors to decrease from Grade 8 to Grade 9 leads us to put forward some conjectures within the unique sociocultural contexts of Hong Kong. Under the new educational system in Hong Kong, all secondary school students are required to study for 3 years in junior secondary school and another 3 years in senior secondary school. By the time they reach Grade 9, they are expected to have already adapted to the school environment. In addition, most adolescents actively select their favorite subjects at Grade 10. Thus, they explore many subjects at Grade 9 and grow increasingly concerned about planning their careers. A focus on academic plans might provide these students with a sense of purpose.

As indicated by the descriptive profile in the study, girls are more prone to self-harm and suicide attempts compared with boys. Puberty causes additional stress for girls during this academic transition. Social comparison and the Hong Kong media exaggerate the importance of physical appearance and body image. These factors contribute to the relatively high prevalence of self-harm and suicidal behaviors among girls because self-harm is related to social stress. Compared with boys, girls are more sensitive to interpersonal relationships such as those with peers and family (Rodham, Hawton, & Evans, 2006). Meanwhile, girls are more inclined to internalize negative emotions compared with boys. The susceptibility to social stress and the internalization of negative emotions may lead to self-destructive behaviors such as self-harm and suicide.

One of the major breakthroughs of the study is the use of a longitudinal approach in exploring the relationships among family functioning, PYD, and self-harm and suicidal behaviors. The major thesis of the revised model is that family functioning influences self-harm and suicidal behaviors via positive youth development attributes. Figure 2 reveals several important observations. First, similar to the findings of Hawton (2005), the most critical predictor of suicidal behavior is self-harm. Second, although mutuality at Wave 1 directly influenced self-harm behavior at Wave 3, a similar path was not found from mutuality at Wave 1 to suicidal behavior at Wave 3. Third, although conflict at Wave 1 directly influenced suicidal behavior at Wave 3, the path from conflict at Wave 1 to self-harm behavior at Wave 3 was not significant. Fourth, only mutuality and communication (but not conflict) at Wave 1 influenced self-harm and suicidal behaviors at Wave 3 in terms of total indirect effects (Table 4).

This longitudinal study is the first to explore how family functioning and PYD influence self-harm and suicidal behaviors among adolescents over time. Self-destructive behaviors among adolescents have long been argued to be influenced by both personal and social factors (Sun & Hui, 2007). This study shows that both family functioning and PYD are important protective factors in reducing self-harm or suicidal behaviors. Using path analysis, we can clearly differentiate the impact of the different components of family functioning (mutuality, conflicts, and communications) on self-harm and suicidal behaviors. The final model suggests that mutuality, conflicts, communication, and PYD exert their influence on self-harm and suicidal behaviors in different manner. This study arrived at two different findings: mutuality directly affects self-harm behaviors, whereas conflicts affect suicidal behaviors. The literature in general (Isacsson & Rich, 2001; Wan et al., 2011) shows that self-harm and suicide attempts operate differently, with self-harm originating from anxiety and suicide attempts originating from depression. In this manner, we can propose that the lack of mutuality or family cohesion can induce internal anxiety in adolescents, and this anxiety may lead to self-harm behaviors. However, overt parent–child conflicts can ultimately lead to adolescent depression, which may result in suicidal behaviors. Further studies can be performed in this direction to distinguish these two types of self-destructive behaviors.

Another contribution of this study is the gender invariance in the proposed model. The descriptive statistics have already shown that girls manifest self-harm and suicidal behaviors more than boys do. The results show that in general, the proposed model was not entirely gender invariant. One path was significantly different, that is, conflicts for girls at Wave 1 led to suicidal behaviors at Wave 3; this path was not significant for boys. Otherwise, all other paths would be gender invariant. One explanation is that girls are more susceptible to social stress than boys (Rodham et al., 2006). Girls take conflicts personally, whereas boys opt to choose other coping methods. This result implies that we should focus on conflicts among girls.

The understanding of self-harm and suicide path models in adolescents in Hong Kong is critical in facilitating the design of culturally sensitive and community-based interventions (Goldston et al., 2008). Both medical and psychosocial interventions are necessary in bringing effective changes to people (Royal College of Psychiatrists, 2010). The prevention of self-harm and suicidal behaviors requires multidisciplinary cooperation among doctors, social workers, and educators. From the findings, we can develop programs that are aimed at enhancing both family functioning and PYD for early adolescents. Several service directions can be taken. First, we should focus on self-harm behaviors because they easily lead to suicidal behaviors. As mentioned previously, this topic is a neglected area in the literature. Second, gender-sensitive practice is in order. The findings suggest that we should focus on family mutuality and communication among boys as well as on family conflicts among girls. Third, psychosocial interventions in schools can come in the form of positive promotional programs or online programs. One example is the Project P.A.T.H.S. in Hong Kong, which is sponsored by the Hong Kong Jockey Club Charities Trust. According to its longitudinal evaluation, the project was able to promote holistic development and reduce risk behavior in adolescents (Shek & Ma, 2012).

Several research directions can be taken in the future. First, although family functioning and PYD come from two earlier waves, self-harm and suicidal behaviors belong to the same wave. As such, we cannot claim that self-harm can lead to suicidal behaviors. Hence, further waves of data are needed. Second, fully understanding the roles of PYD requires the use of the four second-order factors of PYD in model testing. In this sense, we can understand the interaction among the three components of family functioning, the four components of PYD, and two types of self-destructive behaviors. Third, low- and high-risk adolescents should be identified by latent class analysis, and different path models could be tested. We should work not only with low-risk adolescents using early identification strategies and PYD education but also with high-risk adolescents using active interventions and crisis prevention methods.

As Chinese adolescents in Hong Kong were chosen to participate in the study, the findings may not be generalizable to other Chinese communities. Despite this limitation, this study is the first to propose a path model to understand self-harm and suicidal attempts among adolescents in Hong Kong with reference to family functioning, PYD, and gender invariance. The study underscores the alarming prevalence rates of deliberate self-harm and suicidal behaviors and the potential role of family functioning and PYD in promoting the personal well-being of adolescents.

Acknowledgment The preparation for this work and the Project P.A.T.H.S. were financially supported by the Hong Kong Jockey Club Charities Trust. The authorship is equally shared by the authors.

References

Benson, P. L. (1997). *All kids are our kid: What communities must do to raise caring and responsible children and adolescents*. San Francisco: Jossey-Bass.

Blum, R., Sudhinaraset, M., & Emerson, M. R. (2012). Youth at risk: Suicidal thoughts and attempts in Vietnam, China, and Taiwan. *Journal of Adolescent Health, 50*(3 Supple), S37–S44.

Byrne, S., Morgan, S., Fitzpatrick, C., Boylan, C., Crowley, S., Gahan, H., et al. (2008). Deliberate self-harm in children and adolescents: A qualitative study exploring the needs of parents and carers. *Clinical Child Psychology and Psychiatry, 13*(4), 493–504.

Chan, W. S. C., Law, C. K., Liu, K. Y., Wong, P. W. C., Law, Y. W., & Yip, P. S. F. (2009). Suicidality in Chinese adolescents in Hong Kong: The role of family and cultural influences. *Social Psychiatry and Psychiatric Epidemiology, 44*(4), 278–284.

Cheung, G. W., & Rensvold, R. B. (2002). Evaluating goodness-of-fit indexes for testing measurement invariance. *Structural Equation Modeling: A Multidisciplinary Journal, 9*(2), 233–255.

Czyz, E. K., Liu, Z., & King, C. A. (2012). Social connectedness and one-year trajectories among suicidal adolescents following psychiatric hospitalization. *Journal of Clinical Child & Adolescent Psychology, 41*(2), 214–226.

Evans, W., Smith, M., Hill, G., Albers, E., & Neufeld, J. (1996). Rural adolescent views of risk and protective factors associated with suicide. *Crisis Intervention & Time-Limited Treatment, 3*(1), 1–12.

Fox, C., & Hawton, K. (2004). *Deliberate self-harm in adolescence*. London: Jessica Kingsley.

Goldston, D. B., Molock, S. D., Whitbeck, L. B., Murakami, J. L., Zayas, L. H., & Hall, G. C. N. (2008). Cultural considerations in adolescent suicide prevention and psychosocial treatment. *American Psychologist, 63*(1), 14–31.

Hall-Lande, J. A., Eisenberg, M. E., Christenson, S. L., & Neumark-Sztainer, D. (2007). Social isolation, psychological health, and protective factors in adolescence. *Adolescence, 42*(166), 265–286.

Hawton, K. (2005). *What happens to deliberate self harm patients in the long term*. Oxford, UK: University of Oxford Centre for Suicide Research.

Isacsson, G., & Rich, C. L. (2001). Management of patients who deliberately harm themselves. *BMJ, 322*(7280), 213–215.

Law, B. M. F., & Shek, D. T. L. (2013). Self-harm and suicide attempts among young Chinese adolescents in Hong Kong: Prevalence, correlates, and changes. *Journal of Pediatric and Adolescent Gynecology, 26*(3 Suppl), S26–S32.

Lee, S. (2011). Reasons for living and their moderating effects on Korean adolescents' suicidal ideation. *Death Studies, 35*(8), 711–728.

Lubell, K. M., & Vetter, J. B. (2006). Suicide and youth violence prevention: The promise of an integrated approach. *Aggression and Violent Behavior, 11*(2), 167–175.

Maimon, D., Browning, C. R., & Brooks-Gunn, J. (2010). Collective efficacy, family attachment, and urban adolescent suicide attempts. *Journal of Health and Social Behavior, 51*(3), 307–324.

Mota, N., Elias, B., Tefft, B., Medved, M., Munor, G., & Sareen, J. (2012). Correlates of suicidality: Investigation of a representative sample of Manitoba First Nations adolescents. *American Journal of Public Health, 102*(7), 1353–1361.

Mustanski, B., & Liu, R. T. (2013). A longitudinal study of predictors of suicide attempts among lesbian, gay, bisexual, and transgender youth. *Archives of Sexual Behavior, 42*(3), 437–448.

Muthén, L. K., & Muthén, B. O. (1998–2012). *Mplus user's guide* (7th ed.). Los Angeles: Muthén & Muthén.

Pisani, A. R., Wyman, P. A., Petrova, M., Schmeelk-Cone, K., Goldston, D. B., Xia, Y., et al. (2013). Emotion regulation difficulties, youth-adult relationships, and suicide attempts among high school students in underserved communities. *Journal of Youth and Adolescence, 42*(6), 807–820.

Randell, B. P., Wang, W. L., Herting, J. R., & Eggert, L. L. (2006). Family factors predicting categories of suicide risk. *Journal of Child and Family Studies, 15*(3), 255–270. doi:10.1007/s10826-006-9020-6.

Rew, L., Thomas, N., Horner, S. D., Resnick, M. D., & Beuhring, T. (2001). Correlates of recent suicide attempts in a triethnic group of adolescents. *Journal of Nursing Scholarship, 33*(4), 361–367.

Rodham, K., Hawton, K., & Evans, E. (2006). *By their own young hand: Deliberate self-harm and suicidal ideas in adolescent health*. Philadelphia: Jessica Kingsley.

Royal College of Psychiatrists. (2010). *Self-harm, suicide and risk: Helping people who self-harm*. London: Author.

Samuel, D., & Sher, L. (2013). Suicidal behavior in Indian adolescents. *International Journal of Adolescent Medicine and Health, 25*(3), 207–212.

Sharaf, A. Y., Thompson, E. A., & Walsh, E. (2010). Protective effects of self-esteem and family support on suicide risk behaviors among at-risk adolescents: Corrigendum. *Journal of Child and Adolescent Psychiatric Nursing, 23*(1), 45.

Shek, D. T. L., & Ma, C. M. S. (2010). The Chinese Family Assessment Instrument (C-FAI): Hierarchical confirmatory factor analyses and factorial invariance. *Research on Social Work Practice, 20*(1), 112–123.

Shek, D. T. L., & Ma, C. M. S. (2012). Impact of the Project P.A.T.H.S. in the junior secondary school years: Objective outcome evaluation based on eight waves of longitudinal data. *The Scientific World Journal, 2012*, 170345.

Shek, D. T. L., Siu, A. M. H., & Lee, T. Y. (2007). The Chinese positive youth development scale: A validation study. *Research on Social Work Practice, 17*(3), 380–391.

Shek, D. T. L., Sun, R. C. F., & Merrick, J. (2013). Positive youth development constructs: Conceptual review and application. In D. T. L. Shek, R. C. F. Sun, & J. Merrick (Eds.), *Positive youth development: Theory, research and application* (pp. xv–xix). New York: Nova.

Siu, A. M. H., & Shek, D. T. L. (2005). Psychometric properties of the Chinese Family Assessment Instrument in Chinese adolescents in Hong Kong. *Adolescence, 40*(160), 817–830.

Sun, R. C. F., & Hui, E. K. P. (2007). Psychosocial factors contributing to adolescent suicidal ideation. *Journal of Youth and Adolescence, 36*(6), 775–786.

Tuisku, V., Kiviruusu, O., Pelkonen, M., Karlsson, L., Strandholm, T., & Marttunen, M. (2014). Depressed adolescents as young adults – Predictors of suicide attempt and non-suicidal self-injury during an 8-year follow-up. *Journal of Affective Disorders, 152–154*, 313–319.

Wan, Y. H., Hu, C. L., Hao, J. H., Sun, Y., & Tao, F. B. (2011). Deliberate self-harm behaviors in Chinese adolescents and young adults. *European Child & Adolescent Psychiatry, 20*(10), 517–525.

World Health Organization. (2008). *Suicide prevention web release*. Geneva, Switzerland: Author. Retrieved from http://www.who.int/mental_health/prevention/suicide/suicideprevent/en.

Yip, K. S., Ngan, M. Y., & Lam, I. (2003). Pattern of adolescent self-cutting in Hong Kong: Reports from school social workers. *International Journal of Adolescence & Youth, 11*(2), 135–155.

Zhang, J., Li, N., Tu, X. M., Xiao, S., & Jia, C. (2011). Risk factors for rural young suicide in China: A case control study. *Journal of Affective Disorders, 129*(1–3), 244–251.

Zweig, J. M., Phillips, S. D., & Lindberg, L. D. (2002). Predicting adolescent profiles of risk: Looking beyond demographics. *Journal of Adolescent Health, 31*(4), 343–353.

Compensated Dating and Juvenile Prostitution in Early Adolescents in Hong Kong

Tak Yan Lee and Daniel T.L. Shek

Abstract Based on the data matched in 3,239 students across Grade 8 and Grade 9, this study examined the prevalence and change in compensated dating (CD) and juvenile prostitution (JP) behavior in early adolescents in Hong Kong. The related psychosocial correlates and the interrelationships among CD, JP, and other forms of risk behavior were also studied. For the prevalence of CD and JP, about 2 % of the respondents had ever engaged in CD, and less than 0.6 % had engaged in JP. Interestingly, males reported a higher percentage of CD and JP than did females. Results showed that different psychosocial correlates (including positive youth development qualities, family functioning, parental control, and difference in paternal age and maternal age) were related to CD and JP. A moderate relationship was also found between CD and substance abuse.

Keywords Compensated dating • Juvenile prostitution • Chinese adolescents • Positive youth development • Risk behavior • Substance abuse

Introduction

Juvenile prostitution is often understood as a form of child sexual abuse (Yates, MacKenzie, Pennbridge, & Swofford, 1991) and sexual exploitation of children for commercial gain (Louw, 1994). However, young people engaging in juvenile prostitution are not always exploited by others who gain profit from selling them for sex (Mitchell, Finkelhor, & Wolak, 2010). In many cases, these activities are self-initiated. Thus, it is not clear to what extent young people who engage in prostitution are victims or criminals. Similarly, it is not clear if they need protection and/or prosecution (Kittling, 2006). Findings from the United States National Juvenile

T.Y. Lee, Ph.D. (✉)
Department of Applied Social Sciences, City University of Hong Kong,
Tat Chee Avenue, Hong Kong
e-mail: ty.lee@cityu.edu.hk

D.T.L. Shek, Ph.D., B.B.S., S.B.S., J.P.
Department of Applied Social Sciences, The Hong Kong Polytechnic University,
Hunghom, Hong Kong

D.T.L. Shek et al. (eds.), *Chinese Adolescents in Hong Kong*,
Quality of Life in Asia 5, DOI 10.1007/978-981-287-143-5_10

Prostitution Study revealed that based on police statistics, 53 % of the juveniles involved in prostitution were classified as victims, 31 % as delinquents, and 16 % as both victims and delinquents (Mitchell et al., 2010).

The term "compensated dating (CD)" ("enjo-kosai" in Japanese) originated in Japan, but it was not frequently used until the 1990s in Japan. In Japanese, "enjo-kosai" is literally translated as "a relationship with (mainly financial) support" (Ueno, 2003) and can be traced back to Japanese vocabulary used by the male-centered mass media in the 1970s. When "enjo-kosai" is defined separately, "enjo" means "assist" in the sphere of economics, while "kosai" means "socializing and entertaining" in the social and cultural sphere (Lam, 2003). Subsidized dating, assisted relationship, freelance teenage prostitution, and casual teen prostitution are also used interchangeably in the literature to refer to the same phenomenon. Lam stated that the English translation cannot capture the dimension of fun and leisure conveyed by the Japanese expression. Indeed, the juxtaposition of the two terms "enjo" and "kosai" is a way to mock the adult world and make a parody of it. Hence, CD as a phenomenon is deeply affected by culture and may find different expressions in different contexts. For instance, many studies have shown that the main motivation for CD with a girl dating for the purpose of receiving compensation was usually financial remuneration (Kinsella, 2012; Masuzoe, 2000). To some researchers, CD was viewed as a transaction, in which individuals mostly girls sell their sexual services for money or gifts without any control or coercion (Wakabayashi, 2003). Apparently, findings from previous research mainly supported the idea of teenage girls offering their services to older men, whereas teenage males have been very rarely studied. Leheny (2006) reported that cases where older women pay younger males for the same kind of dates are better described as "gyaku enjo kōsai" where "gyaku" means "the other way" (as opposed to the normal way). However, such a phenomenon as it is known may very likely reflect the particular structure of the Japanese society in which CD first appeared and may find different expressions in other cultural contexts. For instance, the Japanese society has been described as "a male-dominated society" (McLelland, 2000), but the same definition may not apply to other societies such as Hong Kong. Besides, there is not much data supporting gender differences in compensated dating out of Japan (Lee & Shek, 2013). However, a study on compensated dating in Taiwan conducted by He (2007) found that in contrast to Japan, CD in Taiwan was associated with the lesbian, gay, bisexual, and transgender (LGBT) world, particularly gay men. Thus, gender differences in juvenile prostitution warrant further investigation. Indeed, this culturally unique phenomenon in Japan (Radford & Tsutsumi, 2004; Wakabayashi, 2003) has influenced other East Asian cultures, including Korea (Kong, 2003), Taiwan (Lam, 2003; Ho, 2003), and Hong Kong (Cheung, Lee, & Li, 2011).

While the term "compensated dating" (CD) has been used in the Asian context, the term "juvenile prostitution" (JP) is widely used in the North American context. JP is the act of engagement in relatively indiscriminate sexual activity in exchange for immediate monetary return or other valuables (Jenkins, 2014). Much of the research in the area of JP has been conducted by criminology researchers because juveniles involved in prostitution are usually considered as delinquents (Gray, 2005; Kreston, 2005). Typically, juvenile prostitution involves sexual intercourse.

The Western phenomenon of JP appears somewhat similar to the practice of CD in the East. However, unlike the Western phenomenon of JP, "enjo-kosai" may consist of a variety of nonsexual services, including having dinner together, watching a movie, or visiting an amusement park. In terms of sexual services, sexual contact may range from allowing the man to touch the girl's body from outside of the clothes to allowing him to touch her body directly without any clothes or demanding that the girl to touch his body (Wakabayashi, 2003). In the Western context, escort services and call girls were identified as one type of JP (McNamara & Bucher, 2012).

Therefore, CD may be undertaken as a temporary state or a transitional stage prior to or even a precursor of JP, where girls make alternative decisions before moving into prostitution in the long run (Kong, 2003). Juveniles involved in CD agree to go on a date with the purpose of receiving financial or material return. Most of them thought that they could choose their clients and the kind of sex service, and they used the term CD to reduce their sense of guilt and the level of social stigma attached to the term prostitute (Cheung et al., 2011). However, the phenomenon of CD calls for attention from the field of child protection for several reasons. First, there is no guarantee what customers will do with juveniles during and after CD. Second, juveniles involved in CD are frequently abused, maltreated, and sometimes raped by customers. Third, it is illegal in Hong Kong for adults having sexual intercourse with children under 16. An ambiguity always occurs when a juvenile has sexual intercourse with an adult in exchange for material returns – the juvenile may have committed an offense, but at the same time they may be a victim of a sex crime. Apparently, juveniles will tend to be treated as victims when they are pimped by adults, but when they take an active role in soliciting sexual activities, they will very likely be seen as offenders (Finkelhor & Ormrod, 2004).

Past research investigating JP has mainly examined female prostitutes, with little research on boys and the pre-JP stage. Mental health and human services practitioners and researchers viewed CD among early adolescents as a growing risk (Cheung et al., 2011). Research showed that female JP in the United States is not uncommon. Studies revealed that several family related factors played a critical role in the determination of a female juvenile's risk for entering prostitution. Primary risk factors such as low economic status in the family, domestic violence and abusive experience, chaotic and ineffective parenting styles, and early sexual experiences are prevalent in the JP literature (Hwang & Bedford, 2004; Seng, 1989). Sexual victimization was found to be strongly related to prostitution (Silbert & Pines, 1981). Runaway teenagers who eventually resort to prostitution in order to support themselves financially were frequently seen in JP (Chesney-Lind & Shelden, 2004; Hwang & Bedford, 2004; Kuntay, 2002; Wakabayashi, 2003). As an escape route of their traumatic familial experiences, drug and alcohol abuse were cited as the primary reasons that juvenile prostitutes remain in the prostitution business in order to fund their substance use (Flowers, 2001; Wakabayashi, 2003).

However, not all juvenile prostitutes have previous traumatic experiences. Opportunities to gain immediate rewards (Brawn & Roe-Sepowitz, 2008) and for sexual excitement (Wakabayashi, 2003) are other reasons for engaging in JP. Like "enjo-kosai" in the East, ineffective parenting appears to be associated with these behaviors. Studies on the family background and history of juvenile prostitutes have been conducted. For example, the Committee on Sexual Offences Against

Children and Youth (C.S.O.A.C.Y., 1984) appointed by the Canadian government found that juvenile prostitutes came from families of a variety of social classes, although a "large portion" of juveniles were from "middle class" homes (p. 973). A noticeable research theme is the relationship between dysfunctional family factors (i.e., intrafamilial substance abuse and sexual, physical, and emotional abuse) and subsequent involvement in prostitution (James & Meyerding, 1978; Vitaliano, James & Boyer, 1981).

As the existing literature on CD and JP is mainly based on Japan, Korea, and Western populations, little is known about the pattern of CD/JP and factors related to this behavior among early adolescents in different Chinese contexts, except that some isolated work was done in Taiwan (He, 2007; Lam, 2003) and Hong Kong (Cheung et al., 2011; Lee & Shek, 2013). There are three reasons why CD and JP should be examined in Chinese contexts. First, as almost one-fifth of the world's population is Chinese people, CD/JP among Chinese adolescents should be investigated. Second, as sex was regarded as a taboo in traditional Chinese culture, it is important to understand CD/JP and related phenomena among contemporary adolescents, who may adopt a more liberal perspective on sex. Third, with growing materialism in adolescents (Shek, Ma, & Lin, 2014), the risk for CD and JP might increase because adolescents may engage in CD and JP simply out of the motivation to gain more material possession.

Against this background, there are four purposes of this paper. First, descriptive profiles on CD, JP, and CD/JP in early Chinese adolescents based on data collected from Grade 9 students are reported. Second, the data collected in Grade 9 were compared with Grade 8. Third, findings on the relationships among CD, JP, and CD/JP and demographic and psychosocial correlates (including basic demographic factors, positive youth development qualities, and perceived family processes) are presented. Finally, interrelationships among CD, JP, and risk behaviors are presented.

Method

The present paper reports findings on the compensated dating and juvenile prostitution behaviors of Grade 9 students collected at the third wave of a 6-year longitudinal study. Compensated dating was not among the study variables of the first wave of data collection (i.e., Grade 7 or Secondary 1 students). The data were collected from 28 secondary schools in Hong Kong. In the 2010–2011 school year, 3,580 Secondary 2 (Grade 8) students responded to the questionnaire. Details about the study can be found in Lee and Shek (2013). One year later, the students were invited again to answer the questionnaire in the third wave of data collection. A total of 4,106 students completed the questionnaire, including 2,185 males (valid percent 53.7 %) and 1,885 females (valid percent 46.3 %). The mean age of participants was 14.65 years (SD=.80). Local students accounted for 77.9 % of the participants; 20.3 % of them were born in Mainland China, and 1.8 % were from other places. The demographic information of the participants is summarized in Table 1. From Wave 2 to Wave 3, data of 3,239 students were successfully matched. The analyses presented in this article are based on this matched sample.

Table 1 The prevalence of compensated dating and juvenile prostitution behaviors across Grade 8 and Grade 9 students in Hong Kong

	Wave 2			*Wave 3*			Related-samples McNemar tests	
	Frequency (valid percent)			Frequency (valid percent)				
	N=3,638			*N*=3,977				
	Yes (%)	No (%)	NA*	Yes (%)	No (%)	NA*	Statistics	*P*
Have you ever accompanied a stranger of either the same or the opposite sex in social activities (e.g., meal, movie, etc.) for the sake of gaining money or material return (e.g., receiving a cell phone as a gift)?	77 (2.1 %)	3,525 (97.9 %)	36	94 (2.4 %)	3,816 (97.6 %)	67	.38	ns
Have you ever had sexual intercourse with a stranger of either the same or the opposite sex for the sake of gaining money or material return (e.g., receiving a cell phone as a gift)?	13 (0.4 %)	3,594 (99.6 %)	31	23 (0.6 %)	3,889 (99.4 %)	65	.19	ns
During the past 12 months, have you ever accompanied a stranger of either the same or the opposite sex in any social activities (e.g., meal, movie, etc.) for the sake of gaining money or material return (e.g., receiving a cell phone as a gift)?	59 (1.6 %)	3,549 (98.4 %)	30	64 (1.6 %)	3,843 (98.4 %)	70	.48	ns
During the past 12 months, have you ever had sexual intercourse with a stranger of either the same or the opposite sex for the sake of gaining money or material return (e.g., receiving a cell phone as a gift)?	16 (0.4 %)	3,597 (99.6 %)	25	25 (0.6 %)	3,889 (99.4 %)	63	.52	ns

Note: Related-samples McNemar tests were conducted to examine whether the difference between the distribution of students with CD and JP behaviors in Wave 2 and Wave 3 is significant.

**NA* no answer, *P* probability, *ns* statistically not significant

Measures of Compensated Dating and Juvenile Prostitution

The same four items were used to assess CD and JP behaviors both in Wave 2 and in Wave 3 (Lee & Shek, 2013). They are (1) Have you ever accompanied a stranger of either the same or the opposite sex in social activities (e.g., meal, movie, etc.) for the sake of gaining money or material return (e.g., receiving a cell phone as a gift)? (2) Have you ever had sexual intercourse with a stranger of either the same or the opposite sex for the sake of gaining money or material return (e.g., receiving a cell phone as a gift)? (3) During the past 12 months, have you ever accompanied a stranger of either the same or the opposite sex in any social activities (e.g., meal, movie, etc.) for the sake of gaining money or material return (e.g., receiving a cell phone as a gift)? (4) During the past 12 months, have you ever had sexual intercourse with a stranger of either the same or the opposite sex for the sake of gaining money or material return (e.g., receiving a cell phone as a gift)? Participants answered a yes-no scale (0 = no; 1 = yes). CD behaviors were measured by averaging the scores of the items (1) and (3) and JP behaviors by items (2) and (4), respectively. The two items assessing "CD" (items 1 and 3) showed strong correlation both in Wave 2 ($r = .72$, $p < .001$) and in Wave 3 ($r = .70$, $p < .001$). Similarly, the two items measuring "JP" (items 2 and 4) also showed strong correlation both in Wave 2 ($r = .78$, $p < .001$) and in Wave 3 ($r = .85$, $p < .001$). In addition, a composite score (CD/JP) was calculated by averaging the scores in the four items. This indicator gives an overall picture on the amount of compensated dating and juvenile prostitution behaviors. In short, the composite score "CD/JP" gives an overall picture of the CD and JP. On the other hand, "CD" and "JP" were considered separately – two items on CD (without sexual intercourse) and JP (with sexual intercourse), to highlight possible differences in the two behaviors. The Cronbach's alpha of the total scale was 0.73 in Wave 2 and 0.78 in Wave 3.

The Chinese Positive Youth Development Scale

The Chinese Positive Youth Development Scale (CPYDS) was developed to assess 15 aspects of positive youth development in Chinese adolescents. The details of the items are reported in Shek, Siu, and Lee (2007). In this study, an abridged version of the CPYDS was used (Lee & Shek, 2013). According to Shek and Ma (2010a), four higher-order factors and 15 dimensions were intrinsic to the scale. These included cognitive-behavioral competencies (CBC), prosocial attributes (PA), positive identity (PID), and general positive youth development qualities (GPYDQ) (Shek & Ma, 2010a). Reliability analyses showed that the total scale and the subscales based on the four higher-order factors were internally consistent.

The Chinese Family Assessment Instrument

The Chinese Family Assessment Instrument (CFAI) was used to assess perceived family functioning in Chinese adolescents. In the present study, three subscales of the CFAI, including mutuality, communication, and conflicts and harmony, were examined. The psychometric properties of the CFAI were supported in previous studies (Shek, 2002a, 2002b, 2003; Shek & Ma, 2010b; Siu & Shek, 2005). Shek and Ma (2010b) showed that the primary and second-order factors had factorial invariance of the CFAI across gender and subgroups. An abridged version of this scale was used in this study. The Cronbach's alpha values of these scales at Wave 3 were mutuality 0.89, communication 0.81, and conflicts and harmony 0.79.

Qualities in the Father-Child and Mother-Child Subsystems

To assess parental control and parent-child relational qualities, 17 items were used in the father-child dyad based on previous findings (Shek, 2007, 2008). These included items on behavioral control, psychological control, and father-child relationship. Similar 17 items were used to measure maternal behavioral control, maternal psychological control, and mother-child relationship. There are research findings showing that these measures were valid and reliable (Shek, 2007, 2008).

Exposure to Pornographic Materials

Twelve items were used to assess the consumption of two types of pornographic materials during the last year (Ma & Shek, 2013). They were Internet pornography (e.g., pornographic picture) and traditional pornography (e.g., pornographic magazines). A composite score was calculated by averaging all 12-item scores in order to obtain the mean of the overall consumption of pornographic materials. The Cronbach's alpha of this scale was 0.91 in Wave 2 and 0.93 in Wave 3.

Substance Use Scale

Eight items were used to assess the participants' frequency of using different types of substance in the past year, such as ketamine and heroin (Shek & Ma, 2011). To give an overall picture on substance abuse, a composite score was calculated by averaging the items in the eight items. The internal consistency of this scale was 0.78 in Wave 2 and 0.68 in Wave 3.

Delinquency Scale

Twelve items were used to assess the frequency of delinquent behaviors of the participants in the past year, such as having sexual relationships with others and breaking into others' places (Shek, Ma, & Tang, 2012). A composite score was calculated by averaging the scores in all items to give an overall picture on delinquency. The Cronbach's alpha of the delinquency scale was 0.80 in Wave 2 and 0.72 in Wave 3.

Perceived Academic and School Competence

Three items were used to test participants' perceptions on their academic and school performance (Shek, 1997). A composite score was calculated by averaging all item scores in order to obtain the mean of the overall academic and school competence. The Cronbach's alpha of the academic and school performance scale was 0.66 in Wave 2 and 0.67 in Wave 3. The mean item-total correlation was 0.47. Given that the scale has only three items, the reliability of this scale is deemed acceptable.

Data Analytic Plan

Firstly, to examine the prevalence of compensated dating and juvenile prostitution among Hong Kong early adolescents, numbers and percentages of CD and JP behaviors at Wave 3 were computed. Secondly, to investigate the stability or change in participants' CD and/or JP behaviors over a 1-year interval, the percentages of adolescents at Wave 3 were compared with the percentages found at Wave 2 by using related samples McNemar tests, a statistical method examining the difference between paired proportions. Participants' CD/JP scale score at the two waves was also compared with a paired-samples *t*-test.

Thirdly, to investigate the predictive effects of different demographic variables and CD/JP at Wave 2 on participants' CD/JP at Wave 3, multiple regression analyses were performed, with participants' composite score on CD/JP scale at Wave 3 serving as the dependent variable. For predictor variables, gender and age were entered in the first block; family background characteristics (i.e., immigrant status, socioeconomic background) in the second block; perceived family functioning at Wave 2 (i.e., mutuality, harmony, communication) in the third block; Wave 2 PYD and academic and school competence in the fourth block; participants' reported CD/JP scores in Wave 2 in the fifth block; parents' age difference in the sixth block; paternal and maternal variables in Wave 2 in the seventh and eighth blocks; and exposure to pornographic materials, drug, and delinquency risk behaviors in Wave 2 and Wave 3 in the ninth and tenth blocks. Finally, since there are important differences between

CD and JP behaviors, they deserve further investigation separately. The above multiple regression analyses were performed with participants' composite scores on CD and JP scale at Wave 3 serving as two distinct dependent variables.

Hypotheses

Based on the existing literature, the following 21 hypotheses were tested:

Hypothesis 1: Age would be positively related to CD/JP behaviors (Cheung et al., 2011; McNamara & Bucher, 2012; Roe-Sepowitz, 2012).

Hypothesis 2: There would be gender differences in CD/JP behaviors (Cheung et al., 2011; Finkelhor & Ormrod, 2004; McNamara & Bucher, 2012), with females displaying more related behaviors.

Hypothesis 3: Compared with students without economic disadvantage, students from families with a poor socioeconomic background would be more likely to be involved in CD/JP behaviors (C.S.O.A.C.Y., 1984).

Hypothesis 4: Students who are immigrants would be more likely to be involved in CD/JP behaviors (Cheung et al., 2011; Hwang & Bedford, 2003).

Hypothesis 5: Perceived family functioning (mutuality, harmony, and good communication within the family) in Wave 2 would be negatively related to CD/JP behaviors (McCuish, Lussier, & Corrado, 2014; McNamara & Bucher, 2012).

Hypothesis 6: Positive youth development attributes in Wave 2 would be negatively related to CD/JP behaviors (Lee & Shek, 2013).

Hypothesis 7: Academic and school competence in Wave 2 would be negatively related to CD/JP behaviors (Lee & Shek, 2013).

Hypothesis 8: Students who were engaged in CD/JP behaviors in Wave 2 would be more likely to engage in these behaviors in Wave 3 (McNamara & Bucher, 2012).

Hypothesis 9: The greater the age differences between the parents, the more likely the students would be engaged in CD/JP behaviors (Brannigan & Van Brunschot, 1997; McNamara & Bucher, 2012; Van Brunschot & Brannigan, 1992).

Hypothesis 10: The higher paternal control (paternal knowledge, paternal expectation, paternal monitoring, satisfaction with paternal control, paternal psychological control) in Wave 2, the less likely the students would be engaged in CD/JP behaviors (McCuish et al., 2014; McNamara & Bucher, 2012).

Hypothesis 11: The higher the maternal control (maternal knowledge, maternal expectation, maternal monitoring, satisfaction with maternal control, maternal psychological control) in Wave 2, the less likely the students would be engaged in CD/JP behaviors (McCuish et al., 2014; McNamara & Bucher, 2012).

Hypothesis 12: The better the father-child relationship in Wave 2, the less likely the students would be engaged in CD/JP behaviors (McCuish et al., 2014; McNamara & Bucher, 2012).

Hypothesis 13: The better the mother-child relationship in Wave 2, the less likely the students would be engaged in CD/JP behaviors (McCuish et al., 2014; McNamara & Bucher, 2012).

Hypothesis 14: Previous exposure to pornographic materials (Internet media) in Wave 2 would be positively related to student engagement in CD/JP behaviors (Clark, Clark, & Adamec, 2007; Mitchell, Jones, Finkelhor, & Wolak, 2011; Wells, Mitchell, & Ji, 2012).

Hypothesis 15: Previous exposure to pornographic materials (traditional mass media) in Wave 2 would be positively related to CD/JP behaviors (Clark et al., 2007; Zillmann, 1989).

Hypothesis 16: The higher the previous level of substance use in Wave 2, the more likely students would be engaged in CD/JP behaviors (Brawn & Roe-Sepowitz, 2008; Cheung et al., 2011; Hagan & McCarthy, 1997; Louw, 1994; McNamara & Bucher, 2012; Wilson & Widom, 2010).

Hypothesis 17: Previous level of delinquency problem behaviors in Wave 2 and CD/JP behaviors would be positively related (Cheung et al., 2011; Flowers, 2001; Hagan & McCarthy, 1997; McNamara & Bucher, 2012; Wilson & Widom, 2010).

Hypothesis 18: Current exposure to pornographic materials (Internet media) in Wave 3 would be positively related to student engagement in CD/JP behaviors (Clark et al., 2007; Mitchell et al., 2011; Wells et al., 2012).

Hypothesis 19: Current exposure to pornographic materials (traditional mass media) in Wave 3 would be positively related to CD/JP behaviors (Clark et al., 2007; Zillmann, 1989).

Hypothesis 20: The higher the current level of substance use, the more likely students would be engaged in CD/JP behaviors (Cheung et al., 2011; Hwang & Bedford, 2004; McNamara & Bucher, 2012; Wilson & Widom, 2010; Yates et al., 1991).

Hypothesis 21: Current level of delinquency problem behaviors and CD/JP behaviors would be positively related (Cheung et al., 2011; Flowers, 2001; Hagan & McCarthy, 1997; McNamara & Bucher, 2012; Wilson & Widom, 2010).

Results

Descriptive Profiles on CD/JP Behavior

Numbers and percentages of participants who reported to have engaged in CD/JP behaviors in the past 1 year are summarized in Table 1. Some observations deserve our attention. First, although CD/JP behaviors were reported both in Wave 2 and Wave 3, the prevalence rates of CD and JP were very low, with only 2.4 % of the respondents had ever engaged in CD and less than 0.6 % had ever engaged in JP. Even though the percentages refer to a limited number of cases, the percentages were quite stable but with a slightly rising trend – the prevalence rates of CD and JP in Wave 2 were 2.1 % and 0.4 %, respectively. Second, the numbers of nonresponses to the four questions on CD and JP in Wave 3 increased when compared to the same questions in Wave 2, although the nonresponse rates of the four questions remained very low ranging from 1.58 to 1.76 %. The nonresponse rates in Wave 2 ranged from 0.69 to 0.98 %. Given the relative small number of participants who reported CD/JP episodes, this might affect the accuracy of the data and subsequent analysis. However, the numbers of respondents not responding in Wave 3 ranged from 63 to 70 which were quite consistent among the four items. It may be the case that participants who decided not to answer skipped the whole section and not just some specific questions.

Mean Differences in the Composite Scores of Compensated Dating and Juvenile Prostitution by Gender and Family Background in Waves 2 and 3

Significant differences in the level of engagement in CD/JP were found between gender in both Waves 2 and 3 (Wave 2: $t=3.116$, $p<0.01$; Wave 3: $t=3.756$, $p<0.001$) with male students showing a slightly higher mean (Table 2). There was no significant difference in CD/JP scores between students from families with or without receiving financial aids in both waves (Table 2). Although significant differences in CD/JP scores were found in two types of parents' marital status in Wave 2 data according to post hoc tests (separated but not remarried: 1.0433; married (first marriage): 1.0094; $F=4.498$, $p<.001$), no significant difference was found in Wave 3 data (Table 2).

Comparison of CD and JP over 1 Year

The differences in percentages of CD and JP were examined between the two waves of data collection. As seen in Table 1, the occurrence rates for the four items were similar among students at Wave 2 and Wave 3. No statistically significant differences were found. In addition, the result of paired-samples t-test ($n=3{,}138$) showed there was no significant difference ($p>.05$) in students' mean composite scores on CD/JP at Wave 2 and Wave 3.

Interestingly, only a few of the participants who reported CD and/or JP behaviors in Wave 2 also reported the same behaviors in Wave 3. Specifically, out of 3,056 respondents, only 5 reported CD both in Wave 2 and Wave 3, and none of them reported to be engaged in sexual intercourses during both years (Table 3). Overall, these figures suggest that adolescent compensated dating and juvenile prostitution are relatively rare and stable phenomena.

Table 2 Mean differences in the composite scores of compensated dating and juvenile prostitution by gender and family background in Waves 2 and 3

	n	Mean	SD	t	Sig. (2-tailed)
Gender (Wave 2)					
Male	1,825	1.0152	0.08921	3.116	0.002
Female	1,692	1.0071	0.06395		
Gender (Wave 3)					
Male	2,085	1.0173	0.10022	3.756	0.000
Female	1,774	1.0073	0.06462		
Receiving financial aids (Wave 2)					
No	2,884	1.0092	0.06970	1.435	ns
Yes	201	1.0211	0.11688		
Receiving financial aids (Wave 3)					
No	3,150	1.0111	0.08223	.930	ns
Yes	198	1.0176	0.09593		
Parents' marital status (Wave 2)					
				F=4.498	0.001
Married (first marriage)[a]	2,938	1.0094	0.07158	Tukey HSD	
Separated but not remarried[a]	75	1.0433	0.17617		ns
Divorced but not remarried	248	1.0192	0.10003		ns
Married (second or above marriage)	161	1.0140	0.07525		ns
Others	121	1.0186	0.08639		ns
Parents' marital status (Wave 3)					
				F=3.987	0.003
Married (first marriage)	2,618	1.0081	0.26962	Tukey HSD	ns
Separated but not remarried	68	1.0735	0.35894		ns
Divorced but not remarried	236	1.0551	0.35898		ns
Married (second or above marriage)	142	1.1197	0.57713		ns
Others	62	1.1290	0.58629		ns

ns statistically not significant

[a]The mean difference between these two groups is significant at the 0.05 level

Table 3 Crosstabs of compensated dating and juvenile prostitution behaviors of Wave 2 and Wave 3

		Compensated dating in Wave 3		
		No	**Yes**	**Total**
Compensated dating in Wave 2	**No**	2,945	58	3,003
	Yes	48	5	53
Total		2,993	63	3,056
		Juvenile prostitution in Wave 3		
		No	**Yes**	**Total**
Juvenile prostitution in Wave 2	**No**	3,042	14	3,056
	Yes	7	0	7
Total		3,049	14	3,063

Multiple Regression Analyses of Compensated Dating and Juvenile Prostitution (CD/JP) Episodes

To further study the influence of individual (i.e., age, gender), family background characteristics (i.e., immigrant status, socioeconomic background), perceived functioning (i.e., mutuality, harmony, good communication within the family), parent-child relationship, PYD, and academic and school performance on compensated dating and juvenile prostitution (as measured by the composite score CD/JP) at Wave 3, multiple regression analyses were performed with the composite score of CD/JP as the dependent variable. The findings based on multiple regression analyses can be seen in Table 4. With reference to the hypotheses put forth in the early part of this chapter, the findings are as follows:

- Hypothesis 1 (i.e., age is related to CD/JP) was supported (Block 1).
- Hypothesis 2 (i.e., gender differences in CD/JP) was supported. However, more male students showed a slightly higher score than female students (Table 2).
- Hypothesis 3 (i.e., students from families with a poor socioeconomic background are more likely to be involved in CD/JP) was not supported (Block 2).
- Hypothesis 4 (i.e., students who are immigrants are more likely to be involved in CD/JP behaviors) was not supported (Block 2).
- Hypothesis 5 (i.e., perceived family functioning in Wave 2 is negatively related to CD/JP behaviors) was not supported (Block 3).
- Hypothesis 6 (i.e., positive youth development as assessed in Wave 2 is negatively related to CD/JP) was partially supported for some of the indicators. While general positive youth development quality was negatively related to CD/JP, positive identity was positively related to CD/JP (Block 4).
- Hypothesis 7 (i.e., academic and school competence in Wave 2 is negatively related to CD/JP) was supported (Block 4).
- Hypothesis 8 (i.e., students who engaged in CD/JP behaviors before are more likely to engage in these behaviors at present) was supported (Block 5).
- Hypothesis 9 (i.e., the greater the age differences between the parents, the more likely students engage in CD/JP behaviors) was supported (Block 6).
- Hypothesis 10 and hypothesis 11 (i.e., the higher the previous level of parental control in Wave 2, the more likely students engage in CD/JP behaviors) were partially supported. Only paternal and maternal psychological control levels measured in Wave 2 were found to be related to CD/JP (Blocks 7 and 8).
- Hypothesis 12 and hypothesis 13 (i.e., the better the parent-child relationship in Wave 2, the less likely students engage in CD/JP behaviors) were not supported (Blocks 7 and 8).
- Hypothesis 14 (i.e., previous level of exposure to pornographic materials through the Internet is positively related to current level of CD/JP) was not supported (Block 9).
- Hypothesis 15 (i.e., previous level of exposure to pornographic materials through traditional mass media is positively related to current level of CD/JP) was supported (Block 9).
- Hypothesis 16 (i.e., previous level of substance use as measured in Wave 2 is positively related to current level of CD/JP) was supported (Block 9).

Table 4 Multiple regression analysis of the composite scores of compensated dating and juvenile prostitution of Wave 3 data

	Composite scores of compensated dating and juvenile prostitution behaviors (CD/JP)				
Predictor	*B*	Beta	Sig.	R^2	R^2 change
Block 1				.004	.003
Age	.02	.047	.008		
Gender					
Block 2				.001	.000
Immigration status			n.s.		
Family economic status			n.s.		
Block 3 (Wave 2)				.002	.001
Family functioning			n.s.		
Mutuality			n.s.		
Harmony			n.s.		
Communication			n.s.		
Block 4 (Wave 2)				.011	.009
Positive youth development					
CBC			n.s.		
PA			n.s.		
GPYDQ	−.054	−.122	.002		
PID	.026	.082	.009		
ASC (Wave 2)	−.019	−.043	.039		
Block 5				.003	.003
CD/JP (Wave 2)	.063	.057	.002		
Block 6				.016	.015
PAD	.006	.128	.000		
Block 7 (Wave 2)				.007	.004
Paternal knowledge			n.s.		
Paternal expectation			n.s.		
Paternal monitoring			n.s.		
Satisfaction with paternal control			n.s.		
Paternal psychological control	.019	.044	.030		
Father-child relationship			n.s.		
Block 8 (Wave 2)				.005	.002
Maternal knowledge			n.s.		
Maternal expectation			n.s.		
Maternal monitoring			n.s.		
Satisfaction with maternal control			n.s.		
Maternal psychological control	.021	.053	.018		
Mother-child relationship			n.s.		
Block 9 (Wave 2)				.031	.030
EPORONI (Wave 2)			n.s.		
EPORONT (Wave 2)	.056	.054	.020		

(continued)

Table 4 (continued)

	Composite scores of compensated dating and juvenile prostitution behaviors (CD/JP)				
Predictor	*B*	Beta	Sig.	R^2	R^2 change
Substance use (Wave 2)	.155	.133	.000		
Delinquency problem behavior (Wave 2)			n.s.		
Block 10 (Wave 3)				.134	.133
EPORONI (Wave 3)					
EPORONT (Wave 3)	.143	.158	.000		
Substance use (Wave 3)	.231	.217	.000		
Delinquency problem behavior (Wave 3)	.047	.080	.000		

n.s. statistically not significant, *ASC* academic and school competence, *CBC* cognitive-behavioral competencies (second-order factor), *PA* prosocial attributes (second-order factor), *GPYDQ* general positive youth development qualities (second-order factor), *PID* positive identity (second-order factor), *PAD* age difference between the parents, *EPORNI* exposure to pornographic materials (Internet), *EPORNT* exposure to pornographic materials (traditional mass media)

- Hypothesis 17 (i.e., previous level of delinquency problem behaviors as measured in Wave 2 is positively related to current level of CD/JP) was not supported (Block 9).
- Hypothesis 18 (i.e., current level of exposure to pornographic materials through the Internet as measured in Wave 3 is positively related to current level of CD/JP) was not supported (Block 10).
- Hypothesis 19 (i.e., current level of exposure to pornographic materials through traditional mass media as measured in Wave 3 is positively related to current level of CD/JP) was supported (Block 10).
- Hypothesis 20 (i.e., current level of substance use as measured in Wave 3 is positively related to current level of CD/JP) was supported (Block 10).
- Hypothesis 21 (i.e., current level of delinquency problem behaviors as measured in Wave 3 is positively related to current level of CD/JP) was supported (Block 10).

Multiple Regression Analyses of Compensated Dating and Juvenile Prostitution Episodes Separately

When considering compensated dating and prostitution separately (Table 5), there were several observations. First, age was found to be positively related to CD (not involving sexual intercourse) but not JP (involving sexual intercourse). Gender difference was found on CD, but not JP. Contrary to the original hypothesis, male students had a higher mean score on CD than female students (Table 5, Block 1). No differences were found between genders on JP. Second, no differences were found between family economic status and immigrant status on both CD and

Table 5 Multiple regression analysis of compensated dating and juvenile prostitution behaviors of Wave 3 data

	Compensated dating behaviors CD (Wave 3)					Juvenile prostitution behaviors JP (Wave 3)				
Predictor	*B*	Beta	Sig.	R^2	R^2 change	*B*	Beta	Sig.	R^2	R^2 change
Block 1				.004	.003				.001	.000
Age	.009	.048	.008							
Gender	−.01	−.036	.048							
Block 2				.009	.005				.004	.000
Immigration status										
Family economic status										
Block 3 (Wave 2)				.005	.004				.002	.001
Family functioning										
Mutuality										
Harmony	−.016	−.105	.006							
Communication										
Block 4 (Wave 2)				.013	.011				.004	.002
Positive youth development										
CBC										
PA										
GPYDQ	−.029	−.145	.000							
PID	.014	.095	.003							
ASC	−.010	−.051	.016							
Block 5 (Wave 2)				.005	.004				.000	.000
CD (Wave 2)	.075	.069	.000							
Block 6 (Wave 2)				.000	.000				.000	.000
JP (Wave 2)										
Block 7				.006	.005				.020	.019
PAD	.002	.080	.014			.002	.141	.000		
Block 8 (Wave 2)				.007	.005				.004	.002
Paternal knowledge										
Paternal expectation										
Paternal monitoring										
Satisfaction with paternal control										
Paternal psychological control	.011	.059	.004							
Father-child relationship										

(continued)

Table 5 (continued)

	Compensated dating behaviors CD (Wave 3)					Juvenile prostitution behaviors JP (Wave 3)				
Predictor	*B*	Beta	Sig.	R^2	R^2 change	*B*	Beta	Sig.	R^2	R^2 change
Block 9 (Wave 2)				.006	.003				.002	.000
Maternal knowledge										
Maternal expectation										
Maternal monitoring										
Satisfaction with maternal control										
Maternal psychological control	.013	.074	.001							
Mother-child relationship										
Block 10 (Wave 2)				.016	.014				.026	.025
EPORONI										
EPORONT						.015	.065	.007		
Substance use	.050	.095	.000			.018	.030	.000		
Delinquency problem behavior										
Block 11 (Wave 3)				.058	.056				.123	.121
EPORONI (Wave 3)	.011	.057	.012							
EPORONT (Wave 3)	.022	0.51	.022			.049	.243	.000		
Substance use (Wave 3)	.072	.142	.000			.033	.146	.000		
Delinquency problem behavior (Wave 3)	.019	.068	.002			.010	.083	.000		

ASC academic and school competence, *CBC* cognitive-behavioral competencies (second-order factor), *PA* prosocial attributes (second-order factor), *GPYDQ* general positive youth development qualities (second-order factor), *PID* positive identity (second-order factor), *PAD* age difference between the parents, *EPORNI* exposure to pornographic materials (Internet), *EPORNT* exposure to pornographic materials (traditional mass media)

JP (Block 2). Third, with regard to perceived family functioning, only one indicator, i.e., family harmony, was found to be negatively related to CD, but not JP (Block 3). Fourth, while general positive youth development qualities (second-order factor) was found to be negatively related to CD (but not JP), positive identity (second-order factor) was positively related to CD (but not JP) (Block 4). Fifth, academic and school competence (ASC) in Wave 2 was negatively related to JP (but not CD) in Wave 3 (Block 4). Sixth, while CD in Wave 2 was a predictor for CD in Wave 3, it was not a predictor for JP in Wave 3 (Block 5). In contrast, JP in

Wave 2 was not a predictor for either CD or JP in Wave 3 (Block 6). Seventh, age difference between father and mother was found to be positively related to both CD and JP in Wave 3 (Block 7). Eighth, both types of parental psychological control, i.e., paternal and maternal, were found to be positively related to CD but not JP (Blocks 8 and 9). Ninth, regarding deviant behaviors measured at Wave 2, it was found that while the previous state of exposure to pornographic materials (traditional mass media) was positively related to JP but not CD, the previous amount of substance abuse was associated with both CD and JP measured in Wave 3 (Block 10). The previous state of exposure to pornographic materials (Internet) and the previous level of delinquency problem behaviors were not related to CD and JP (Block 10). Finally, while the current state of exposure to pornographic materials (Internet) at Wave 3 was positively related to CD but not JP, the current state of exposure to pornographic materials (traditional mass media), the current amount of substance abuse, and the current level of delinquency problem behaviors were associated with both CD and JP measured in Wave 3 (Block 11).

In summary, several interesting observations were highlighted from the findings. First, signs of CD and JP were still relatively uncommon among Secondary 3 (Grade 9) students in Hong Kong, although the prevalence should not be underestimated. Second, in line with findings from Wave 2 of the same research, it showed that more boys reported having experience in CD/JP and CD than girls did. Third, there are some slight differences in the factors associated with CD, JP, and CD/JP behaviors. Fourth, while some youths who previously engaged in CD with strangers continued to do so after 1 year, none of those who had sexual intercourse reported to do so in both waves of data collection. Fifth, the age difference between parents was found to be positively associated with CD, JP, and CD/JP behaviors. On the contrary, receiving welfare support was not associated with CD, JP, and CD/JP behaviors. Sixth, CD and JP were weakly associated with the previous level of substance use, while only JP was found to be positively related to the previous exposure to pornographic materials (traditional mass media). Finally, the current states of CD and JP were also weakly associated with some current risk behaviors.

Discussion

The aims of this longitudinal study were to examine the prevalence and psychosocial correlates of CD/JP among Hong Kong Chinese early adolescents and to assess how these behaviors changed after 1 year. There are several unique characteristics of the present study. First, this is the first known scientific study of compensated dating and juvenile prostitution in the Chinese context of Hong Kong adopting a longitudinal research design, and a large sample was employed to provide a broader and comprehensive understanding of these phenomena. Second, validated measures of positive youth development (Shek & Ma, 2010a) and family functioning in the Chinese contexts (Shek, 2002a, 2002b, 2003; Shek & Ma, 2010b; Siu & Shek, 2005) were used. Given the majority of research in this area was conducted in

Western societies, this study adds to the growing literature on compensated dating and juvenile prostitution in the Chinese cultural context (Cheung et al., 2011; Lee & Shek, 2013). It also sheds light on our understanding of both CD and JP phenomena and design of appropriate preventive programs for Chinese adolescents. Third, to examine the differences between CD and JP, the present study adopted a new analytic strategy to consider CD and JP separately, and interesting findings were observed. With regard to socioeconomic variables, age was positively related to CD/JP and CD but not JP (hypothesis 1). Similarly, gender differences were found in CD/JP and CD but not JP. Chinese boys reported a higher level of CD/JP and CD than Chinese girls (hypothesis 2). The differentiation between CD and JP reconfirmed the finding of our previous study using Wave 2 data, while no gender difference was found for the involvement in JP. This phenomenon may be related to the growing trend of rising homosexual and pedophilia activities in Hong Kong which needs further exploration (Cheung et al., 2011; Lee & Shek, 2013). This finding reconfirms the importance of providing help for adolescents, particularly males.

Financial situation and immigrant status were not related to the current states of CD/JP, CD, and JP (hypotheses 3 and 4). This finding was different from the results found in analyzing Wave 2 data that adolescents from families receiving financial assistance had a slightly higher chance of getting involved in CD (Lee & Shek, 2013). However, the finding of the present study was consistent with the current literature that adolescents may be willing to engage in CD to earn quick and easy money to satisfy their urges for fashionable consumption (Ueno, 2003). Research in Japan has found that many adolescents engaging in CD come from well-off or middle-class families (Ueno, 2003). They find CD attractive because they believe that they can choose clients freely. Ironically, they are subject to conformist pressure created by the popular culture. Girls who engaged in CD may be likely to be in search of affection in the absence of attention at home and to have extra spending power in purchasing fashionable items (McCoy, 2004). The problem becomes more serious when teenagers expose themselves to an expensive consumer culture and to an environment in which pornographic materials are easily available. Consumption is not only to fulfill personal needs but also to enhance one's own identity and status in Asian societies. Tempted by curiosity and risked by the lack of proper sex education, early adolescents might get involved in CD and probably JP in a later stage. A comprehensive positive youth development program that incorporates the cultivation of proper values and attitude toward sexual behavior (Shek, 2013) and concepts of money and success is important (Lee & Law, 2011). It is noteworthy that new teaching units on sex education and concepts of money and success were designed for use in the extension phase of the Project P.A.T.H.S. in Hong Kong, a preventive program which adopted the positive youth development framework (Lee & Law, 2011; Shek, Ma, & Merrick, 2012). Interestingly, family conflict was the only significant perceived family functioning predictor of CD, but not CD/JP and JP. This finding supported the importance of family harmony in the prevention of CD among adolescents (hypothesis 5). These observations suggest that CD and JP might be distinct phenomena with different underlying processes, and CD could be an important risk factor for JP.

With regard to the positive youth development attributes (hypothesis 6), general positive youth development qualities (second-order factor) was negatively related to CD/JP and CD, but not JP. This is consistent with the theoretical assertions that positive youth development will help prevent students from engaging in adolescent risk behavior and it can be considered a protective factor. However, in contrast to our prediction, positive identity measured in Wave 2 was found to be positively related to CD/JP and CD, but not JP. This is a puzzling finding of the present study. Although the Positive Identity Subscale score was able to discriminate the well and poor adjustment groups (Shek et al., 2006) and the subscale has been successfully used in previous studies based on early adolescents (Lee & Shek, 2013; Shek, 2013; Sun & Shek, 2012), the present findings do not seem to be in line with previous results. How is it possible that a positive identity goes in the same direction of CD/JP behaviors? One interpretation is that for engaging in CD and/or JP, one should have some self-confidence and feel attractive. At the same time, engaging in such activities may receive some rewards in return, a sense of achievement and a sense of being in control, which may reflect a higher positive identity.

Indeed, the perception of CD behaviors may be quite positive among some youths. A survey conducted by Yates, MacKenzie, Pennbridge, & Swofford (2009) indicated that 82 % of students are willing to go shopping, dining, and entertaining with a stranger who will pay for all expenses and 48 % of the participants were willing to do so for some form of compensation. Analyzing the change in social discourse in Taiwan, Ho (2003) noticed that image of female sexuality was no longer geared toward a desire to please men, but was highly energetic as well as obnoxiously provocative instead. On the contrary, the image of males changed to more aesthetic, fragile, and vulnerable. This may partially explain why CD was perceived quite positively by a large number of interviewees and sometimes spread among youths after they have learned that some of their friends are involved in this risky behavior. Contrary to the common idea of compensated dating as sexual exploitation of adolescents, it may be that some adolescents involved are sometimes more capable of managing the delicate multiplicities and complexities of sexual desires than most adults, born and raised in completely different social-sexual contexts, who instead are much less experienced. Paradoxically, a lower sense of self-confidence may be a protective factor for preventing youth to engage in such behaviors. Thus, this may be the case when a positive feeling (positive identity) is positively related to a questionable behavior. However, it has to be also reminded that positive identity is statistically significant for CD but not for JP. Adolescents who engaged in CD might have a stronger feeling (might be disguised feeling) on what they do are on their free will, and thus they accept their own identities in engaging in socially undesirable behaviors like compensated dating. This may explain why they perceived that they had a higher level of positive identity. It is suggested that future studies should be carried out to examine this issue further.

Consistent with our prediction, previous perceived level of academic and school competence (ASC) measured in Wave 2 showed negative relationships with CD/JP and CD but not JP behaviors (Block 4 in Tables 4 and 5). Actually, this may well reflect the complexity of the causes which lead to CD and JP behaviors and may serve to debunk some myths. Indeed, while one may think that adolescents who engage in CD and/or JP behaviors are simply those who fail in school, this is not completely true. On the contrary, previous research (Hagan & McCarthy, 1997; Wilson & Widom, 2010) found that school problems can be a protective factor of CD behaviors, suggesting that this may refer to school involvement. In some cases, adolescents who engage in CD and/or JP behaviors perform well in schools and may even score above average. Findings from similar research in Taiwan (Ho, 2003) showed that girls involved in CD/JP come from perfectly functional families and have good grades in school. To some adolescents, being engaged in CD/JP behaviors may even be a sign of being particularly smart and more able than other peers of the same age to handle such situations. According to Ho (2003), some girls have become quite adept in reading people and handling complicated human interaction: "they have learned to target only middle-aged men, not because these men are more lustful, but because these men, according to these girls […] would not make trouble for the girls should the transaction go awry" (p. 332).

An interesting result is that early adolescents, who previously engaged in CD, and particularly in JP, rarely continue to do so in the following year (hypothesis 8), meaning that CD/JP history is not always a good predictor. The composite score of CD/JP behaviors from Wave 2 proved to be a predictor for the composite score of CD/JP and CD behaviors in Wave 3 (Table 4, Block 5), but when considering CD and JP behaviors in Wave 2 separately, both behaviors had no relationship with either CD or JP in Wave 3 (Table 5, Blocks 5 and 6). It may be because the composite score was largely affected by the weight of CD in Wave 2 as a predictor for CD in Wave 3, whereas JP in Wave 2 was not a predictor for JP in Wave 3. As already mentioned, CD and JP behaviors are inconsistent from 1 year to the next, and thus it is difficult to identify an underlying pattern. However, it is noteworthy that this finding was affected by missing responses in the questionnaire (i.e., students who completed the questionnaire but skipped this specific question) and by the fact that some students did not take part in Wave 3 of the survey. Indeed, a considerable number of students who reported CD/JP behaviors in Wave 2 did not respond to the same questionnaire in the following year, and the reasons for this are not clear. It may be the case that some of these adolescents might not want to take part in the study. It is also possible that such students might be more at risk and they might have left the school. Thus, an important data source may be lost.

Moreover, another variable which was associated to CD and JP behaviors was parents' age difference (PAD). This variable is a risk factor of both CD and JP behaviors (Table 4, Block 6 and Table 5, Block 7). One plausible explanation is that a wider age difference between the parents may be associated with weakened family functioning, higher parental conflicts, and lower levels of parental support and control. Large age difference between father and mother is a phenomenon commonly found in some economically advanced cities with surrounding rural areas or countries. Many young females from rural areas in southern part of China were attracted to get married with older singleton males living in a capitalistic urban city of Hong

Kong. This was particularly the case when China began its open door policy in early 1980s. The cross-border marriage was typically old husband with young wife in the last few decades.

The present findings revealed that parental psychological control was another risk factor for CD behaviors. Previous research (Cheung et al., 2011) found that excessive control within the family was a risk factor of CD and JP behaviors because CD or JP may be a reaction to such pressure from the family. It was argued that excessive parental control was not necessarily as effective as previously thought (Stättin & Kerr, 2000), and it could even produce a result contrary to expectations (Albrecht, Galambos, & Jansson, 2007). Shek (2006) argued that psychological control was part of the parenting characteristics in Chinese parents. Hence, it is theoretically and practically important to examine this issue in future.

Furthermore, while exposure to pornographic materials through traditional mass media (EPORONT) and substance abuse measured in Wave 2 were significant predictors to CD/JP behaviors (Table 4, Block 9), exposure to pornographic traditional materials, substance abuse, and together with parental age difference were the only three significant predictors to JP behaviors (Table 5, Blocks 7 and 10). To examine the relationships between the current levels of involvement in risk behaviors and current involvement in CD/JP behaviors, correlation analyses showed that exposure to traditional pornographic materials (EPORONT), substance abuse, and delinquency behaviors were positively related to CD/JP, CD, and JP (Table 4, Block 10 and Table 5, Block 11). Such results are unsurprising, given that consumption of pornography, delinquency, marijuana use in particular, alcohol drinking, cigarette smoking, and conduct disorder are well known for being risk factors (Cavanagh, 2007; Davila et al., 2009; Little & Rankin, 2001; Paul, Fitzjohn, Herbison, & Dickson, 2000; So & Chan, 1992; South, Latz, & Baumer, 2005; Zillmann, 1989). However, when analyzing CD behaviors alone, the significance of EPORONT faded away (Table 5, Block 10). In this case, substance use was the only predictor, while EPORONT was no longer statistically significant. Moreover, when analyzing JP behavior independently, the variable EPORONT was one of the three significant predicators. This could probably be explained by the fact that exposure to pornographic materials on the Internet is easier given that such materials are readily available to the public, so it does not play a significant role. Instead, pornographic materials on traditional mass media (e.g., DVDs, printed magazines, etc.) require an additional effort for buying and require adolescents to go on-site. This would require some planning and cost, and it is less likely to be an occasional or casual activity. Finally, exposure to pornographic materials through traditional mass media plays an important role in the case of JP, while it is relatively marginal in CD behaviors.

Altogether, 10 blocks of variables were tested for CD/JP (Table 4) and 11 blocks for CD and JP separately (Table 5). The difference was due to the use of CD and JP as separate variables in the analysis of CD and JP (Table 5, Blocks 5 and 6). Although statistically significant results were found, it must be added that the magnitude of the relationships is small probably due to the low prevalence rate of CD, JP, and CD/JP behaviors among early adolescents in Hong Kong. Nevertheless, the present findings could help social scientists to construct models on compensated dating and juvenile prostitution in Chinese adolescents in Hong Kong and contribute to the understanding of the risky behaviors of CD and JP.

Although the present study is pioneering in different Chinese communities, this study has several limitations. First, it was based only on respondents' self-report. Although anonymity was guaranteed, respondents may not be willing to disclose their private lives. Second, as the present findings were based on early adolescents in Hong Kong, they may not be easily generalized to other Chinese cultures, such as Mainland China and Taiwan, as well as adolescents in different age groups. Third, we only used four items for investigating CD and JP. It would be helpful if more items could be added in future studies. For example, information on the number of dating, their frequency, actual sexual activities involved, reward received, and personal motivation to do so could be added. Fourth, participants reported a rather inconsistent CD behavior from 1 year to another; only in five cases participants reported such behavior in both waves, and none of the 7 cases involving JP behavior reported similar behaviors in Wave 3. This finding is quite surprising and leaves the door open to further examination. Given that the study studied socially undesirable behaviors, difficulties in data collection are understandable. At the same time, this poses a serious limitation for the predictive power of the statistical model, as such inconsistent behavior may not show through any specific pattern, and thus may result difficult to explain. Fifth, only 986 students reported the age of both parents, while in 2,253 cases they failed to report at least one of them or both. It is quite striking that a large majority of students did not know their parents' age. Not only this affects the statistical analysis of the results on age difference between parents, but it also leaves the door open to discussion about the parent-child relationship and how much they know (or not) each other.

Despite the above limitations and the exploratory nature of the present study, it is able to examine the psychosocial and family functioning correlates of different CD and JP behaviors among Hong Kong early adolescents. This emergent phenomenon involves early adolescents and even children under 14. Thus, more effort in promoting money literacy and sex education among this population should be emphasized. However, money and sex are not necessarily the main causes of such behaviors. The findings of this study suggest that different factors in the personal and family systems are related to such behaviors. CD and JP behaviors seem to be more complex than just a business trade. For example, the current study suggested some differences between CD and JP. Future research should investigate more the grounds for CD and JP from both parties involved.

Acknowledgment The preparation for this chapter and the Project P.A.T.H.S. were financially supported by the Hong Kong Jockey Club Charities Trust.

References

Albrecht, A. K., Galambos, N. L., & Jansson, S. M. (2007). Adolescents' internalizing and aggressive behaviors and perceptions of parents' psychological control: A panel study examining directions of effects. *Journal of Youth and Adolescence, 36*, 673–684.

Brannigan, A., & Van Brunschot, E. G. (1997). Youthful prostitution and child sexual trauma. *International Journal of Law and Psychiatry, 20*(3), 337–354.

Brawn, K. M., & Roe-Sepowitz, D. (2008). Female juvenile prostitutes: Exploring the relationship to substance use. *Children and Youth Services Review, 30*, 1395–1402.

C.S.O.A.C.Y. (Committee on Sexual Offences Against Children and Youth). (1984). *Sexual offences against children*. Ottawa, ON: Department of Supply and Services.

Cavanagh, S. E. (2007). The social construction of romantic relationships in adolescence: Examining the role of peer networks, gender, and race. *Sociological Inquiry, 77*(4), 572–600.

Chesney-Lind, M., & Shelden, R. G. (2004). *Girls, delinquency, and juvenile justice* (3rd ed.). Belmont, CA: Wadsworth/Thomson Learning.

Cheung, J. C. K., Lee, T. Y., & Li, J. C. M. (2011). *Family-centered prevention of adolescent girls' and boys' prostitution: Final report submitted to the Central Policy Unit, Government of the Hong Kong Special Administrative Region, H.K.* Social Capital and Impact Assessment Research Unit and Department of Applied Social Studies, City University of Hong Kong, Hong Kong. Retrieved from https://www.google.com.hk/#q=Family-centered+prevention+of+adolescent+girls%E2%80%99+and+boys%E2%80%99+prostitution:+Final+report+submitted+to+the+Central+Policy+Unit

Clark, R. E., Clark, J. F., & Adamec, C. (2007). *The encyclopedia of child abuse* (3rd ed.). New York: Facts On File, Inc.

Davila, J., Stroud, C. B., Starr, L. R., Miller, M. R., Yoneda, A., & Hershenberg, R. (2009). Romantic and sexual activities, parent-adolescent stress, and depressive symptoms among early adolescent girls. *Journal of Adolescence, 32*(4), 909–924.

Finkelhor, D. & Ormrod, R. (2004). Prostitution of juveniles: Patterns from NIBRS. *Juvenile Justice Bulletin*. Retrieved from https://www.oconnorhouse.org/ngo/tool-kit/research_articles/prostitution/Prostitution%20of%20Juveniles%20-%20Patterns.pdf

Flowers, R. B. (2001). *Runaway kids and teenage prostitution: America's lost, abandoned, and sexually exploited children*. Westport, CT: Praeger.

Gray, E. S. (2005). Juvenile courts and sexual exploitation: A judge's observations. In S. W. Cooper, R. J. Estes, A. P. Giardino, N. D. Kellogg, & V. I. Vieth (Eds.), *Medical, legal, & social science aspects of child sexual exploitation: A comprehensive review of pornography, prostitution, and internet crime* (pp. 711–714). St. Louis, MO: G.W. Medical Publishing.

Hagan, J., & McCarthy, B. (1997). *Mean streets: Youth crime and homelessness*. Cambridge, UK: Cambridge University Press.

He, T. (2007). Cyberqueers in Taiwan: Locating histories of the margins. *Journal of International Women's Studies, 8*(2), 55–73.

Ho, J. (2003). From spice girls to enjos kosai: Formations of teenager girls' sexualities in Taiwan. *Inter-Asia Cultural Studies, 4*(2), 325–336.

Hwang, S. L., & Bedford, O. (2003). Precursors and pathways to adolescent prostitution in Taiwan. *Journal of Sex Research, 40*(2), 201–211.

Hwang, S. L., & Bedford, O. (2004). Juveniles' motivations for remaining in prostitution. *Psychology of Women Quarterly, 28*(2), 136–146.

James, J., & Meyerding, J. (1978). Early sexual experience as a factor in prostitution. *Archives of Sexual Behaviour, 7*(1), 31–42.

Jenkins, J. P. (2014). Prostitution. In *Encyclopaedia Britannica*. Retrieved from http://www.britannica.com/EBchecked/topic/479546/prostitution

Kinsella, S. (2012). Narratives and statistics: How compensated dating (enjo kōsai) was sold. In R. Goodman, Y. Imoto, & T. Toivonen (Eds.), *A sociology of Japanese youth: From returnees to NEETs* (pp. 54–80). Abingdon, UK: Routledge.

Kittling, N. (2006). God bless the child: The United States' response to domestic juvenile prostitution. *Nevada Law Journal, 6*, 913–926.
Kong, M. H. (2003). Material girls: Sexual perceptions of Korean teenage girls who have experienced compensated dates. *Asian Journal of Women's Studies, 9*(2), 67–94.
Kreston, S. S. (2005). Investigation and prosecution of the prostitution of children. In S. W. Cooper, R. J. Estes, A. P. Giardino, N. D. Kellogg, & V. I. Vieth (Eds.), *Medical, legal, & social science aspects of child sexual exploitation: A comprehensive review of pornography, prostitution, and internet crimes* (pp. 745–788). St. Louis, MO: G.W. Medical Publishing.
Kuntay, E. (2002). Family backgrounds of teenage female sex workers in Istanbul metropolitan area. *Journal of Comparative Family Studies, 33*(3), 345–358.
Lam, O. W. (2003). Why did enjo kosai anchor in Taiwan but not in Hong Kong? Or the convergence of "enjo" and "kosai" in teenage sex work. *Inter-Asia Cultural Studies, 4*(2), 353–363.
Lee, T. Y., & Law, B. M. F. (2011). Teaching money literacy in a positive youth development program: The project P.A.T.H.S. in Hong Kong. *The Scientific World Journal, 11*, 2287–2298.
Lee, T. Y., & Shek, D. T. L. (2013). Compensated dating in Hong Kong: Prevalence, psychosocial correlates, and relationships with other risky behaviors. *Journal of Pediatric and Adolescent Gynecology, 26*(3S), S42–S48.
Leheny, D. (2006). *Think global, fear local: Sex, violence, and anxiety in contemporary Japan*. Ithaca, NY: Cornell University Press.
Little, C. B., & Rankin, A. (2001). Why do they start it? Explaining reported early-teen sexual activity. *Sociological Forum, 16*(4), 703–729.
Louw, S. (1994). *Juvenile prostitution: An investigation*. Retrieved from https://www.google.com.hk/#q=Juvenile+prostitution:+An+investigation.
Ma, C. M. S., & Shek, D. T. L. (2013). Consumption of pornographic materials in early adolescents in Hong Kong. *Journal of Pediatric and Adolescent Gynecology, 26*(3S), S18–S25.
Masuzoe, Y. (Ed.). (2000). *Years of trial Japan in the 1990s*. Tokyo: Echo Inc.
McCoy, A. (2004). Blaming children for their own exploitation: The situation in East Asia. In *ECPAT report on the implementation of the agenda for action against the commercial sexual exploitation of children* (pp. 36–43). Bangkok, Thailand: ECPAT International.
McCuish, E. C., Lussier, P., & Corrado, R. R. (2014). Examining antisocial behavioral antecedents of juvenile sexual offenders and juvenile non-sexual offenders. *Sex Abuse*. Advanced online publication. doi: 10.1177/1079063213517268.
McLelland, M. J. (2000). *Male homosexuality in modern Japan: Cultural myths and social realities*. Richmond, VA: Corson Press.
McNamara, R. H., & Bucher, C. C. (2012). *Problem children: Special problems in delinquency*. Durham, NC: Carolina Academic Press.
Mitchell, K. J., Finkelhor, D., & Wolak, J. (2010). Conceptualizing juvenile prostitution as child maltreatment: Findings from the National Juvenile Prostitution Study. *Child Maltreatment, 15*(1), 18–36.
Mitchell, K. J., Jones, L. M., Finkelhor, D., & Wolak, J. (2011). Internet-facilitated commercial sexual exploitation of children: Findings from a nationally representative sample of law enforcement agencies in the United States. *Sexual Abuse, 23*(1), 43–71.
Paul, C., Fitzjohn, J., Herbison, P., & Dickson, N. (2000). The determinants of sexual intercourse before age 16. *Journal of Adolescent Health, 27*(2), 136–147.
Radford, L., & Tsutsumi, K. (2004). Globalization and violence against women: Inequalities in risks, responsibilities, and blame in the UK and Japan. *Women's Studies International Forum, 27*(1), 1–12.
Roe-Sepowitz, D. E. (2012). Juvenile entry into prostitution: The role of emotional abuse. *Violence Against Women, 18*(5), 562–579.
Seng, M. J. (1989). Child sexual abuse and adolescent prostitution: A comparative analysis. *Adolescence, 24*(95), 665–675.
Shek, D. T. L. (1997). The relation of parent-adolescent conflict to adolescent psychological well-being, school adjustment, and problem behavior. *Social Behavior and Personality, 25*(3), 277–290.

Shek, D. T. L. (2002a). Assessment of family functioning: The Chinese version of the family assessment device. *Research on Social Work Practice, 12*, 502–524.

Shek, D. T. L. (2002b). Assessment of family functioning Chinese adolescents: The Chinese family assessment instrument. In N. N. Singh, T. Ollen-Dick, & A. N. Singh (Eds.), *International perspectives on child and adolescent mental health* (pp. 297–316). Amsterdam: Elsevier.

Shek, D. T. L. (2003). Family functioning and psychological well-being, school adjustment, and substance abuse in Chinese adolescents: Are findings based on multiple studies consistent? In S. P. Shohov (Ed.), *Advances in psychology research* (pp. 163–184). New York: Nova Science.

Shek, D. T. L. (2006). Assessment of perceived parental psychological control in Chinese adolescents in Hong Kong. *Research on Social Work Practice, 16*(4), 382–391.

Shek, D. T. L. (2007). A longitudinal study of perceived differences in parental control and parent-child relational qualities in Chinese adolescents in Hong Kong. *Journal of Adolescent Research, 22*(2), 156–188.

Shek, D. T. L. (2008). Economic disadvantage, perceived family life quality, and emotional well-being in Chinese adolescents: A longitudinal study. *Social Indicators Research, 85*(2), 169–189.

Shek, D. T. L. (2013). Sexual behavior and intention to engage in sexual behavior in junior secondary school students in Hong Kong. *Journal of Pediatric and Adolescent Gynecology, 26*(3S), S33–S41.

Shek, D. T. L., & Ma, C. M. S. (2010a). Dimensionality of the Chinese positive youth development scale: Confirmatory factor analyses. *Social Indicators Research, 98*(1), 41–59.

Shek, D. T. L., & Ma, C. M. S. (2010b). The Chinese family assessment instrument (C-FAI): Hierarchical confirmatory factor analyses and factorial invariance. *Research on Social Work Practice, 20*(1), 112–123.

Shek, D. T. L., & Ma, C. M. S. (2011). Substance abuse in junior secondary school students in Hong Kong: Prevalence and psychosocial correlates. *International Journal of Child Health and Human Development, 4*(4), 433–442.

Shek, D. T. L., Ma, C. M. S., & Lin, L. (2014). The Chinese adolescent materialism scale: Psychometric properties and normative profiles. *International Journal on Disability and Human Development, 13*(2), 285–295.

Shek, D. T. L., Ma, H. K., & Merrick, J. (2012). Effectiveness of the project P.A.T.H.S. in Hong Kong: Evaluation based on different strategies and different studies over time. *The Scientific World Journal, 2012*. Retrieved from http://www.hindawi.com/journals/tswj/2012/427801/

Shek, D. T. L., Ma, C. M. S., & Tang, C. Y. P. (2012). Delinquency and problem behavior intention among early adolescents in Hong Kong: Profiles and psychosocial correlates. *International Journal on Disability and Human Development, 11*(2), 151–158.

Shek, D. T. L., Siu, A. M. H., & Lee, T. Y. (2007). The Chinese Positive Youth Development Scale: A validation study. *Research on Social Work Practices, 17*(3), 380–391.

Shek, D. T. L., Siu, A. M. H., Lee, T. Y., Cheng, H., Tsang, S., Lui, J., et al. (2006). Development and validation of a positive youth development scale in Hong Kong. *International Journal of Adolescent Medicine and Health, 18*(3), 547–558.

Silbert, M. H., & Pines, A. M. (1981). Sexual child abuse as an antecedent to prostitution. *Child Abuse & Neglect, 5*, 407–411.

Siu, A. M., & Shek, D. T. L. (2005). Psychometric properties of the Chinese family assessment instrument in Chinese adolescents in Hong Kong. *Adolescence, 40*(160), 817–830.

So, C. Y. K., & Chan, J. M. (1992). *Mass media and youth in Hong Kong: A study of media use, youth archetype, and media influence*. Hong Kong: Commission on Youth.

South, S. J., Lutz, A., & Baumer, E. P. (2005). Adolescent residential mobility and premature life-course transitions: The role of peer networks. *Sociological Studies of Children & Youth, 11*, 23–52.

Stättin, H., & Kerr, M. (2000). Parental monitoring: A reinterpretation. *Child Development, 71*(4), 1072–1085.

Sun, R. C. F., & Shek, D. T. L. (2012). Positive youth development, life satisfaction and problem behavior among Chinese adolescents in Hong Kong: A replication. *Social Indicators Research, 105*(3), 541–559. Retrieved from http://link.springer.com/article/10.1007/s11205-011-9786-9

Ueno, C. (2003). Self-determination on sexuality? Commercialization of sex among teenage girls in Japan. *Inter-Asia Cultural Studies, 4*(2), 317–324.

Van Brunschot, E. G., & Brannigan, A. (1992). *Childhood correlates of career prostitution.* Calgary, Canada: Mimeo, University of Calgary.

Vitaliano, P. P., James, J., & Boyer, D. (1981). Sexuality of deviant females: Adolescent and adult correlates. *Social Work, 26*, 468–472.

Wakabayashi, T. (2003). Enjokosai in Japan: Rethinking the dual image of prostitutes in Japanese and American law. *UCLA Women's Law Journal, 13*, 143–184.

Wells, M., Mitchell, K. J., & Ji, K. (2012). Exploring the role of the internet in juvenile prostitution cases coming to the attention of law enforcement. *Journal of Child Sexual Abuse, 21*(3), 327–342.

Wilson, H. W., & Widom, C. S. (2010). The role of youth problem behaviors in the path from child abuse and neglect to prostitution: A perspective examination. *Journal of Research on Adolescence, 20*(1), 210–236. doi:10.1111/j.1532-7795.2009.00624.x.

Yates, G. L., MacKenzie, R. G., Pennbridge, J., & Swofford, A. (1991). A risk profile comparison of homeless youth involved in prostitution and homeless youth not involved. *Journal of Adolescent Health, 12*(7), 545–548.

Yau, K. S., Ng, W. Y., & Leung, P. Y. (2009). *Cognition and values of compensated dating among secondary schools in Hong Kong*. Hong Kong, China: The Hong Kong Association of Sexuality Educators, Researchers & Therapists Limited (In Chinese).

Zillmann, D. (1989). Effects of prolonged consumption of pornography. In D. Zillmann & J. Bryant (Eds.), *Pornography: Research advances and policy considerations* (pp. 127–157). Hillsdale, NJ: Erlbaum.

Intention to Gamble Among Junior Secondary School Students in Hong Kong: Changes and Predictors

Daniel T.L. Shek and Lu Yu

Abstract Adolescent gambling is a growing problem in the global context. In this chapter, intention to engage in gambling among junior secondary school students is examined using the data based on a 3-year longitudinal study. Results showed that intention to engage in gambling behavior increased in the junior secondary school years. Based on the Wave 3 data, concurrent prediction analyses showed that age, gender, parental marital status, family functioning, and positive youth development attributes predicted intention to engage in gambling at the same time. Longitudinal analyses further showed that gender, family communication, and positive youth development at Wave 1 predicted intention to gamble at Wave 3. While being male and growing up in non-intact families can be regarded as risk factors for adolescent intention to engage in gambling, good family functioning and possession of positive youth development attributes are factors protecting junior secondary school students from engaging in gambling.

Keywords Positive youth development • Intention to gamble • Adolescent gambling • Early adolescents • Chinese

Introduction

Gambling as a popular leisure activity for adults has been well received in the Chinese culture and is generally considered as an acceptable form of social interaction. It is said in Chinese that "a little gambling cheers the heart and is good for one's health" ("xiao du yi qing"). Such positive social acceptance about gambling activities potentially increases people's vulnerability to problematic gambling in Chinese society which further leads to various adverse outcomes (Korn & Shaffer, 1999). As far as the detrimental effects of problem gambling are concerned, researchers showed that it decreased working performance, destroyed family

D.T.L. Shek, Ph.D., B.B.S., S.B.S., J.P. (✉) • L. Yu, Ph.D.
Department of Applied Social Sciences, The Hong Kong Polytechnic University, Hunghom, Hong Kong
e-mail: daniel.shek@polyu.edu.hk

D.T.L. Shek et al. (eds.), *Chinese Adolescents in Hong Kong*,
Quality of Life in Asia 5, DOI 10.1007/978-981-287-143-5_11

relationship, and created financial crisis, physical problems, as well as mental health issues (Fisher, 1993; Kourgiantakis, Saint-Jacques, & Tremblay, 2013; Potenza, Fiellin, Heninger, Rounsaville, & Mazure, 2002; Roy, Custer, Lorenz, & Linnoila, 1988). It has also been reported that gambling participation was associated with other risky behaviors in college students, such as substance abuse, drinking, and unprotected sexual behaviors (Dickson, Derevensky, & Gupta, 2004; Gupta & Derevensky, 1998; Ladouceur, Dubé, & Bujold, 1994). Considering the harmful consequences of uncontrollable gambling behaviors, the American Psychiatric Association (APA) first included "pathological gambling" as an impulse control disorder in the third version of the Diagnostic and Statistical Manual of Mental Disorders in 1980 (DSM-III; American Psychiatric Association, 1980). Pathological gambling was defined as an individual's progressive loss of control on gambling behaviors which causes damage and disruption to the individual's family, personal or vocational pursuits, and money-related issues. In the most recent version of the Diagnostic and Statistical Manual (DSM-V), the diagnosis "pathological gambling" has been changed to "gambling disorder" and listed in the group "addiction and related disorders" as the first formal recognition as a behavioral addiction in the psychiatry literature (DSM-V; American Psychiatric Association, 2013).

During the past few decades, many prevalence studies have been conducted to estimate gambling behaviors and problematic gambling in the global context (Derevensky, Shek, & Merrick, 2011). In the United States, it was reported that the rate of lifetime problem gambling ranged from 0.9 to 2.3 % in the general population (Kessler et al., 2008; Petry, Stinson, & Grant, 2005; Shaffer, Labrie, LaPlante, Nelson, & Stanton, 2004). Similarly, researchers in European countries have found a rate of 0.5–3 % for problem gambling (European Gaming and Betting Association, 2012; Wardle et al., 2007). In a recent worldwide report on gambling activities (Williams, Volberg, & Stevens, 2012), it was revealed that Asian countries had higher rates of problem gambling compared to North America, Europe, and Australia, with the highest rates being observed in Singapore, Macau, and Hong Kong, possibly due to the relatively favorable social norms regarding gambling activities in these areas.

Among different age groups, researchers have found that the prevalence rates of pathological gambling tend to be higher in adolescents than in adult populations (Griffiths & Wood, 2000; Gupta & Derevensky, 1998), suggesting that children and young people are more vulnerable to developing gambling problems. Based on a meta-analysis, Shaffer and Hall (1996) found that 4.4–7.4 % of youth (aged 13–20) displayed symptoms of pathological gambling behavior, which were significantly higher than the rate for adults (ranging from 1 to 2 %). Similarly, the National Research Council (NRC, 1999) estimated that the rate of pathological gambling in adolescents ranged from 1.2 to 11.2 % in the United States based on a comprehensive review and concluded that the proportion of pathological gamblers in youth could be more than three times that of adults. This observation is puzzling because persons under 18 years of age are usually not permitted to gamble in many jurisdictions.

With particular reference to Hong Kong, the Hong Kong Polytechnic University conducted a large-scale study on local people's participation in gambling activities in 2001 and found that almost four-fifths of the respondents (78 %) had participated in at least 1 of the 13 gambling activities listed in the survey. Mark Six (64.2 %), social gambling (e.g., playing mahjong and cards with friends and relatives) (45.9 %), and horse racing (30.4 %) were the three most popular forms of gambling. Using telephone interviews with 2,004 local residents, it was reported that 4.0 % and 1.8 % of the respondents could be classified as problem and pathological gamblers, respectively. Based on a representative sample of 2,000 secondary school students, the same group of researchers reported that 54.0 % of the adolescent respondents had engaged in gambling behaviors in the past year, 20.0 % reported themselves as having exhibited one or more of the diagnostic criteria of pathological gambling, and 7.1 % and 2.6 % of the entire sample could be diagnosed as problem gamblers and pathological gamblers, respectively. These figures suggest that gambling and problem gambling are severe public health issues in Hong Kong, particularly for the youth. As it is well documented that starting gambling at an early age is associated with an increased risk of developing subsequent problem gambling (Gupta & Derevensky, 1998; Kaminer, Burleson, & Jadamec, 2002), there is an urgent need to prevent gambling behaviors in youth as early as possible.

To effectively prevent and treat problem gambling, a number of theories have been proposed to explain the etiology of gambling behaviors among which the theory of planned behavior (TPB, Ajzen & Fishbein, 1980) has been given increasing attention. According to TPB, gambling behavior is influenced by one's intention to perform that behavior, and one's intention is affected by three independent factors: attitude toward the behavior, perceived subjective norms regarding that behavior, and perceived behavioral control. When an individual's attitude, subjective norm, and perceived behavioral control regarding the behavior become more favorable, an individual would have a higher intention to perform the behavior, which further predicts the individual's participation in that behavior (Ajzen, 1991). This theory has been examined in a few empirical studies based on different populations, and supporting evidence was generally found. For example, a study based on college students showed that the intention to gamble correlated strongly and positively with both gambling frequency and problem gambling (Moore & Ohtsuka, 2002). A more recent research revealed that both attitudes and subjective norms were significantly associated with one's intention to gambling, and perceived behavioral control positively predicted gambling frequency (Martin et al., 2010). Given the high social acceptance about gambling behavior in different Chinese societies (i.e., favorable social norms), this theory well explains the higher rate of gambling in Chinese populations.

Another popular perspective that is often used in public health prevention to explain adolescent risky behaviors including gambling is the socio-ecological theory (Bronfenbrenner, 1979). It is believed that adolescent development is affected by the interdependent systems of influence at individual, family, school, neighborhood, and community levels. Problem behaviors occur when the impact of risk factors overwhelmed the effect of protective factors. Therefore, by reducing the risk factors while strengthening the protective factors involved in the development of problem behaviors, such behaviors could be prevented. A number of studies have been conducted to identify the risk and protective factors at different ecological levels that contribute to gambling behaviors. First, some demographic factors have been associated with gambling behaviors in youth. Two most consistent findings regarding the risk factors for youth gambling are gender and age. Boys have been found to gamble more frequently and show more social and emotional problems related to their gambling than girls (Wardle et al., 2007; Welte, Barnes, Tidwell, and Hoffman 2008). Besides, older adolescents gamble more than their younger counterparts. These findings are similar to the patterns of other types of addictive behaviors, such as drug use and Internet addiction observed in different studies (Barnes, Welte, Hoffman, & Dintcheff, 1997; Yu & Shek, 2013). Regarding the relationship between gambling and other demographic factors, relatively few studies have been conducted and the findings are inconsistent. For example, Winters, Bengston, Door, and Stinchfield (1998) reported that minority adolescents had higher rates of gambling compared to White youth, while similar rates in adolescents of different ethical groups were found in another study (Volberg, Abbott, Rönnberg, & Munck, 2001).

Second, at family level, parental gambling behavior and gambling cognition have been identified as significant predictors of adolescent gambling (Oei & Raylu, 2004). Researchers consistently found that adolescents who reported excessive parental gambling showed higher rates of pathological gambling themselves (e.g., Jacobs, 2000). Parental gambling cognitions were also positively related to offspring cognitions about gambling (Oei & Raylu). In contrast, less has been reported in the literature about the extent to which family structure and family functioning may influence adolescent gambling behaviors and/or intention, although a substantial amount of research has shown the importance of parental support and monitoring in the prevention of drug use and other problem behaviors in adolescence (Barnes, 1990; Shek & Yu, 2012). Existing research findings were also inconsistent. For example, Langhinrichsen-Rohling, Rohde, Seeley, and Rohling (2004) reported that both family composition (live with both parents versus not living with them) and family cohesion failed to predict adolescent gambling. As there are methodological issues in the studies in the field such as overrepresentation of non-intact families in some studies, the relationship between adolescent gambling and family functioning as well as family structure remains unclear.

Third, based on a positive youth development approach, different internal developmental assets have been proposed to be important protective factors that prevent various risk behaviors and problems in youth (Catalano, Berglund, Ryan, Lonczak, and Hawkins 2004). For example, the occurrence of Internet addiction in adolescents is positively associated with low self-esteem, lack of social and emotional skills, and shyness, while negatively associated with effective time management skills, positive coping style, and good problem-solving skills (Amiel & Sargent, 2004; Armstrong, Phillips, & Saling, 2000; Kraut et al., 1998; Morahan-Martin, & Schumacher, 2003). A 5-year longitudinal study based on a large-scale positive youth development program in Hong Kong (the Project P.A.T.H.S.) also revealed that participants of the program demonstrated significantly lower levels of delinquent behaviors than did the control group. However, direct evidence showing linkages between positive youth development constructs and adolescent gambling is very limited. An exception is the work by Shek (2010) who studied positive youth development and gambling intention in a sample of secondary school students in Hong Kong based on a 2-year longitudinal study. The findings revealed that positive youth development indexed by different indicators was negatively related to adolescent behavioral intention to gamble; positive youth development measures predicted adolescent gambling and their changes over time. This study provides important evidence for the protective role of positive youth development attributes in the development of gambling behaviors in youth. Nonetheless, one limitation of the study is that other factors at different ecological levels, such as the family, were not included in the data analyses so that the possible influences of these factors cannot be controlled. Consistent with the propositions of the ecological perspective, to have a more accurate understanding about how positive youth development may contribute to youth gambling, demographic, individual, and family factors must be taken into account simultaneously.

In addition to the above-mentioned research gaps, there are three limitations intrinsic to the existing literature on youth problem gambling behaviors. First, while a large amount of studies have examined the prevalence of problem gambling and pathological gambling in young people, limited research investigates adolescent gambling intention. In fact, adolescents are usually banned legally from gambling and most of them are financially dependent on family. It is reasonable to assume that there are more youth who have behavioral intentions to engage in gambling activities than those who really show gambling behaviors due to the limited social availability and financial capability. This group of young people should be investigated and provided with effective prevention services, as gambling intention has been proved to be an important precedent of gambling behaviors. Second, compared to studies conducted in Western countries, relatively few studies on youth gambling were carried out on Chinese populations (Shek & Ma, 2011). Given the high level of social acceptance (i.e., favorable social norms) toward gambling in different Chinese societies, it is important to examine the prevalence rate and the sociodemographic and psychosocial correlates of this phenomenon in Chinese adolescents. Third, most studies on youth gambling adopted cross-sectional design which cannot identify the cause and effect relationship between gambling and different psychosocial correlates. Longitudinal studies are needed to enable researchers to find out causal factors of gambling in adolescents.

Against the above background, the present study has three purposes. First, we aimed to estimate the rates of behavioral intention to engage in gambling activities in junior secondary school students in Hong Kong based on a large sample of secondary school students. Second, the study will further examine how different demographic factors and family factors may predict one's gambling intention using a longitudinal design. Based on literature review, it was hypothesized that (1) males would report more gambling intentions than did females, (2) age would be positively related to youth gambling intention, (3) adolescents living in non-intact families would be more likely to have gambling intention than do those from intact families, and (4) high family functioning would predict low level of gambling intention. Third, the relationship between positive youth development and adolescent gambling intention will be investigated after controlling for demographic factors and family factors. Generally speaking, it was hypothesized that different positive youth development constructs would be negatively correlated with youth gambling intention both cross-sectionally and longitudinally.

Methods

Participants and Procedures

This study is part of a large-scale longitudinal project on youth development in Hong Kong (Shek & Yu, 2012). A total of 28 secondary schools were randomly selected from all secondary schools in Hong Kong to participate in this research. Starting from the 2009/2010 school year, all secondary 1 students from the selected schools were invited to participate in the study, and they were followed up for 3 consecutive years during their junior secondary school time. As such, in the school years of 2010/2011 and 2011/2012, the same cohort of students in the selected 28 schools who were participants for the first wave of data collection in the school year of 2009/2010 (Wave 1: 3,325 students, age = 12.59 ± 0.74 years) was invited to attend the second and third waves of data collection (Wave 2: 3,638 students, age = 13.64 ± 0.75 years; Wave 3: 4,106 students, age = 14.65 ± 0.80 years). The demographic information of the participants is summarized in Table 1. From Wave 1 through Wave 3, data of 2,667 students were successfully matched, indicating an acceptable attrition rate of 19.8 %.

After obtaining consent from the school, students, and their parents, the participants were invited to complete a comprehensive youth development questionnaire including both existing instruments and scales developed by the first author. The questionnaire survey was conducted by a trained research assistant in classroom settings with standardized instructions. At each measurement occasion, the students were assured of the confidentiality of the data collected. Participants responded to the questionnaires in a self-administered format. The research assistant was present throughout the administration process to answer possible questions from the participants.

Instruments

The questionnaire used in this study comprises questions about participants' problem behavior intention, demographic information, participants' family environment, different measures of youth development constructs, and other problem behaviors. Students' intention to engage in gambling behavior was measured by asking a question about the possibility that the adolescent would involve in any

Table 1 Demographic profile of the participants

	Wave 1		Wave 2		Wave 3	
	N	Percentage (%)	*N*	Percentage (%)	*N*	Percentage (%)
Gender						
Male	1,719	52.2	1,864	52.1	2,185	53.7
Female	1,572	47.8	1,716	47.9	1,885	46.3
Place of birth						
Hong Kong	2,590	78.3	2,806	78.6	3,195	79.4
Mainland	655	19.3	690	19.3	762	18.9
Others	64	1.9	73	2.0	68	1.7
Parents' marital status						
First marriage	2,781	84.4	2,985	82.7	3,372	82.5
Divorced	209	6.3	256	7.1	345	8.4
Separated	73	2.2	78	2.2	95	2.3
Remarried	129	3.9	168	4.7	189	4.6
Others (not first marriage)	104	3.2	122	3.4	86	2.1
Family economic status						
Receiving CSSA	225	6.8	208	5.8	212	5.2
Not receiving CSSA	2,606	78.3	2,932	81.2	3,308	81.4
Others (don't know)	465	13.9	472	13.1	545	13.4

gambling activities in the coming 2 years from now on, with 4 response options (1 = absolutely will not; 2 = probably will not; 3 = probably will; 4 = absolutely will). Higher score represents a high level of intention to engage in gambling behavior. Other instruments related to the present paper are introduced below.

The Chinese Positive Youth Development Scale (CPYDS)

The Chinese Positive Youth Development Scale (CPYDS) was designed to assess positive youth development attributes of the participants. There are 15 dimensions of the scale, including bonding (3 items), resilience subscale (3 items), social competence (3 items), emotional competence (3 items), cognitive competence (3 items), behavioral competence (3 items), moral competence (3 items), self-determination (3 items), self-efficacy (2 items), beliefs in the future (3items), clear and positive identity (3 items), spirituality (3 items), prosocial involvement (3 items), prosocial norms (3 items), and recognition for positive behavior (3 items).

Utilizing confirmatory factor analyses, Shek and Ma (2010a) further proposed that the 15 subscales in the CPYDS could be reduced to four dimensions. The first dimension is cognitive behavioral competence (CBC) which is the mean score of the mean subscale scores of cognitive competence, self-determination, and behavioral competence.

Table 2 Descriptive statistics and internal consistency of the scales

	Mean			Standard deviation			Cronbach's α		
	W1	W2	W3	W1	W2	W3	W1	W2	W3
Family functioning									
Mutuality (CFAIM)	3.89	3.80	3.82	0.89	0.90	0.87	0.87	0.88	0.89
Conflict (CFAIC)	2.19	2.27	2.30	0.92	0.93	0.92	0.76	0.78	0.79
Communication (CFAICOM)	3.51	3.41	3.43	1.01	0.96	0.93	0.81	0.81	0.81
Total score of family functioning (CFAIALL)	3.73	3.65	3.65	0.81	0.81	0.79	0.90	0.90	0.90
Positive youth development									
Cognitive-behavioral competencies (CBC)	4.45	4.42	4.43	0.75	0.74	0.70	0.87	0.89	0.89
Prosocial attributes (PA)	4.50	4.38	4.39	0.89	0.86	0.82	0.83	0.84	0.83
General positive youth development (GPYDQ)	4.58	4.51	4.52	0.71	0.71	0.67	0.93	0.93	0.93
Positive identity (PIT)	4.24	4.16	4.14	0.96	0.96	0.93	0.87	0.89	0.89
Total score of positive youth development (PYD)	4.51	4.43	4.44	0.70	0.69	0.65	0.96	0.96	0.96
Intention of engaging in gambling	1.27	1.38	1.43	0.67	0.78	0.83	–	–	–

W1 Wave 1, *W2* Wave 2, *W3* Wave 3

The second dimension is prosocial attributes (PA) which is computed by averaging the total mean scores of the prosocial involvement and prosocial norms subscales. The third dimension is positive identity (PIT). The dimension score is computed by averaging mean scores of beliefs in the future and clear and positive identity subscales. The final dimension is general positive youth development qualities (GPYDQ). Its scale score equals to the mean score of resilience, social competence, self-efficacy, moral competence, bonding, recognition for positive behavior, spirituality, and emotional competence subscales. In the present study, the four composite scores and the total score of the CPYDS were used as indicators of positive youth development attributes. Higher scores represent higher levels of developmental assets. Reliability coefficients of these scales at each wave are summarized in Table 2.

Chinese Family Assessment Instrument (CFAI)

Nine items of the Chinese Family Assessment Instrument (Shek & Ma, 2010b) were used to assess three aspects of perceived family functioning, including family mutuality (CFAIM), family conflicts (CFAIC), and family communication (CFAICOM). Students were asked to respond to a 5-point Likert scale on their perceptions of their family lives. Average score across all nine items was used as the indicator of general family functioning (CFAIALL), with high scores representing for high levels of family functioning. Reliability analysis showed that the scale was internally consistent (Cronbach's $\alpha = 0.90$ at each of the three waves).

Data Analytic Plan

First, to examine adolescents' intention to engage in gambling behaviors over time, descriptive statistical analyses were used. Specifically, numbers and percentages of adolescents who reported different possibilities of having gambling activities in the coming 2 years were computed at each wave of data collection. To compare students' gambling intention across three waves, a repeated measures ANOVA was performed to test the effect of time on students' scores of the gambling intention item.

Second, to examine the sociodemographic correlates of adolescent intention to engage in gambling, a one-way ANOVA was conducted based on Wave 3 data, with gender, grade, economic status, and intactness of the family being independent variables while participants' scores on the question about the possibility of engaging in gambling behavior being the dependent variable.

Third, to investigate the concurrent relationship between positive youth development, family functioning, and students' gambling intention, a hierarchical regression model was tested based on Wave 3 data. Specifically, participants' scores on gambling intention served as the dependent variable, with age and gender entered in the first block, parental marital status and family functioning indicators (CFAIM, CFAIC, CFAICOM) entered in the second block, and different positive youth development indicators (CBC, PIT, PA, GPYDQ) entered in the third block. To further investigate the roles of overall family functioning and positive youth development in adolescents' gambling intention, another regression model was tested, with the general indictors of family functioning (CFAIALL) and positive youth development (PYD) being used to replace their respective individual indictors, i.e., CFAIALL replaced CFAIM, CFAIC, and CFAICOM in the second block, and PYD replaced CBC, PIT, PA, and GPYDQ in the third block.

Fourth, to test the longitudinal effects of different predictors on gambling intention in youth, two regression models were further fitted. The two models were basically the same as the ones testing concurrent relationships described above, except that all the independent variables were measured at Wave 1 while the dependent variable was measured at Wave 3.

Results

Prevalence of Gambling Intention and Its Demographic Correlates

Descriptive statistics about the variables under study at three waves of data collection are presented in Table 2. Numbers and percentages of participants who showed different intentions to engage in gambling behaviors in the coming 2 years are summarized in Table 3. As mentioned, a repeated measures ANOVA was conducted to examine differences in participants' gambling intention item scores across time.

Table 3 Numbers and percentage of participants expressing intention to engage in gambling at different levels

From now on, would you involve in any gambling activities in the coming 2 years?	Participants					
	W1		W2		W3	
	No.	%	No.	%	No.	%
1. Absolutely will not	2,742	82.8	2,825	77.8	2,962	75
2. Probably will not	295	8.9	357	9.8	408	10.3
3. Probably will	208	6.3	334	9.2	431	10.9
4. Absolutely will	65	2.0	115	3.2	146	3.7

W1 Wave 1, *W2* Wave 2, *W3* Wave 3

Table 4 Descriptive statistics of participants' scores on gambling intention by gender and parental marital status

	Mean	SD
Gender		
Male	1.52	0.90
Female	1.34	0.73
Parents' marital status		
First marriage	1.41	0.81
Divorced	1.58	0.96
Separated	1.60	0.88
Remarried	1.45	0.85
Others (not first marriage)	1.63	1.04

Note: Results were based on Wave 3 data

The effect of time was significant, Wilks' lambda=0.97, $F(2, 2{,}548)=43.00$, $p<.001$. Post hoc analyses showed that participants' intention to engage in gambling behavior increased every year. Students' scores on this item at Wave 3 were significantly higher than those at Wave 2 ($p<.001$), which was also significantly higher than the scores at Wave 1 ($p<.001$). Such a tendency can also be observed from the percentages of participants with different gambling intention. As shown in Table 3, with age increased, more and more students indicated that they would probably (Wave 1=6.3 %; Wave 2=9.2 %; Wave 3=10.9 %) or absolutely (Wave 1=2.0 %; Wave 2=3.2 %; Wave 3=3.7 %) engage in gambling behaviors in the coming 2 years.

Based on Wave 3 data, the results of ANOVA showed significant main effects of gender ($p<.05$) and parental marital status ($p<.03$) on students' gambling intention. Boys displayed more gambling intentions than did girls; participants from intact families were less likely to indicate intention to engage in gambling behaviors than were students from non-intact families. Specifically, students whose parents were in their first marriage scored significantly lower than did students with parents who were divorced, separated, or in other non-marriage status. Table 4 showed the means and standard deviations of the item score on gambling intention by gender and parental marital status.

Concurrent Prediction of Intention to Gamble by Sociodemographic and Psychosocial Factors

The concurrent predictive effects of participants' family functioning and positive youth development on their intention to engage in gambling behaviors were examined based on Wave 3 data. Table 5 presents the results of multiple regression analysis which showed several interesting phenomena. First, both participants' age ($\beta = .09$, $p < .01$) and gender ($\beta = .09$, $p < .01$) significantly predicted gambling intention. With increase in age, students tended to show more gambling intentions; boys expressed higher level of intention to engage in gambling than did girls. These findings are consistent with the results of ANOVA reported earlier. Second, having divorced parents increased

Table 5 Concurrent prediction on students' gambling intention

	B	Beta	Sig	R^2	R^2 change
First block					
Age	.08	.09	.00		
Gender	.15	.09	.00	.02	.02**
Second block					
Parental marital status					
Divorced	.12	.04	.02		
Separated	.17	.03	.07		
Remarried	.04	.01	.50		
Others	.13	.02	.19		
Family functioning					
CFAIM	−.03	−.03	.30		
CFAIC	.02	.03	.26		
CFAICOM	−.08	−.10	.00	.04	.02**
Third block					
CBC	.06	.05	.07		
PA	−.15	−.15	.00		
PIT	.04	.05	.09		
GPYDQ	−.10	−.08	.02	.06	.02**
Supplementary analysis					
Second block					
CFAIALL	−.13	−.13	.00	.04	.02**
Third block					
PYD	−.14	−.11	.00	.05	.01**

Notes: Both predictors and the dependent variable were measured at Wave 3
Gender: 1 = male; 0 = female
Parental marital status: Others = other situation of non-intact family
CFAIM family mutuality, *CFAIC* family conflict, *CFAICOM* family communication, *CFAIALL* general indicator of family functioning, *CBC* cognitive behavioral competence, *PA* prosocial attributes, *GPYDQ* general positive youth development qualities, *PIT* positive and clear identity, *PYD* mean score of the Chinese Positive Youth Development Scale
**$p < .001$

the risk of showing gambling intention in adolescents ($\beta = .04$, $p < .05$). Third, family communication was negatively related to gambling intention ($\beta = -.10$, $p < .001$). Fourth, after controlling for the demographic variables and family factors, higher levels of prosocial attributes (PA) and general positive youth development qualities (GPYDQ) significantly predicted lower level of gambling intention in adolescents ($\beta = -.15$, $p < .001$ for PA; $\beta = -.08$, $p < .05$). In the supplementary analyses, it was found that general indicators of family functioning (CFAIALL) and positive youth development (PYD) both served as protective factors in adolescent gambling intention ($\beta = -.13$, $p < .001$ for CFAIALL; $\beta = -.11$, $p < .001$ for PYD). In other words, good family functioning and positive youth development were related to decreased intention to engage in gambling behaviors in youth.

Prediction of Gambling Intention over Time

The longitudinal predictive effects of participants' demographic variables, family factors, and positive youth development constructs at Wave 1 on adolescent gambling intention at Wave 3 were examined using hierarchical multiple regression. As shown in Table 6, several predictors showed significant longitudinal effects on youth gambling intention. First, gender was positively correlated with the dependent variable ($\beta = -.15$, $p < .001$); boys showed stronger intention to engage in gambling than girls. Second, after controlling for the demographic factors and parental marital status, family communication still played a role in preventing students developing gambling intention ($\beta = -.10$, $p < .001$). Third, higher level of general positive youth development qualities (GPYDQ) predicted lower level of gambling intention in adolescents ($\beta = -.11$, $p < .001$). For the supplementary analyses, both CFAIALL ($\beta = -.10$, $p < .001$) and PYD ($\beta = -.08$, $p < .001$), the two general indicators of family functioning and positive youth development, were significantly related to adolescents' intention to engage in gambling behaviors in a negative way. These findings are basically consistent with the results based on cross-sectional data at Wave 3. However, an unexpected finding is the positive relationship between youth gambling intention and positive and clear identity (PIT, $\beta = .10$, $p < .001$). In other words, the higher the individual's positive identity, the more likely he or she would express the intention to engage in gambling behaviors in the next 2 years.

Discussion

The present study examined the prevalence rate of behavioral intention to engage in gambling activities in Hong Kong adolescents and investigated both the concurrent and longitudinal effects of different sociodemographic and psychosocial factors on this phenomenon over 2 years. This is the first study examining the prevalence of youth gambling intention in Hong Kong based on a large and representative sample

Table 6 Longitudinal prediction of students' gambling intention

	B	Beta	Sig	R^2	R^2 change
First block					
Age	.04	.03	.16		
Gender	.15	.09	.00	.01	.01**
Second block					
Parental marital status					
Divorced	.06	.02	.39		
Separated	−.01	.00	.93		
Remarried	.05	.01	.61		
Others	.17	.04	.10		
Family functioning					
CFAIM	−.05	−.05	.17		
CFAIC	−.01	−.01	.68		
CFAICOM	−.10	−.12	.00	.04	.03**
Third block					
CBC	−.02	−.02	.66		
PA	−.05	−.06	.09		
PIT	.08	.10	.01		
GPYDQ	−.11	−.10	.04	.04	.01*
Supplementary analysis					
Second block					
CFAIALL	−.10	−.10	.00	.03	.02**
Third block					
PYD	−.10	−.08	.00	.04	.01*

Notes: Predictors were all measured at Wave 1 while the dependent variable was measured at Wave 3
Gender: 1 = male; 0 = female
Parental marital status: Others = other situation of non-intact family
CFAIM family mutuality, *CFAIC* family conflict, *CFAICOM* family communication, *CFAIALL* general indicator of family functioning, *CBC* cognitive behavioral competence, *PA* prosocial attributes, *GPYDQ* general positive youth development qualities, *PIT* positive and clear identity, *PYD* mean score of the Chinese Positive Youth Development Scale
*$p < .01$; **$p < .001$

of adolescents over a period of 3 years. Such epidemiological data are essential for developing programs that will meet the needs of junior secondary school students in Hong Kong. The present findings underscore the important role of family and positive youth development in preventing adolescent gambling intention. Both cross-sectional and longitudinal data analyses showed that good family functioning and high levels of positive youth development predicted low gambling intention after controlling for the effects of the sociodemographic factors. These findings raise both theoretical and practical implications in the prevention of gambling behaviors in young people.

Collapsing the "possible" and "absolute" behavioral intention for gambling responses together, the results showed that 8.3 % (secondary one) to 14.6 % (secondary three) of the responding students intended to gamble in the next 2 years.

This observation suggests that gambling intention in Hong Kong adolescents is a rising behavioral phenomenon in adolescents in Hong Kong. From secondary 1 to secondary 3, the percentage of participants who reported having the intention to engage in gambling activities increased by year (from 8.3 %, 12.4 %, to 14.6 %). Similar results were found when comparing the mean scores of gambling intention across 3 years. This finding is consistent with our hypothesis that age would be positively correlated with gambling intention in youth. With increase in age, more adolescents report behavioral intention to participate in gambling activities. This indicates the importance of early intervention/prevention targeting gambling behaviors and intentions. Researchers showed that a high proportion (90.0 %) of social gamblers started to gamble for recreational and social purposes since they were just children and young adolescents, from the age of 10–16 (The Hong Kong Polytechnic University, 2001). Therefore, effective prevention strategies must be taken for youth with gambling intentions before they really engage in gambling activities.

In line with our initial hypothesis, the results of ANOVA showed that being male and having a non-intact family structure increase the intention to gamble. This finding was also consistent with the results of multiple regression analyses based on cross-sectional data, in which gender and family structure significantly predicted participants' scores on their intention to engage in gambling behaviors in the next 2 years. However, when longitudinal data were employed, family structure indicated by parental marital status failed to predict gambling intention in adolescents. Participants from non-intact families did not show higher behavioral intention to gamble than did those whose parents were in their first marriage. As such, the present results may not be able to provide a clear answer to the question about whether and to what extent family structure would influence youth gambling intention and behaviors. It is recommended that this issue should further be examined in future studies such as using multiple indicators that can measure family structure in a more comprehensive way.

Family functioning was found to have significant effects on youth gambling intention. Both concurrent and longitudinal data analyses suggest that more frequent family communication and overall positive family functioning were associated with lower level of gambling intention. In other words, adolescents having high quality of family life tend to display a lower level of intention to gamble. This supports previously reported research findings that there were positive relationships between family dysfunction and various types of adolescent problem behaviors such as substance abuse, suicidal intention, and Internet addiction in different populations (Barrera, Biglan, Ary, & Li, 2001; Doherty & Allen, 1994; Shek, 2005; Shek & Yu, 2012). The present study is also in line with the theoretical prediction that poor family functioning is conducive to impaired youth functioning (Beavers, Hampson, & Hulgus, 1985; Epstein, Bishop, Ryan, Miller, & Keitner, 1993). The longitudinal findings of the present study provide sound and direct evidence for the important role of family in the development of adolescents' behavioral intention to engage in gambling. Based on the findings, it is suggested that when designing preventive interventions targeting adolescent gambling intentions and behaviors, helping professionals and researchers should consider how to improve family functioning in terms of facilitating communication among family members, strengthening family cohesion, and resolving family conflicts effectively. Unfortunately, as pointed out by Shek (2013), relevant family quality of life promotion programs are grossly inadequate in different Chinese contexts.

The finding that positive youth development constructs are directly related to adolescent gambling intention is consistent with earlier reports about other types of youth risky behaviors (Catalano et al., 2004). After controlling for the demographic factors and family factors, the influence of positive youth development on adolescent gambling intention was still significant. While the influence of developmental assets/positive youth development on a range of adolescent problem behaviors has been demonstrated in many publications in the past (Hawkins, Catalano, & Miller, 1992; Pollard, Hawkins, & Arthur, 1999; Sun & Shek, 2010), the present study is the first that clearly supports the prediction of positive youth development on youth gambling intention, which adds to the literature. The implication is that to prevent and reduce gambling behaviors and intentions in adolescents, future programs need to incorporate components that can promote healthy development in participants and foster their positive qualities. As many adolescent problem gamblers show a lack of psychosocial competencies such as emotional and behavioral competencies, Shek and Sun (2011) suggested that the use of positive youth development constructs in prevention programs for adolescent problem gambling would be helpful. Adopting this approach, the basic argument is that through strengthening of the inner strengths and resources of adolescents, adolescent risk behavior (including problem gambling) would disappear.

An unexpected finding is the positive correlation between "positive and clear identity" factor and adolescent gambling intention. Longitudinal data analyses showed that participants who had a high level of positive identity at Wave 1 were more likely to indicate their intention of gambling in the next 2 years. This seems to be contradicting with our initial hypothesis that positive youth development constructs should have protective effects on youth development. However, this finding may be well explained by the theory of planned behavior (Ajzen & Fishbein, 1980) in which perceived behavioral control is believed to be positively related to one's gambling intention. It is possible that adolescents with high level of positive and clear identity have more confidence in their ability to control their own behaviors (i.e., overconfidence) and thus tend to show more intention for gambling in the future. Similar findings were reported by Taormina (2009) based on a sample of 500 Chinese residents of Macau. In this study, participants' illusion of control was positively related with both gambling attitudes and gambling behaviors. The present finding seems to suggest that while it is important to foster a positive self-identity in adolescents, it is equally important to help them establish a realistic attitude toward gambling and rational evaluation about one's behavioral control, particularly in programs that aim at preventing/intervening gambling intention and behaviors. As this is an odd finding, there is a need to further examine the relationship between self-identity and intention to engage in gambling.

Although this is a pioneering work in the field, there are several limitations of this study. First, adolescent gambling intention was measured at three time points in three consecutive years of junior secondary school. More waves of data should be collected to have a more complete understanding about the developmental tendency of gambling intention in the high school years of adolescents in Hong Kong. Second, only behavioral intention was measured in the present study. Future studies should also assess participants' real gambling behavior and see how different psychosocial correlates predict actual gambling behavior. Third, as one single item was used to measure gambling intention, this may produce a less discriminating response profile. More comprehensive measures on behavioral intention to gambling in the future may be employed in future research. Fourth, the assessment was based on self-reported questionnaire. Information from other informants such as parents and teachers should also be collected in future studies. Despite the limitations, the present findings help youth researchers and practitioners understand the prevalence rate of gambling intention and its demographic, family, and positive youth development correlates in Hong Kong adolescents. The present findings have important implications for future research and practice on preventing gambling behavior in Hong Kong youth.

Acknowledgment The preparation for this work and the Project P.A.T.H.S. were financially supported by the Hong Kong Jockey Club Charities Trust. The authorship is equally shared by the first author and second author.

References

Ajzen, I. (1991). The theory of planned behavior. *Organizational Behavioral and Human Decision Processes, 50*(2), 179–211.

Ajzen, I., & Fishbein, M. (1980). *Understanding attitudes and predicting social behavior.* Englewood Cliffs, NJ: Prentice-Hall.

American Psychiatric Association. (1980). *Diagnostic and statistical manual of mental disorders* (3rd ed.). Washington, DC: Author.

American Psychiatric Association. (2013). *Diagnostic and statistical manual of mental disorders* (5th ed.). Arlington, VA: American Psychiatric Publishing.

Amiel, T., & Sargent, S. L. (2004). Individual differences in Internet usage motives. *Computers in Human Behavior, 20*(6), 711–726.

Armstrong, L., Phillips, J. G., & Saling, L. L. (2000). Potential determinants of heavier internet usage. *International Journal of Human-Computer Studies, 53*, 537–550.

Barnes, G. M. (1990). Impact of the family on adolescent drinking patterns. In R. L. Collins, K. E. Leonard, & J. S. Searles (Eds.), *Alcohol and the family: Research and clinical perspectives* (pp. 137–161). New York: The Guilford Press.

Barnes, G. M., Welte, J. W., Hoffman, J. H., & Dintcheff, B. A. (1997). Changes in alcohol use and alcohol-related problems among 7th to 12th grade students in New York State, 1983–1994. *Alcoholism: Clinical and Experimental Research, 21*(5), 916–922.

Barrera, M., Jr., Biglan, A., Ary, D., & Li, F. (2001). Replication of a problem behavior model with American Indian, Hispanic, and Caucasian youth. *Journal of Early Adolescence, 21*(2), 133–157.

Beavers, W. R., Hampson, R. B., & Hulgus, Y. F. (1985). Commentary: The Beavers systems approach to family assessment. *Family Process, 24*(3), 398–405.

Bronfenbrenner, U. (1979). *The ecology of human development.* Cambridge, MA: Harvard University Press.

Catalano, R. F., Berglund, M. L., Ryan, J. A. M., Lonczak, H. S., & Hawkins, J. D. (2004). Positive youth development in the United States: Research findings on evaluations of positive youth development programs. *Annals of the American Academy of Political and Social Science, 591*, 98–124.

Derevensky, J. L., Shek, D. T. L., & Merrick, J. (Eds.). (2011). *Youth gambling: The hidden addiction*. Berlin, Germany: de Gruyter.

Dickson, L. M., Derevensky, J. L., & Gupta, R. (2004). Harm reduction for the prevention of youth gambling problems: Lessons learned from adolescent high-risk behavior prevention programs. *Journal of Adolescent Research, 19*(2), 233–263.

Doherty, W. J., & Allen, W. (1994). Family functioning and parental smoking as predictors of adolescent cigarette use: A six-year prospective study. *Journal of Family Psychology, 8*(3), 347–353.

Epstein, N. B., Bishop, D., Ryan, C., Miller, I. W., & Keitner, G. I. (1993). The McMaster model view of healthy family functioning. In F. Walsh (Ed.), *Normal family processes* (pp. 138–160). New York: The Guilford Press.

European Gaming and Betting Association. (2012). *Problem gaming, factsheet*. Retrieved from http://www.egba.eu/pdf/EGBA_FS_ProblemGaming.pdf

Fisher, S. (1993). Gambling and pathological gambling in adolescents. *Journal of Gambling Studies, 9*(3), 277–288.

Griffiths, M., & Wood, R. T. A. (2000). Risk factors in adolescence: The case of gambling, videogame playing and the Internet. *Journal of Gambling Studies, 16*(2–3), 199–225.

Gupta, R., & Derevensky, J. L. (1998). Adolescent gambling behavior: A prevalence study and examination of the correlates associated with problem gambling. *Journal of Gambling Studies, 14*(4), 319–345.

Hawkins, J. D., Catalano, R. F., & Miller, J. Y. (1992). Risk and protective factors for alcohol and other drug problems in adolescence and early adulthood: Implications for substance abuse prevention. *Psychological Bulletin, 112*(1), 64–105.

Jacobs, D. F. (2000). Juvenile gambling in North America: An analysis of long term trends and future prospects. *Journal of Gambling Studies, 16*(2–3), 119–152.

Kaminer, Y., Burleson, J. A., & Jadamec, A. (2002). Gambling behavior in adolescent substance abuse. *Substance Abuse, 23*(3), 191–198.

Kessler, R. C., Hwang, I., LaBrie, R., Petukhova, M., Sampson, N. A., Winters, K. C., et al. (2008). DSM-IV pathological gambling in the National Comorbidity Survey Replication. *Psychological Medicine, 38*(9), 1351–1360.

Korn, D. A., & Shaffer, H. J. (1999). Gambling and the health of the public: Adopting a public health perspective. *Journal of Gambling Studies, 15*(4), 289–365.

Kourgiantakis, T., Saint-Jacques, M. C., & Tremblay, J. (2013). Problem gambling and families: A systematic review. *Journal of Social Work Practice in the Addictions, 13*(4), 353–372.

Kraut, R., Patterson, M., Lundmark, V., Kiesler, S., Mukopadhyay, T., & Scherlis, W. (1998). Internet paradox: A social technology that reduces social involvement and psychological well-being? *American Psychologist, 53*, 1017–1031.

Ladouceur, R., Dubé, D., & Bujold, A. (1994). Prevalence of pathological gambling and related problems among college students in the Quebec metropolitan area. *Canadian Journal of Psychiatry, 39*(5), 289–293.

Langhinrichsen-Rohling, J., Rohde, P., Seeley, J. R., & Rohling, M. L. (2004). Individual, family and peer correlates of adolescent gambling. *Journal of Gambling Studies, 20*(1), 23–46.

Martin, R. J., Usdan, S., Nelson, S., Umstattd, M. R., LaPlante, D., Perko, M., et al. (2010). Using the theory of planned behavior to predict gambling behavior. *Psychology of Addictive Behaviors, 24*(1), 89–97.

Moore, S., & Ohtsuka, K. (2002). Gambling activities of young Australians: Developing a model of behaviour. In J. J. Marotta, J. A. Cornelius, & W. R. Eadington (Eds.), *The downside: Problem and pathological gambling* (pp. 429–453). Reno, NV: Institute for the Study of Gambling & Commercial Gaming.

Morahan-Martin, J., & Schumacher, P. (2003). Loneliness and social uses of the internet. *Computers in Human Behavior, 19*(6), 659–671.
National Research Council. (1999). *Pathological gambling: A critical review*. Washington, DC: The National Academies Press.
Oei, T. P., & Raylu, N. (2004). Familial influence on offspring gambling: A cognitive mechanism for transmission of gambling behavior in families. *Psychological Medicine, 34*(7), 1279–1288.
Petry, N. M., Stinson, F. S., & Grant, B. F. (2005). Comorbidity of DSM-IV pathological gambling and other psychiatric disorders: Results from the National Epidemiologic Survey on Alcohol and Related Conditions. *Journal of Clinical Psychiatry, 66*(5), 564–574.
Pollard, J. A., Hawkins, J. D., & Arthur, M. W. (1999). Risk and protection: Are both necessary to understand diverse behavioral outcomes in adolescence? *Social Work Research, 23*(3), 145–158.
Potenza, M. N., Fiellin, D. A., Heninger, G. R., Rounsaville, B. J., & Mazure, C. M. (2002). Gambling: An addictive behavior with health and primary care implications. *Journal of General Internal Medicine, 17*(9), 721–732.
Roy, A., Custer, R., Lorenz, V., & Linnoila, M. (1988). Depressed pathological gamblers. *Acta Psychiatrica Scandinavica, 77*(2), 163–165.
Shaffer, H. J., & Hall, M. N. (1996). Estimating the prevalence of adolescent gambling disorders: A quantitative synthesis and guide toward standard gambling nomenclature. *Journal of Gambling Studies, 12*(2), 193–214.
Shaffer, H. J., LaBrie, R. A., LaPlante, D. A., Nelson, S. E., & Stanton, M. V. (2004). The road less travelled: Moving from distribution to determinants in the study of gambling epidemiology. *Canadian Journal of Psychiatry, 49*(8), 504–516.
Shek, D. T. L. (2005). A longitudinal study of perceived family functioning and adolescent adjustment in Chinese adolescents with economic disadvantage. *Journal of Family Issues, 26*(4), 518–543.
Shek, D. T. L. (2010). Positive youth development and behavioral intention to gamble among Chinese adolescents in Hong Kong. *International Journal of Adolescent Medicine and Health, 22*(1), 163–172.
Shek, D. T. L. (2013). *Development and evaluation of youth and family life education programs: Back to the basics*. Paper presented at the Family Life Education Conference 2013 organized by the Ministry of Social and Family Development, Singapore Government.
Shek, D. T. L., & Ma, C. M. S. (2010a). Dimensionality of the Chinese Positive Youth Development Scale: Confirmatory factor analyses. *Social Indicators Research, 98*, 41–59.
Shek, D. T. L., & Ma, C. M. S. (2010b). The Chinese Family Assessment Instrument (C-FAI): Hierarchical confirmatory factor analyses and factorial invariance. *Social Indicators Research, 20*, 112–123.
Shek, D. T. L., & Ma, C. M. S. (2011). Positive youth development and intention to gamble. In J. L. Derevensky, D. T. L. Shek, & J. Merrick (Eds.), *Youth gambling: The hidden addiction* (pp. 99–111). Berlin, Germany: de Gruyter.
Shek, D. T. L., & Sun, R. C. F. (2011). Relationship between positive youth development and intention to gamble among Chinese adolescents in Hong Kong. In J. L. Derevensky, D. T. L. Shek, & J. Merrick (Eds.), *Youth gambling: The hidden addiction* (pp. 113–122). Berlin, Germany: de Gruyter.
Shek, D. T. L., & Yu, L. (2012). Internet addiction in Hong Kong adolescents: Profiles and psychosocial correlates. *International Journal of Disability and Human Development, 11*(2), 133–142.
Sun, R. C. F., & Shek, D. T. L. (2010). Life satisfaction, positive youth development, and problem behaviour among Chinese adolescents in Hong Kong. *Social Indicators Research, 95*, 455–474.
Taormina, R. J. (2009). Social and personality correlates of gambling attitudes and behaviour among Chinese residents of Macau. *Journal of Social and Personal Relationships, 26*(8), 1047–1071.
The Hong Kong Polytechnic University. (2001). *A study on Hong Kong peoples' participation in gambling activities*. Hong Kong: The Home Affairs Bureau of the Hong Kong Government.
Volberg, R. A., Abbott, M. W., Rönnberg, S., & Munck, I. M. E. (2001). Prevalence and risks of pathological gambling in Sweden. *Acta Psychiatrica Scandinavica, 104*(4), 250–256.

Wardle, H., Sproston, K., Orford, J., Erens, B., Griffiths, M., Constantine, R., et al. (2007). *British gambling prevalence survey 2007*. London: The Stationery Office.

Welte, J. W., Barnes, G. M., Tidwell, M. C., & Hoffman, J. H. (2008). The prevalence of problem gambling among U.S. adolescents and young adults: Results from a national survey. *Journal of Gambling Studies, 24*(2), 119–133.

Williams, R. J., Volberg, R. A., & Stevens, R. M. G. (2012). *The population prevalence of problem gambling: Methodological influences, standardized rates, jurisdictional differences, and worldwide trends*. Report prepared for the Ontario Problem Gambling Research Centre and the Ontario Ministry of Health and Long Term Care. Retrieved from http://hdl.handle.net/10133/3068

Winters, K. C., Bengston, P., Door, D., & Stinchfield, R. (1998). Prevalence and risk factors of problem gambling among college students. *Psychology of Addictive Behaviors, 12*(2), 127–135.

Yu, L., & Shek, D. T. L. (2013). Internet addiction in Hong Kong adolescents: A three-year longitudinal study. *Journal of Pediatric and Adolescent Gynecology, 26*(3 Suppl), S10–S17.

Promotion of Positive Youth Development and Family Quality of Life in Chinese Adolescents

Daniel T.L. Shek and Rachel C.F. Sun

Abstract According to the ecological perspective, adolescent behavior is influenced by processes in different systems. With reference to the individual system, developmental assets such as psychosocial competencies protect adolescents from risk behavior. Regarding the family system, positive family functioning and dyadic parent-child relational quality are also protective factors for adolescent problem behavior. Besides protecting adolescents from risk behavior, protective factors in these two domains also promote adolescent holistic development. In this chapter, ecological influences with reference to individual developmental assets and family social capital on adolescent personal well-being with particular reference to adolescent risk behavior are outlined. Positive youth development programs with particular focus on the Project P.A.T.H.S. in Hong Kong and programs that can be used to promote family quality of life are also examined. The chapter ends by discussing the possible directions for developing positive youth development and family quality of life enhancement programs in the Chinese contexts.

Keywords Personal well-being • Positive youth development • Family quality of life • Early adolescents • Chinese

Introduction

Research findings showed that poor adolescent well-being is a growing problem in the global context. As far as mental health problem (i.e., negative personal well-being) is concerned, Burnett-Zeigler et al. (2012) showed that among 1,076 adolescents seeking help from urban clinics, 14.3 % showed mental health problems and 42.8 % of them used mental health services in the previous 3 months. Risks factors for adolescent female mental health problems included poor academic performance,

D.T.L. Shek, Ph.D., B.B.S., S.B.S., J.P. (✉)
Department of Applied Social Sciences, The Hong Kong Polytechnic University, Hunghom, Hong Kong
e-mail: daniel.shek@polyu.edu.hk

R.C.F. Sun, Ph.D.
Faculty of Education, The University of Hong Kong, Hong Kong, Hong Kong

D.T.L. Shek et al. (eds.), *Chinese Adolescents in Hong Kong*,
Quality of Life in Asia 5, DOI 10.1007/978-981-287-143-5_12

low parental monitoring, and drug abuse. In another study examining the prevalence, risk factors, and risk behaviors (e.g., substance abuse) among 9,863 students in the United States, Saluja et al. (2004) showed that about 18 % of adolescents reported depressive symptoms, with growing prevalence rates across age. The risk factors identified included being a female, involvement in bullying as perpetrators or victims, substance abuse, and reports of somatic symptoms.

Besides mental health problems, adolescents also exhibit other risk behavior. As far as adolescent substance abuse is concerned, Conway et al. (2013) examined the prevalence and demographic correlates of substance use among 2,524 10th grade American students. Marijuana (26.3 %) was the most commonly used in the past year, followed by misuse of medication (8.7 %) and other illicit drugs (8.3 %). Alcohol consumption (35.3 %) and smoking (18.9 %) were also prevalent in young people. Substance abusers also reported higher levels of somatic symptoms and depression. Based on the responses of adolescents in Nigeria, Atilola, Ayinde, and Adeitan (2013) showed that the 12-month prevalence of alcohol use and other substance use was 21.4 %, followed by 11.5 % for alcohol, 7.0 % for tobacco, 3.9 % for other substances, and 1.0 % for marijuana. The risk factors for substance abuse included being male, parental alcohol and substance use, and poor academic performance.

Another example of adolescent risk behavior is bullying and school violence. Kubwalo, Muula, Siziya, Pasupulati, and Rudatsikira (2013) examined the prevalence and correlates of school bullying in Grade 7 and Grade 8 students in Malawi. Roughly 44.5 % of the students reported that they had been bullied in the month before the study. Risk factors for school bullying were loneliness, having no close friends, smoking, and drinking. Celbis, Karaoglu, Egri, and Ozdemir (2012) examined school bullying in 22,343 students in Malatya. About one-fourth of the students had been involved in a physical fight at least once in the past year and 5.7 % had carried a weapon on school premises. Having exposed to physical violence on school property, neighborhood and home settings were predictors of violence-related behaviors.

With specific reference to Hong Kong, Shek, Ma, and Sun (2011) highlighted several developmental issues in young people, including adolescent drug abuse, Internet use problems, adolescent sexuality problems, bullying, and adolescent materialistic orientation. For example, ketamine abuse was very serious among adolescents in 2009. In fact, Hong Kong has the highest number of ketamine abuse in young people in the global context. Although the numbers of ketamine abusers have dropped in the past few years, the hidden nature of adolescent substance abuse has intensified. Besides, mental health problems in adolescents in Hong Kong have also been reported. Leung et al. (2008) examined the prevalence of DSM-IV disorders among 541 Chinese adolescents from Hong Kong. The overall prevalence rate of DSM-IV disorders was 16.4 % and the prevalence estimates for anxiety disorders and depressive disorders were 6.9 % and 1.3 %, respectively.

With reference to the above-mentioned adolescent developmental problems in the Western and Chinese contexts, there are two questions which policy-makers, academics, youth workers, and the allied professionals should address. The first question is how to make sense of these adolescent developmental issues. In other words, how do we explain these phenomena particularly from a "scientific" perspective? The second question is how to tackle and prevent these adolescent developmental issues. Besides treating the problems (e.g., substance abuse treatment), early identification of adolescents at risk and primary prevention programs are also important issues for consideration.

Ecological Perspective of Adolescent Personal Well-Being

How can we explain adolescent well-being such as mental health problems and risk behavior? What are the factors influencing adolescent well-being? Besides academic understanding, scientific understanding and related perspectives are important as far as intervention and prevention are concerned. Theoretically, different perspectives on the micro and macro levels have been proposed in the scientific literature to explain adolescent risk behavior as follows:

- Biological perspective: Problem "genes" and faulty physiological mechanisms contribute to adolescent risk behavior. The recommended intervention approaches include genetic engineering, operations such as brain lesion, and drug therapy.
- Freudian and neo-Freudian perspectives: Early traumas and socialization problems (e.g., attachment problem) contribute to adolescent risk behavior. Psychoanalysis, resolution of unconscious conflicts, and psychoeducation are proposed to be the intervention foci.
- Behavioral approach: Learning and conditioning problems contribute to adolescent risk behavior. Changing in the environment via behavioral modification helps to reduce adolescent risk behavior.
- Cognitive approach: Distorted thinking such as irrational beliefs and dysfunctional attitudes contributes to adolescent risk behavior. Cognitive therapies such as reframing and development of new beliefs would be the intervention foci.
- Cognitive-behavioral approach: Both environmental and cognitive processes lead to adolescent risk behavior. Through changing the behavior and thinking of an individual, the related risk behavior will be changed.
- Humanistic perspective: Lack of love, authentic experience, or unconditional positive regard creates adolescent risk behavior. Rebuilding of self and developing more positive encounters would be helpful.
- Interpersonal perspective: Interpersonal problems such as social skill deficits contribute to adolescent risk behavior. Promotion of interpersonal skills and interaction is an intervention focus.
- Family perspective: Faulty systemic and/or dyadic family processes lead to adolescent risk behavior. Family intervention such as family therapy is the preferred intervention approach.
- Sociocultural perspective: Problematic social processes such as inequality, discrimination, and poverty lead to adolescent risk behavior. Macro changes in social policies and structures are solutions to reduce adolescent risk behavior.
- Social constructionist perspective: Adolescent risk behavior as a "problem" does not exist because it is "constructed" by the mainstream discourses only. The focus of "intervention" in this perspective is to use narratives to "reconstruct" the meanings and discourses about adolescent risk behavior.

Although there are many psychological and sociological accounts of adolescent personal well-being such as adolescent risk behavior, there is a growing view suggesting that there is a need to transcend the "person" (i.e., micro influences) and "environment" (i.e., macro influences). As such, understanding of the influences of different ecological systems, including the personal and environmental systems (including the interpersonal, family, community, and global systems), on adolescent development is important (Parker & Buriel, 1998).

For example, according to Shek (2007), risk factors in the personal system (such as lack of resilience and low emotional intelligence), interpersonal system (such as loneliness or undesirable peer influence), family system (such as overstrict or overloose parental control), and community system (such as loose legislation and lack of norms) contribute to adolescent substance abuse. Besides, some ecological theorists proposed that the microsystem (i.e., person within a system), mesosystem (mutual influences among different systems), exosystem (influence from an outside system), macrosystem (such as social influences), and chronosystem (influences across time) shape individual behavior, such as adolescent risk behavior (Bronfenbrenner, 1988).

There are different forms of the ecological approach. Nevertheless, the common thesis intrinsic to the different models is that protective factors in the individual (such as self-efficacy and self-confidence) and the environment (such as support from school and the family) would "protect" a person from risk behavior. In reality, protective factors are major pillars in the youth enhancement programs: Protective factors were strongly emphasized in the Social Development Model (Catalano & Hawkins, 2002); Granger (2002) argued that changes in individuals would be triggered by the capacity of individuals, organizations, systems, and communities; Felner and Felner (1989) also proposed different intervention strategies based on the transactional-ecological framework.

In the 3-year longitudinal study covered in this book, there are findings showing that positive youth development (i.e., individual system) and family functioning (i.e., family system) protect adolescents from risk behavior. For example, research findings showed that while family functioning was positively related to positive youth development, it was negatively related to Internet addiction, consumption of pornographic materials, and intention to engage in risk behavior (Ma & Shek, 2013; Shek & Yu, 2012; Yu & Shek, 2013). Hence, discussion on these two areas will be carried out in the following sections.

Positive Youth Development Qualities and Developmental Assets

Under the influence of the notion of "storm and stress," adolescent development has been viewed in terms of problems and pathologies in the West in the past decades. Besides, youth work has focused on the reduction or prevention of youth problems. While focusing on adolescent problems and their remedial actions are important topics, there are views suggesting that this "pathological" approach limits our understanding of the potentials and abilities of adolescents. For example, Pittman, Irby, Tolman, Yohalem, and Ferber (2001) argued that "prevention alone is not enough" and "problem-free is not fully prepared." In other words, the absence of developmental problems does not necessarily imply that an adolescent successfully transits to adulthood. Without whole person development, an adolescent without problems would still encounter difficulties in their development.

Damon (2004) stated that contrary to the traditional approach to adolescent development which emphasizes pathologies of young people, the positive youth development approach focuses on talents and potentials of adolescents. For example, Benson (1997) developed a developmental model with 40 adolescent developmental assets. Similar emphases can be found in the positive youth development models in the literature (Benson, Mannes, Pittman, & Ferber, 2004; Lerner & Benson, 2003).

Regarding the specific components of holistic adolescent development, Lerner, Fisher, and Weinberg (2000) suggested that the five "Cs" (caring/compassion, competence, character, connection, confidence) are important developmental outcomes. Similarly, Pittman et al. (2001) suggested five developmental components in holistic youth development. The first attribute is "confidence" which refers to self-worth (e.g., one's ideas and contributions are perceived to be meaningful), mastery, and future orientation (e.g., awareness of one's progress in life and future projection). The second attribute is "character" which refers to responsibility and autonomy (e.g., accountability and obligations) and spirituality (e.g., connection to families, cultural groups, communities, and higher beings). The third attribute is "connection" which refers to safety and structure (e.g., having access to security), membership, and belonging (e.g., intimate relationship with at least one relationship). The fourth attribute is "competence" which includes knowledge; skills in the health, civic, physical, social, emotional, cognitive, and personal domains; and behavior such as applying and practicing new life skills and new roles. The final attribute is "contribution" which refers to participation and influence, such as making a difference and advocating for a cause. In their reflections on the work regarding positive youth development, Pittman, Irby, and Ferber (2000) also suggested four "Cs" (competence, confidence, character, connectedness) and three "Ls" (learning to be productive, learning to connect, learning to navigate) as indicators for optimal adolescent development.

One developmental asset commonly emphasized by researchers in different positive youth development models is psychosocial competencies in young people. Many researchers suggested that building psychosocial competencies (particularly, cognitive, academic, social, and emotional competence) is a fundamental task in adolescence. For example, Eccles and Gootman (2002) proposed several personal and social competencies that are fundamental to positive youth development. With reference to the specific assets to be developed, Weissberg and O'Brien (2004) suggested that there are five core social-emotional competencies including self-awareness, social awareness, self-management, relationship skills, and responsible actions. According to Graczyk et al. (2000), promotion of social and emotional learning of adolescents (SEL) can serve as a unifying framework that can integrate the risk and protective factors paradigm and the competence enhancement paradigm.

Are there any contradictions between the prevention science perspective (i.e., focus on adolescent pathologies and problems) and the positive youth development paradigm? The answer by Catalano, Berglund, Ryan, Lonczak, and Hawkins (2002) is "no." According to them, searching for risk and protective factors, adoption of a developmental perspective, upholding the belief that problem behaviors share many common antecedents, and the proposal that youth developmental outcomes are determined by risk and protective factors are the basic assertions of the prevention science perspective. On the other hand, the idea that it is important to focus on diverse youth developmental possibilities and problems rather than dealing with a single youth problem relates to the assertion that "problem-free is not fully prepared." Emphasis should also be placed on how both personal and environmental factors influence human behavior and how the utilization of developmental models focuses on growing, learning, and changing in young people. They argued that the prevention science approach and the positive youth development approach are compatible and complementary.

Empirically, there are research findings showing that positive youth development influences adolescent developmental outcomes. Studies showed that positive youth development attributes such as competence and character were negatively related to adolescent problem behavior such as depression, delinquency, and substance abuse (Jelicic, Bobek, Phelps, Lerner, & Lerner, 2007; Lerner et al., 2005). In a longitudinal study conducted in Hong Kong, Sun and Shek (2010) examined the relationships among life satisfaction, positive youth development, and problem behavior in 7,975 Secondary 1 students. As predicted, positive youth development was positively related to life satisfaction but negatively with adolescent problem behavior. Results from structural equation models showed that adolescents having higher levels of positive youth development were more satisfied and showed less problem behavior, with a bidirectional relationship between life satisfaction and problem behavior. The above findings were replicated in the study of Sun and Shek (2012) based on the responses of 7,151 Chinese Secondary 2 students. Again, findings based on structural equation models showed that adolescents with higher levels of positive youth development were more satisfied with life and had lesser problem behavior, with life satisfaction and problem behavior mutually influencing each other. In another study using three waves of data, the cross-sectional and longitudinal influences of positive youth development and life satisfaction on adolescent problem behavior were examined in 4,523 Chinese students followed from Grade 7, Grade 9 to Grade 11 (Sun & Shek, 2013). Results showed the influence of positive youth development on adolescent problem behavior, and the mediating effect of life satisfaction on the relationship was also found.

Family Quality of Life and Adolescent Well-Being

Different systemic and dyadic family processes have been proposed to influence adolescent development. According to the family-ecological models, different subsystems have influences on adolescent developmental outcomes such as risk behavior (Kotchick, Shaffer, Forehand, & Miller, 2001). Parenting and family characteristics were also found to influence children's problem behavior and achievement strategies (Amato & Fowler, 2002; Aunola & Nurmi, 2005; Aunola, Stattin, & Nurmi, 2000).

As far as family functioning is concerned, different "desired" systemic family functioning qualities are proposed in different family models: clear boundaries, balanced power structure, intimacy, autonomy, pleasant relationship, and skilled negotiation are characteristics proposed in the Beavers Systems Model (Beaver & Hampson, 1990); "optimal" levels of cohesion, adaptability, and communication are postulated in the Circumplex Model (Olson, Russell, & Sprenkle, 1989); and problem solving, communication, roles, affective responsiveness, affective involvement, and behavioral control are proposed in the McMaster Family Functioning Model (Epstein, Bishop, Ryan, Miller, & Keitner, 1993; Epstein, Ryan, Bishop, Miller, & Keitner, 2003). Research in the global and Chinese contexts has shown that family functioning is positively related to adolescent well-being (Gorman-Smith, Tolan, & Henry, 2000; Shek, 2002).

Besides systemic family functioning, different dyadic parent-child processes also influence adolescent development. Primarily, parenting styles have been proposed to shape adolescent development. In the pioneer work of Schaefer (1959, 1965), parents with the attributes of "warmth" and "autonomy" facilitated the development of children and adolescents. Baumrind (1971, 1991) proposed the authoritarian, authoritative, and permissive types of parenting and argued that authoritative parenting was the "optimal" form of parenting. In the model proposed by Maccoby and Martin (1983), authoritative parenting was regarded as facilitating youth development as compared to authoritarian, permissive, and indulgent parenting.

Regarding parental control, there are views suggesting that while behavioral control such as parental monitoring promotes adolescent development (Chen, Liu, & Li, 2000; Dishion & McMahon, 1998), psychological control leads to negative adolescent developmental outcomes (Barber, 1996, 2002). Furthermore, the quality of parent-child relationship was positively related to adolescent development (Kwok-Lai & Shek, 2010; Liu, Fang, Deng, & Zhang, 2012; Shek & Lee, 2007). For example, there are research findings showing that parent-adolescent conflict was positively related to adolescent developmental problems (Wierson, Forehand, & McCombs, 1988). In short, theories and research suggest that positive family quality of life is an important factor promoting the development of adolescents.

Positive Youth Development Programs

In the Western contexts, there are many intervention programs that have utilized positive youth development constructs in the program design. For example, Guerra and Williams (2003) described the development, implementation, and evaluation of a multiyear project with integrated health promotion and prevention programs. In the project, five core competencies for healthy young development were emphasized, including positive identity, personal agency, self-regulation, social relationship skills, and prosocial system of beliefs. Catalano et al. (2002) reviewed 77 programs on positive youth development in the United States. They showed that 25 programs were successful and 15 positive youth development constructs could be identified in the successful programs, including bonding, psychosocial competencies (such as emotional competence), spirituality, optimism, and prosocial attributes.

Regarding the different systems and ecological contexts that could generate changes in adolescents, an important context for creating changes in adolescents is the school system. It is assumed that by carefully designing curricula-based positive youth development programs for students, their psychosocial competence would be promoted. There are numerous examples in the West that school-based positive youth development programs generated positive changes in students (e.g., Durlak, Weissberg, Quintana, & Perez, 2004; Lafferty, Mahoney, & Thombs, 2003). Durlak, Weissberg, Dymnicki, Taylor, and Schellinger (2011) reviewed more than 200 psychosocial competence programs for students. Their review showed that compared with control participants, students in the experimental group generally showed significant improvements in skills, attitudes, and behavior in the social and emotional domains. The experimental subjects also showed an 11-percentile-point gain in academic achievement. Similar review was conducted by Catalano et al. (2012). The review showed that there were evidence-based positive youth development programs in the scientific literature.

Programs Promoting Family Quality of Life

Besides generating changes in the school context, others have asserted that family processes such as parenting and parent-child relational qualities are important influences of adolescent development (Kerr, Beck, Shattuck, Kattar, & Uriburu, 2003; Kumpfer & Alvarado, 2003). In fact, many family theorists believe that youth problems are simply a reflection of family problems. A review of the literature shows that parenting and family intervention programs have been designed to promote the quality of family life in families with adolescents (Bunting, 2004; Cedar & Levant, 1990; Collins & Fetsch, 2012; Mejia, Calam, & Sanders, 2012). Some examples of family quality of life promotion programs are as follows:

- *Parent Effectiveness Training* (*PET*): This parenting program was built upon the humanistic principles intrinsic to the work of Thomas Gordon and Carl Rogers. The program focuses on the promotion of democratic and collaborative relationships in the family. With this objective in mind, parents are trained in listening, communication, and child-parent problem solving techniques. In particular, emphasis is put on active listening, messages about the issues but without judgments (I-messages), and identification of solutions that are acceptable to both people (i.e., win-win solutions) (Rinn & Markle, 1977).

- *Systematic Training for Effective Parenting* (*STEP*): This parenting program is based on the ideas of Individual Psychology identified by Alfred Adler and Rudolf Dreikurs. In the program, parents are trained to identify four goals of misbehavior: attention, power, revenge, and inadequacy. They also discovered ways to build children's self-esteem through encouragement and develop an effective discipline system based on parental firmness and kindness. Parents are helped to deal with emotional problems and promote positive emotional growth of their children. The topics in this parenting program include understanding oneself and their children, giving encouragement to oneself and one's children, building up the courage to be imperfect, listening and talking to one's children, enabling children to learn to cooperate and behave reasonably, and choosing one's parenting approach (Adams, 2001; McInnis-Dittrich, 1996; Snow, Kern, & Penick, 1997). The evaluation findings of the STEP Program can be seen in SAMHSA's National Registry of Evidence-Based Programs and Practices.
- *Positive Parenting Program* (*Triple P*): The Triple P is based on integrative theoretical model with building blocks derived from the social learning theory, child and family behavior therapy, applied behavioral analyses, developmental research, social information processing models, developmental psychopathology, and ecological models. The program is based on a self-regulatory model on parental competence, with elements of self-sufficiency, parental self-sufficiency, self-management, and personal agency. The principles of positive parenting include creating a safe and engaging environment, fostering a positive learning environment, using assertive discipline, having realistic expectations, and taking care of oneself as a parent (Martin & Sanders, 2003; Ralph & Sanders, 2003; Sanders, Markie-Dadds, Tully, & Bor, 2000; Sanders, Markie-Dadds, & Turner, 2003).

Several observations can be highlighted from this brief review. First, most of the existing family quality of life enhancement programs are designed for parents, with relatively fewer programs developed for adolescents. From the family-ecological perspective, changes in parents alone are not adequate because of the interactive and dynamic nature of the parent-adolescent relationship. Hence, family quality of life enhancement programs should also be designed for adolescents. Second, there is a growing tendency to endorse a multisystem and ecological framework in parenting and family quality of life enhancement programs. That is, instead of focusing on a single set of principles (such as humanistic principles), factors in other systems should also be taken into account.

Third, while some parenting programs are popular and well received by the public, few evaluation studies have been conducted. In fact, it is not common for researchers and practitioners in the field to conduct rigorous evaluation studies. In fact, some of the popular programs are simply employed by workers because of "word of mouth" instead of empirical evidence. Finally, compared with programs in the West, there are very few Chinese family intervention programs. In addition, there are few published studies on family enhancement programs in different Chinese contexts.

Evidence-Based PYD and Family Quality of Life Enhancement Programs for Chinese People

Shek and Yu (2011) reviewed adolescent prevention and positive youth development programs in Asia. They concluded that with the notable exception of the Project P.A.T.H.S. in Hong Kong, there were very few validated youth enhancement programs in different Chinese societies, as compared to the observation that there was much effort to develop prevention and enhancement programs for young people in Western societies. There are several strengths of the Project P.A.T.H.S.. First, academics in five universities were involved. Second, The Hong Kong Jockey Club Charities Trust injected an enormous amount of money into the project. Third, a systematic curriculum in both Chinese and English was developed by the research team. Fourth, more than 210,000 students participated in the project in the initial implementation phase. Fifth, multiple evaluation strategies including a randomized group trial were used to assess the effectiveness of the project. Sixth, data collected from multiple evaluation methods suggest that different people such as program participants and implementers perceived the project positively; students in the experimental schools perform better than do those in the control schools. Finally, the Project P.A.T.H.S. was listed as an effective program which can promote holistic development in Chinese adolescents (Catalano et al., 2012). Obviously, the Project P.A.T.H.S. can be employed as a prototype positive youth development program for Chinese adolescents. Nevertheless, there are several issues on the theoretical, implementation, and evaluation levels that should be considered as far as the development of positive youth development programs for Chinese adolescents is concerned.

Theoretically speaking, several questions on the nature of positive youth development require further thoughts. First, while positive youth development is desirable, it is important to ask whether the positive traits must necessarily result in better adolescent developmental outcomes. For example, an adolescent who is overconfident about one's ability to control drugs would easily become addicted to drugs. Similarly, an adolescent who has very good social skills may have dating problems in a premature manner. Hence, it is interesting to ask whether there is a linear relationship between positive youth development attributes and adolescent developmental outcomes. The second issue concerns the possible relationships among different components of positive youth development. For example, how is spirituality related to other psychosocial competencies and prosocial behavior? This is still an underdeveloped area which needs further investigation.

The final theoretical question is how Western PYD constructs are related to Chinese ideals for adolescent development (Shek, Yu, & Fu, 2013). As there are different emphases of Confucian, Buddhist, and Taoist thoughts, the integration would be complex and challenging. For example, how can the Confucian concept of "ren" be related to caring disposition? Besides, as "doctrine of the mean" and "interpersonal harmony" are emphasized by Confucianism, how can this be reconciled with the Western notion of striving for excellence is another interesting question to be considered. Finally, how to reconcile the "individualistic" focus in the Western contexts and the "collectivistic" focus in the Chinese culture is a challenging task faced by theorists in positive youth development.

On the level of program development and implementation, how the above-mentioned theoretical issues are incorporated on the program level is an important issue to be addressed. For example, how to deal with the concept of "filial piety" in the context of promotion of bonding is an interesting challenge for the program developers. "Respect for authority" and "interpersonal harmony" are also topics requiring integration of different concepts across cultures. Another issue concerns the "ideal" teaching modes adopted in positive youth development programs. While didactic and vertical teacher-student relationships are commonly adopted in the Chinese contexts, interactive and horizontal teacher-student relationships are preferred in positive youth development programs. Besides, as Chinese people are reserved in expressing their emotions and thoughts, how to encourage and facilitate students to express their thoughts and emotions is a thought-provoking issue for frontline teachers. Finally, how adequate time can be allocated in the current overloading curriculum is another question for reflection. Teaching time is always a structural problem facing positive youth development programs. Whether adequate time is allocated largely depends on the vision of the schools about the importance of positive youth development and holistic youth development and about whether those should be treated as a priority.

On the level of evaluation, although the evaluation findings from the Project P.A.T.H.S. are groundbreaking in different Chinese communities, the evaluation was conducted by the research team rather than independent research groups. Hence, evaluation studies conducted by independent research groups should be attempted. In addition, long-term follow-up evaluation studies adopting randomized group trials are indispensable. In particular, long-term case studies examining the changes in the program participants are helpful, especially regarding the degree to which adolescents applied the concepts and materials learned in the program.

As far as family quality of life enhancement programs are concerned, there are several issues that should be considered. Similar to the notion of positive youth development, researchers and practitioners should be sensitive to the characteristics of Chinese families. First, traditional Chinese families were more collectivistic than individualistic where the focus was put more on the family than on the individual, and family members were expected to sacrifice for the family. Second, a structured power hierarchy was emphasized in traditional Chinese culture where younger members were submissive to the elder members. Finally, the authority of the father was of paramount importance in traditional Chinese families. These characteristics are intrinsic to the "Family Letters" in the traditional Chinese culture where children were taught to observe the family rules and expectations. Shek and Sun (2014) pointed out there were gradual changes from the collectivistic emphasis to individualistic emphasis in contemporary Chinese families which suggests that the design of family quality of life enhancement programs should take note of these cultural attributes.

In view of the unique characteristics of Chinese families, it is important to ask several conceptual questions. First, to what extent family quality of life enhancement programs developed in the West are applicable to Chinese families? Second, to what extent traditional Chinese family values and emphases are still relevant to contemporary Chinese families? Finally, how to integrate traditional Chinese family values and contemporary family theories and intervention programs? One example is how to encourage Chinese adolescents to express their views in a filial manner without creating unnecessary conflicts. Another example is how to express emotions in a healthy manner in front of family members.

In the Project P.A.T.H.S., there are some units which are family related, such as understanding the emotions of and seeking help from family members. However, as the focus of the Project P.A.T.H.S. is more related to individual competence, there is a need to reinforce the family competences of adolescents. One suggestion is to develop additional teaching units in the project. Some topics are as follows:

- Understanding of one's development, including developmental tasks and personal well-being
- Understanding of the family: Systemic family functioning attributes such as family communication and emotional expression, dyadic parent-child relational qualities, and relationships among individual, dyadic, and systemic factors
- Factors affecting family quality of life: Macro factors (e.g., poverty) affecting family quality of life, micro factors affecting family quality of life, and risk and protective factors on family quality of life
- Knowledge on family quality of life: Role of the family on adolescent personal well-being, family life cycle, and related developmental tasks
- Skills on family quality of life: Interpersonal skills within the family context, handling emotions and conflict resolution in the family, and skills to nurture family competence
- Attitudes on family quality of life: Attitude toward filial piety, family intactness, parental marital disruption, Chinese family values, and family issues
- Family values such as love, concern, communication, harmony, respect, and responsibility
- Dealing with family crises: Family resilience and conflict resolution
- Building a harmonious family: Responsibilities of different family members

While the above topics are also applicable to parents, there are additional topics that should be incorporated in family quality of life enhancement programs designed for parents. They are listed as follows:

- Knowledge about how parents influence adolescent behavior, such as how parental marital disruption impairs adolescent development
- Reflection on one's developmental history and how such history influences one's development
- Understanding one's parenting characteristics and beliefs about parenting and parent-child relationship with particular reference to Chinese cultural beliefs
- Interaction with adolescent children: Issues, skills, and principles
- Dealing with adolescent problem behavior: Role of discipline and parental control

- Looking academic excellence in a proper context: Traditional Chinese values and contemporary challenges and helping children to realize their academic potentials
- Growing with children together: Importance of personal growth in parenting and reflections about personal growth

In conclusion, individual competence and family social capital are important developmental assets in adolescent development. Theoretically speaking, there are models proposing that personal well-being indexed by positive youth development attributes and family quality of life indexed by family functioning are protective factors for adolescent development. Empirically, the findings presented in the various chapters in this book underscore the importance of positive youth development and family functioning in the development of junior secondary school students in Hong Kong. Practically speaking, evaluation findings of the Project P.A.T.H.S. in Hong Kong show that positive youth development programs are able to promote the holistic development of adolescent development in Hong Kong. To strengthen personal well-being and family quality of life in Chinese adolescents, several issues are highlighted for further consideration.

Acknowledgments The preparation for this work and the Project P.A.T.H.S. were financially supported by The Hong Kong Jockey Club Charities Trust. The authorship is equally shared by the first author and second author.

References

Adams, J. F. (2001). Impact of parent training on family functioning. *Child & Family Behavioral Therapy, 23*(1), 29–42.

Amato, P., & Fowler, F. (2002). Parenting practices, child adjustment, and family adversity. *Journal of Marriage and Family, 64*, 703–716.

Atilola, O., Ayinde, O., & Adeitan, O. (2013). Beyond prevalence and pattern: Problematic extent of alcohol and substance use among adolescents in Ibadan South-West Nigeria. *African Health Sciences, 13*(30), 777–784.

Aunola, K., & Nurmi, J. E. (2005). The role of parenting styles in children's problem behavior. *Child Development, 76*(6), 1144–1159.

Aunola, K., Stattin, H., & Nurmi, J. E. (2000). Parenting styles and adolescents' achievement strategies. *Journal of Adolescence, 23*, 205–222.

Barber, B. K. (1996). Parental psychological control: Revisiting a neglected construct. *Child Development, 67*, 3296–3319.

Barber, B. K. (2002). *Intrusive parenting: How psychological control affects children and adolescents*. Washington, DC: American Psychological Association.

Baumrind, D. (1971). Types of adolescents life-styles. *Developmental Psychology Monographs, 4*, 1–102.

Baumrind, D. (1991). The influence of parenting style on adolescent competence and substance use. *Journal of Early Adolescence, 11*(1), 56–95.

Beaver, R. W., & Hampson, R. B. (1990). *Successful families: Assessment and intervention.* New York: Norton.

Benson, P. L. (1997). *All kids are our kids: What communities must do to raise caring and responsible children and adolescents*. San Francisco: Jossey-Bass.
Benson, P. L., Mannes, M., Pittman, K., & Ferber, T. (2004). Youth development, developmental assets, and public policy. In R. M. Lerner & L. Steinberg (Eds.), *Handbook of adolescent psychology* (pp. 781–814). Hoboken, NJ: Wiley.
Bronfenbrenner, U. (1988). Interacting systems in human development. Research paradigms: Present and future. In N. Bolger, A. Caspi, G. Downey, & M. Moorehouse (Eds.), *Persons in context: Development processes* (pp. 25–49). Cambridge, UK: Cambridge University Press.
Bunting, L. (2004). Parenting programmes: The best available evidence. *Child Care in Practice, 10*(4), 327–343.
Burnett-Zeigler, I., Walton, M. A., Ilgen, M., Barry, K. L., Chermack, S. T., Zucker, R. A., et al. (2012). Prevalence and correlates of mental health problems and treatment among adolescent seen in primary care. *Journal of Adolescent Health, 50*(6), 559–564.
Catalano, R. F., Berglund, M. L., Ryan, J. A. M., Lonczak, H. S., & Hawkins, J. D. (2002, June 24). Positive youth development in the United States: Research findings on evaluations of positive youth development programs. *Prevention & Treatment, 5*, Article 15.
Catalano, R. F., Fagan, A. A., Gavin, L. E., Greenberg, M. T., Irwin, C. E., Jr., Ross, D. A., et al. (2012). Worldwide application of prevention science in adolescent health. *Lancet, 379*(9826), 1653–1664.
Catalano, R. F., & Hawkins, J. D. (2002, June 24). Response from authors to comments on "positive youth development in the United States: Research findings on evaluations of positive youth development programs". *Prevention & Treatment, 5*(1), Article 20.
Cedar, B., & Levant, R. F. (1990). A meta-analysis of the effects of parent effectiveness training. *The American Journal of Family Therapy, 18*(4), 373–384.
Celbis, O., Karaoglu, L., Egri, M., & Ozdemir, B. (2012). Violence among high school students in Malatya: A prevalence study. *Turkish Journal of Medical Sciences, 42*(2), 343–350.
Chen, X., Liu, M., & Li, D. (2000). Parental warmth, control, and indulgence and their relations to adjustment in Chinese children: A longitudinal study. *Journal of Family Psychology, 14*(3), 401–419.
Collins, C. L., & Fetsch, R. J. (2012). A review and critique of 16 major parent education programs. *Journal of Extension, 50*(4), Article #4FEA8.
Conway, K. P., Vullo, G. C., Nichter, B., Wang, J., Compton, W. M., Iannotti, R. J., et al. (2013). Prevalence and patterns of polysubstance use in a nationally representative sample of 10th graders in the United States. *Journal of Adolescent Health, 52*(6), 716–723.
Damon, W. (2004). What is positive youth development? *The Annals of the American Academy of Political and Social Science, 591*, 13–24.
Dishion, T. J., & McMahon, R. J. (1998). Parental monitoring and the prevention of child and adolescent problem behavior: A conceptual and empirical formulation. *Clinical Child and Family Psychology Review, 1*(1), 61–75.
Durlak, J. A., Weissberg, R. P., Dymnicki, A. B., Taylor, R. D., & Schellinger, K. B. (2011). The impact of enhancing students' social and emotional learning: A meta-analysis of school-based universal interventions. *Child Development, 82*(1), 405–432.
Durlak, J. A., Weissberg, R. P., Quintana, E., & Perez, F. (2004). Primary prevention: Involving schools and communities in youth health promotion. In L. A. Jason, C. B. Keys, Y. Suarez-Balcazar, R. R. Taylor, & M. I. Davis (Eds.), *Participatory community research: Theories and methods in action* (pp. 73–86). Washington, DC: American Psychological Association.
Eccles, J. S., & Gootman, J. A. (Eds.). (2002). *Community programs to promote youth development*. Washington, DC: National Academy Press.
Epstein, N. B., Bishop, D., Ryan, C., Miller, I., & Keitner, G. (1993). The McMaster model: View of healthy family functioning. In F. Walsh (Ed.), *Normal family processes* (pp. 138–160). New York: The Guilford Press.
Epstein, N. B., Ryan, C. E., Bishop, D. S., Miller, I. W., & Keitner, G. (2003). The McMaster model: View of healthy family functioning. In F. Walsh (Ed.), *Normal family processes: Growing diversity and complexity* (3rd ed., pp. 581–607). New York: The Guilford Press.

Felner, R. D., & Felner, T. Y. (1989). Primary prevention programs in the educational context: A transactional-ecological framework and analysis. In L. A. Bond & B. E. Compas (Eds.), *Primary prevention and promotion in the schools* (pp. 13–49). Newbury, CA: Sage.

Gorman-Smith, D., Tolan, P. H., & Henry, D. B. (2000). A developmental-ecological model of the relation of family functioning to patterns of delinquency. *Journal of Quantitative Criminology, 16*(2), 169–198.

Graczyk, P. A., Weissberg, R. P., Payton, J. W., Elias, M. J., Greenberg, M. T., & Zins, J. E. (2000). Criteria for evaluating the quality of school-based social and emotional learning programs. In R. Bar-On & J. D. A. Parker (Eds.), *The handbook of emotional intelligence* (pp. 391–409). San Francisco: Jossey-Bass.

Granger, R. C. (2002). Creating conditions linked to positive youth development. In R. M. Lerner, C. S. Taylor, & A. von Eye (Eds.), *Pathways to positive development among diverse youth* (pp. 149–164). San Francisco: Jossey-Bass.

Guerra, N. G., & Williams, K. R. (2003). Implementation of school-based wellness centres. *Psychology in the Schools, 40*, 473–487.

Jelicic, H., Bobek, D. L., Phelps, E., Lerner, J. V., & Lerner, R. M. (2007). Using positive youth development to predict contribution and risk behaviors in early adolescence: Findings from the first two waves of the 4-H study of positive youth development. *International Journal of Behavioral Development, 31*(3), 263–273.

Kerr, M. H., Beck, K., Shattuck, T. D., Kattar, C., & Uriburu, D. (2003). Family involvement, problem and prosocial behaviour outcomes of Latino youth. *American Journal of Health Behavior, 27*(Suppl. 1), S55–S65.

Kotchick, B. A., Shaffer, A., Forehand, R., & Miller, K. S. (2001). Adolescent sexual risk behavior: A multi-system perspective. *Clinical Psychology Review, 21*(4), 493–519.

Kubwalo, H. W., Muula, A. S., Siziya, S., Pasupulati, S., & Rudatsikira, E. (2013). Prevalence and correlates of being bullied among in-school adolescents in Malawi: Results from the 2009 Global School-Based Health Survey. *Malawi Medical Journal, 25*(1), 12–14.

Kumpfer, K. L., & Alvarado, R. (2003). Family-strengthening approaches for the prevention of youth problem behaviors. *American Psychologist, 58*(6–7), 457–465.

Kwok-Lai, S. Y. C., & Shek, D. T. L. (2010). Personal and family correlates of suicidal ideation among Chinese adolescents in Hong Kong. *Social Indicators Research, 95*(3), 407–419.

Lafferty, C. K., Mahoney, C. A., & Thombs, D. L. (2003). Diffusion of a developmental asset-building initiative in public schools. *American Journal of Health Behavior, 27*(Suppl. 1), S35–S44.

Lerner, R. M., & Benson, P. L. (Eds.). (2003). *Developmental assets and asset-building communities: Implications for research, policy, and practice*. New York: Kluwer Academic/Plenum.

Lerner, R. M., Fisher, C. B., & Weinberg, R. A. (2000). Toward a science for and of the people: Promoting civil society through the application of developmental science. *Child Development, 71*(1), 11–20.

Lerner, R. M., Lerner, J. V., Almerigi, J. B., Theokas, C., Phelps, E., Gestsdottir, S., et al. (2005). Positive youth development, participation in community youth development programs, and community contributions of fifth-grade adolescents: Findings from the first wave of the 4-H study of positive youth development. *Journal of Early Adolescence, 25*(1), 17–71.

Leung, P. W. L., Hung, S. F., Ho, T. P., Lee, C. C., Liu, W. S., Tang, C. P., et al. (2008). Prevalence of DSM-IV disorders in Chinese adolescents and the effects of an impairment criterion: A pilot community study in Hong Kong. *European Child & Adolescent Psychiatry, 17*(7), 452–461.

Liu, Q. X., Fang, X. Y., Deng, L. Y., & Zhang, J. T. (2012). Parent-adolescent communication, parental Internet use and Internet-specific norms and pathological Internet use among Chinese adolescents. *Computers in Human Behavior, 28*(4), 1269–1275.

Ma, C. M. S., & Shek, D. T. L. (2013). Consumption of pornographic materials in early adolescents in Hong Kong. *Journal of Pediatric and Adolescent Gynecology, 26*, S18–S25.

Maccoby, E. E., & Martin, J. (1983). Socialization in the context of the family: Parent-child interaction. In E. M. Hetherington (Vol. Ed.) & P. H. Mussen (Series Ed.), *Handbook of child psychology: Vol. 4. Socialization, personality, and social development* (pp. 1–101). New York: Wiley.

Martin, A. J., & Sanders, M. R. (2003). Balancing work and family: A controlled evaluation of the Triple P-Positive Parenting Program as a work-site intervention. *Child and Adolescent Mental Health, 8*(4), 161–169.
McInnis-Dittrich, K. (1996). Violence prevention: An ecological adaptation of Systematic Training for Effective Parenting. *Families in Society, 77*(7), 414–422.
Mejia, A., Calam, R., & Sanders, M. R. (2012). A review of parenting programs in developing countries: Opportunities and challenges for preventing emotional and behavioral difficulties in children. *Clinical and Child Family Psychology Review, 15*(2), 163–175.
Olson, D. H. L., Russell, C. S., & Sprenkle, D. H. (1989). *Circumplex model: Systemic assessment and treatment of families*. New York: The Haworth Press.
Parker, R. D., & Buriel, R. (1998). Socialization in the family: Ethnic and ecological perspectives. In N. Eisenberg (Ed.), *Handbook of child psychology: Vol. 3. Social, emotional and personality development* (pp. 463–552). New York: Wiley.
Pittman, K., Irby, M., & Ferber, T. (2000). Unfinished business: Further reflections on a decade of promoting youth development. *Youth Development: Issues, Challenges, and Directions*, 17–64. Retrieved November 17, 2004, from https://www.google.com.hk/#q=youth+development+issues+challenges+and+directions
Pittman, K. J., Irby, M., Tolman, J., Yohalem, N., & Ferber, T. (2001). *Preventing problems, promoting development, encouraging engagement: Competing priorities or inseparable goals?* Retrieved November 17, 2004, from http://www.google.com.hk/url?sa=t&rct=j&q=&esrc=s&source=web&cd=1&ved=0CC8QFjAA&url=http%3A%2F%2Fforumfyi.org%2Ffiles%2FPreventing%2520Problems%2C%2520Promoting%2520Development%2C%2520Encouraging%2520Engagement.pdf&ei=4c7dUt2fM-KyiAerl4GoAg&usg=AFQjCNESCcFvQMiW9Ho-uPQVPPcmpn9jpA&bvm=bv.59568121,d.aGc
Ralph, A., & Sanders, M. R. (2003). Preliminary evaluation of the Group Teen Triple P program for parents of teenagers making the transition to high school. *Australian e-Journal for the Advancement of Mental Health, 2*(3), 1–10.
Rinn, R. C., & Markle, A. (1977). Parent effectiveness training: A review. *Psychological Reports, 41*, 95–109.
Saluja, G., Iachan, R., Scheidt, P. C., Overpeck, M. D., Sun, W. Y., & Giedd, J. N. (2004). Prevalence of and risk factors for depressive symptoms among young adolescents. *Archives of Pediatrics and Adolescent Medicine, 158*, 760–765.
Sanders, M. R., Markie-Dadds, C., Tully, L. A., & Bor, B. (2000). The Triple P-Positive Parenting Program: A comparison of enhanced, standard, and self-directed behavioral family intervention for parents of children with early onset conduct problems. *Journal of Consulting and Clinical Psychology, 68*(4), 624–640.
Sanders, M. R., Markie-Dadds, C., & Turner, K. M. T. (2003). Theoretical, scientific and clinical foundations of the Triple P-Positive Parenting Program: A population approach to the promotion of parenting competence. *Parenting Research and Practice Monograph No. 1*, 1–24. Retrieved October 15, 2013, from http://www.cimharchive.trilogyir.com/downloads/handouts/Theoret%20Scientific%20Clinical%20Foundation%20for%20Triple%20P.pdf
Schaefer, E. S. (1959). A circumplex model for maternal behavior. *Journal of Abnormal and Social Psychology, 59*, 226–235.
Schaefer, E. S. (1965). Children's reports of parental behavior: An inventory. *Child Development, 36*(2), 413–424.
Shek, D. T. L. (2002). Family functioning and psychological well-being, school adjustment, and problem behavior in Chinese adolescents with and without economic disadvantage. *Journal of Genetic Psychology, 163*(4), 497–502.
Shek, D. T. L. (2007). Tackling adolescent substance abuse in Hong Kong: Where we should and should not go. *TheScientificWorldJOURNAL: TSW Child Health & Human Development, 7*, 2021–2030.
Shek, D. T. L., & Lee, T. Y. (2007). Perceived parental control processes, parent-child relational qualities and psychological well-being of Chinese adolescents in intact and non-intact families in Hong Kong. *International Journal of Adolescent Medicine and Health, 19*(2), 167–175.

Shek, D. T. L., Ma, H. K., & Sun, R. C. F. (2011). A brief overview of adolescent developmental problems in Hong Kong. *TheScientificWorldJOURNAL, 11*, 2243–2256.

Shek, D. T. L., & Sun, R. C. F. (2014). Parenting in Hong Kong: Traditional Chinese cultural roots and contemporary phenomena. In H. Selin (Ed.), *Parenting across cultures: Childrearing, motherhood and fatherhood in non-western cultures* (pp. 25–38). Heidelberg, Germany: Springer.

Shek, D. T. L., & Yu, L. (2011). A review of validated youth prevention and positive youth development programs in Asia. *International Journal of Adolescent Medicine and Health, 23*(4), 317–324.

Shek, D. T. L., & Yu, L. (2012). Longitudinal impact of the Project PATHS on adolescent risk behavior: What happened after five years? *TheScientificWorldJOURNAL, 2012*, 13 pp. doi:10.1100/2012/316029.

Shek, D. T. L., Yu, L., & Fu, X. (2013). Confucian virtues and Chinese adolescent development: A conceptual review. *International Journal of Adolescent Medicine and Health, 25*(4), 335–344.

Snow, J. N., Kern, R. M., & Penick, J. (1997). The effects of STEP on patient progress in an adolescent day hospital. *Individual Psychology, 53*(4), 388–395.

Sun, R. C. F., & Shek, D. T. L. (2012). Positive youth development, life satisfaction and problem behaviour among Chinese adolescents in Hong Kong: A replication. *Social Indicators Research, 105*(3), 541–559.

Sun, R. C. F., & Shek, D. T. L. (2010). Life satisfaction, positive youth development, and problem behavior among Chinese adolescents in Hong Kong. *Social Indicators Research, 95*(3), 455–474.

Sun, R. C. F., & Shek, D. T. L. (2013). Longitudinal influences of positive youth development and life satisfaction on problem behavior among adolescents in Hong Kong. *Social Indicators Research, 114*, 1171–1197.

Weissberg, R. P., & O'Brien, M. U. (2004). What works in school-based social and emotional learning programs for positive youth development. *The Annals of the American Academy of Political and Social Science, 591*, 86–97.

Wierson, M., Forehand, R., & McCombs, A. (1988). The relationship of early adolescent functioning to parent-reported and adolescent-perceived inter-parental conflict. *Journal of Abnormal Child Psychology, 16*(6), 707–718.

Yu, L., & Shek, D. T. L. (2013). Internet addiction in Hong Kong adolescents: A three-year longitudinal study. *Journal of Pediatric and Adolescent Gynecology, 26*(3), S10–S17.

Index

D.T.L. Shek et al. (eds.), *Chinese Adolescents in Hong Kong*, Quality of Life in Asia 5, DOI 10.1007/978-981-287-143-5

Q

MIX
Papier aus verantwortungsvollen Quellen
Paper from responsible sources
FSC® C105338

If you have any concerns about our products,
you can contact us on
ProductSafety@springernature.com

In case Publisher is established outside the EU,
the EU authorized representative is:
Springer Nature Customer Service Center GmbH
Europaplatz 3, 69115 Heidelberg, Germany

Printed by Libri Plureos GmbH
in Hamburg, Germany